50 LANDMARK PAPERS

every

Plastic Surgeon Should Know

This book identifies key scientific papers in the field of Plastic Surgery and explains why these papers are important in contemporary clinical management.

The text includes commentaries on landmark papers in a wide range of clinical areas within Plastic, Reconstructive, and Aesthetic Surgery. These are not necessarily the most cited in their field, though many of them are. Reviewers were asked to pick a paper in their field of expertise that, in their view, should be read more carefully, and they have selected papers that they are passionate about – and may have (co)authored – and which underpin the care of patients. Further, the insights offered will stimulate further reading and will facilitate a deeper understanding of a topic and, of course, be useful in examinations.

This an invaluable reference for Plastic Surgery trainees, fellows, and surgeons studying for exams, as well as for seasoned clinicians who want to stay current in their field.

50 Landmark Papers Series

50 Landmark Papers every Spine Surgeon Should Know
Alexander R Vaccaro, Charles G Fisher and Jefferson R Wilson

50 Landmark Papers every Trauma Surgeon Should Know
Stephen M Cohn and Ara J Feinstein

50 Landmark Papers every Acute Care Surgeon Should Know
Stephen M Cohn and Peter Rhee

50 Landmark Papers every Vascular and Endovascular Surgeon Should Know
Juan Carlos Jimenez and Samuel Eric Wilson

50 Landmark Papers every Oral and Maxillofacial Surgeon Should Know
Niall MH McLeod and Peter A Brennan

50 Landmark Papers every Intensivist Should Know
Stephen M Cohn, Alan Lisbon and Stephen Heard

50 Landmark Papers every Thyroid and Parathyroid Surgeon Should Know
Sam Wiseman and Sebastian Aspinall

50 Landmark Papers every Pediatric Surgeon Should Know
Mark Davenport, Bashar Aldeiri and Joseph Davidson

50 Landmark Papers every Breast Surgeon Should Know
Lynda Wyld, Ramsey Cutress and Jenna Morgan

50 Landmark Papers every Plastic Surgeon Should Know
Tor Wo Chiu

For more information about this series, please visit www.routledge.com/50-Landmark-Papers/book-series/50LP

50 LANDMARK PAPERS

every

Plastic Surgeon Should Know

Edited by

Tor Wo Chiu

Specialist in Plastic Surgery
Chief of Division of Plastic Reconstructive and Aesthetic Surgery
Prince of Wales Hospital
Hong Kong

CRC Press
Taylor & Francis Group
Boca Raton London New York

CRC Press is an imprint of the
Taylor & Francis Group, an **informa** business

First edition published 2026
by CRC Press
2385 NW Executive Center Drive, Suite 320, Boca Raton, FL 33431

and by CRC Press
4 Park Square, Milton Park, Abingdon, Oxon, OX14 4RN

CRC Press is an imprint of Taylor & Francis Group, LLC

ISBN: 978-1-032-53810-5 (hbk)
ISBN: 978-1-032-53684-2 (pbk)
ISBN: 978-1-003-41373-8 (ebk)

DOI: 10.1201/9781003413738

Typeset in Times LT Std
by Deanta Global Publishing Services, Chennai, India

Contents

Contributors

Rajeev B. Ahuja
Sir Ganga Ram Hospital
Asia Pacific Burn Association
New Delhi, India

Asim Ali
University of Toronto
Hospital for Sick Children
Toronto, Ontario, Canada

Robert J. Allen Sr.
Louisiana State University Health Sciences Centre
New Orleans, Louisiana

Claudio Angrigiani
Buenos Aires, Argentina

Rachel Bluebond-Langner
NYU Langone Health
New York, New York

Gregory H. Borschel
Indiana University School of Medicine
Plastic Surgery
Riley Children's Hospital
Indianapolis, Indiana

Jevan Cevik
Monash University
Melbourne, Australia

Pallab Chatterjee
Plastic Surgery
Armed Forces Medical Services
New Delhi, India

Velda Chow
University of Hong Kong
Hong Kong SAR, China

Whitney T.H. Chow
John Radcliffe Hospital
Oxford University Hospitals NHS Foundation
    Trust
United Kingdom

Peter G. Cordeiro
Plastic and Reconstructive Surgery Service
Memorial Sloan Kettering Cancer Center
New York, New York

Jordan R. Crabtree
Indiana University School of Medicine
Plastic Surgery
Riley Children's Hospital
Indianapolis, Indiana

Andrea Donoso-Samper
Universidad El Bosque
Bogotá, Colombia

Alp Ercan
Plastic Surgery
Istanbul University–Cerrahpasa Hospital
Istanbul, Turkey

Nicola Fleming
Department of Plastic and Reconstructive Surgery
Western Health
Melbourne, Australia

Paola Ghione
Lymphoma Service
Memorial Sloan Kettering Cancer Center
New York, New York

Geoffrey G. Hallock
Sacred Heart Hospital
Allentown, Pennsylvania

Curtis Hanba
Department of Otolaryngology – Head and Neck
  Surgery
University of Minnesota
Minneapolis, Minnesota
Chang Gung Memorial Hospital
Taoyuan City, Taiwan

Valerie Ho Wai Yee
University of Hong Kong
Hong Kong SAR, China

Joon Pio Hong
University of Ulsan
Seoul, South Korea

Chao-Hsin Huang
Kaohsiung Medical University Hospital
Kaohsiung, Taiwan

Chenyu Huang
Beijing Tsinghua Changgung Hospital
Tsinghua University
Beijing, China

Marco Innocenti
Plastic Surgery
University of Bologna
Orthoplastic Department
Rizzoli Orthopaedic Institute
Bologna, Italy

Hiro Ishii
Oxford University Hospitals NHS Foundation Trust
Oxford, United Kingdom

Anna Rose Johnson
Washington University in St. Louis
St. Louis, Missouri

Kidakorn Kiranantawat
Division of Plastic and Maxillofacial Surgery
Department of Surgery
Ramathibodi Hospital
Mahidol University
Bangkok, Thailand

Yur-Ren Kuo
Kaohsiung Medical University Hospital
Kaohsiung, Taiwan

Chia-Chun Lee
Kaohsiung Medical University Hospital
Kaohsiung, Taiwan

Lianne N.Y. Leung
Chinese University of Hong Kong
Prince of Wales Hospital
Hong Kong SAR, China

Michael Leung
Department of Plastic and Reconstructive
  Surgery
Monash Health
Melbourne, Australia

Cheng Hean Lo
Victorian Adult Burns Service
Alfred Health
Melbourne, Australia

Steven Lo
Canniesburn Plastic Surgery Unit
University of Glasgow
Glasgow, United Kingdom

Nelson Low
Monash Health
Melbourne, Australia

Susan E. Mackinnon
Center for Nerve Injury and Paralysis
  Plastic and Reconstructive Surgery
Division of Plastic and Reconstructive Surgery
Washington University School of Medicine
St. Louis, Missouri

Eldon Mah
St Vincent's Hospital
University of Melbourne
Melbourne, Australia

Jaume Masia
Plastic Surgery Department
Hospital de la Santa Creu i Sant Pau / Hospital
    del Mar
Barcelona, Spain

Rei Ogawa
Nippon Medical School
Tokyo, Japan

Terence Tai-lun Poon
Tuen Mun Hospital
Hong Kong SAR, China

Savitha Ramachandran
Sengkang General Hospital
Plastic Aesthetic and Reconstructive Surgery
Duke NUS Medical School
Singapore

Sanathorn Ratanapoompinyo
Division of Plastic and Reconstructive Surgery
Department of Surgery
Panyananthaphikkhu Chonprathan Medical
    Center
Srinakharinwirot University
Bangkok, Thailand

Sophie Ricketts
St Vincent's Hospital
University of Melbourne
Melbourne, Australia

Isabel S. Robinson
NYU Langone Health
New York, New York

Warren M. Rozen
Monash University,
Melbourne, Australia

Marcela Sánchez-Vargas
Clínica Colsanitas
Fundación CTIC
Bogota, Colombia

Eric Santamaria
Department of Plastic and Reconstructive
    Surgery
Hospital General Dr. Manuel Gea Gonzalez
Universidad Nacional Autónoma de México
Mexico City, Mexico

Dajiang Song
Hunan Cancer Hospital
Changsha, China

Francois Stapelberg
New Zealand National Burn Service
Auckland, New Zealand

Wen Shien Tai
Department of Plastic and Reconstructive
    Surgery
Western Health
Melbourne, Australia

Akihiko Takushima
Kyorin University
Tokyo, Japan

Jeannette W.C. Ting
The Chinese University of Hong Kong
Hong Kong SAR, China

Wing-Lim Tse
Prince of Wales Hospital
The Chinese University of Hong Kong
Shatin, Hong Kong SAR, China

Karen Vuong
Department of Plastic & Reconstructive Surgery
Western Health
Melbourne, Australia

Marcus J.D. Wagstaff
Plastic and Reconstructive Surgery
Unit Adult Burns Service
Skin Engineering Laboratory
Royal Adelaide Hospital
Adelaide, Australia

Wei Wang
Department of Plastic and Reconstructive
  Surgery
Shanghai Ninth People's Hospital
Shanghai Jiao Tong University
School of Medicine
Shanghai, China

Fu-Chan Wei
Department of Plastic and Reconstructive Surgery
Chang Gung Memorial Hospital
Chang Gung University and Medical College
Taoyuan City, Taiwan

Stuart Winter
Nuffield Department of Surgical Sciences
University of Oxford
Oxford University NHS Foundation Trust
Oxford, United Kingdom

Luccie M. Wo
Department of Surgery
Division of Plastic Surgery
Yale School of Medicine
New Haven, Connecticut

Kitty Wu
Mayo Clinic
Rochester, Minnesota

Wenjing Xi
Shanghai Ninth People's Hospital
Shanghai Jiao Tong University School of
  Medicine
Shanghai, China

Josephine Yip
University of Hong Kong
Hong Kong SAR, China

CHAPTER 1

The Accuracy of Computed Tomographic Angiography for Mapping the Perforators of the Deep Inferior Epigastric Artery: A Blinded, Prospective Cohort Study

Rozen WM, Ashton MW, Stella DL, Phillips TJ, Grinsell D, Taylor GI.
Plast Reconstr Surg. 2008 Oct;122(4):1003–1009

METHODS

A prospective, single-blind, cohort study was undertaken on 60 consecutive patients for whom deep inferior epigastric artery perforator flap surgery had been planned. Patients who did not undergo the procedure during the study period were excluded, with 42 patients ultimately included in the study. All computed tomographic angiography scans were obtained at a single institution. Perforators were mapped both on angiography and intraoperatively using a grid of 4-mm squares centered on the umbilicus. Only perforators larger than 1 mm were included in the study. All imaging findings were recorded by a single operator, and all intraoperative findings were recorded by the operating surgeon.

RESULTS

Computed tomographic angiography identified 280 major perforators in 42 patients. It was highly accurate, demonstrating 279 perforators recorded accurately, with one false-positive and one false-negative. Its sensitivity for mapping perforators was thus 99.6%, with a positive predictive value of 99.6%.

CONCLUSION

Computed tomographic angiography is highly accurate in identifying and mapping the perforators of the deep inferior epigastric artery. Its accuracy is superior to that of the previous modalities used in this role and suggests the usefulness of this technique before deep inferior epigastric artery perforator flap surgery for breast reconstruction.

EXPERT COMMENTARY

Jevan Cevik and Warren M. Rozen

Study Design

Single-blinded, prospective cohort study of 42 patients planned for deep inferior epigastric artery perforator flap breast reconstruction. Computed tomographic angiography (CTA) scans were performed, and perforators were mapped on angiography and compared with intraoperative findings.

Follow-Up

Data regarding perforator presence and location was collected at the time of surgery. Patients were followed up for 2 months postoperatively.

Inclusion/Exclusion Criteria

Patients planned for deep inferior epigastric artery perforator flap breast reconstruction within the study period were included. Only perforators greater than 1 mm in diameter were included in the statistical analysis. Patients whose operation did not occur within the study period, or those who did not receive a deep inferior epigastric artery perforator flap, were excluded.

RESULTS

Computed tomography angiography of the deep inferior epigastric artery preoperatively identified 280 major perforators in 42 patients, with a sensitivity of 99.6% and a positive predictive value of 99.6% for mapping perforators. The study found that CTA was highly accurate, demonstrating 279 accurately recorded perforators with only one false-positive and one false-negative result. All flaps were successful with no total or complete flap losses; the incidence of fat necrosis was 7% and the incidence of donor site morbidity within the 2-month follow-up period was 0%.

Study Limitations

A greater sample size may offer further validity to these results. There are limitations to the use of CTA such as the potential for contrast reactions, nephrotoxicity, and claustrophobia. Additionally, radiation exposure is a consideration, although the study describes techniques for minimizing this exposure. Specificity was unable to be determined in the study as there is no "true-negative" for evaluating the absence of a perforator.

Relevant Studies

In 2006, Masia et al.[1] performed a similar study comparing CTA results with intraoperative findings; however, this study focused on only the best three perforators rather than considering all suitable perforators (>1 mm diameter). The present study built upon this work, conducting a blinded assessment of all suitable perforators.

Study Impacts

The abdominal wall has become one of the most popular donor sites for autologous tissue for breast reconstructive procedures. Numerous reasons for this choice exist, including the common presence of excess tissue and a similarity to natural breast tissue.[2,3] Initially, free flaps based on the anterolateral abdominal wall were musculocutaneous in nature, including the deep muscle. Yet, as our understanding of surgical vascular anatomy evolved, it became evident that sacrificing the abdominal wall muscle was not necessary – leading to the development of perforator-based fasciocutaneous flaps.[4,5]

One such flap is the deep inferior epigastric artery perforator flap (DIEP).[2] Unlike muscle-based musculocutaneous flaps, the DIEP flap spares the abdominal musculature, resulting in reduced donor site morbidity postoperatively. Yet, perforator location and vascular anatomy remain highly variable, differing greatly between each individual patient.[6-8] Thus, surgeons faced challenges in executing the flap given the unpredictable nature of the vascular anatomy.

To combat this challenge, surgeons developed preoperative imaging techniques to help them navigate this complex anatomical landscape. Initially, visualization was performed using handheld Doppler (HHD) ultrasound. This technology allowed surgeons to assess the location of blood vessels preoperatively, guiding them when performing intraoperative dissection.[9-11] Yet, HHD ultrasound remained rudimentary in its ability to visualize the abdominal wall vasculature and its findings are inconsistent between users.[12] Another imaging modality, color duplex ultrasonography (CDU), allowed surgeons the ability to visualize perforators with images and could represent the flow in such vessels.[13] However, like HHD ultrasound, it is largely user dependent, and, depending on the user's skill, false negatives and false positives can be common.

Given the limitations of its predecessors, CTA represented a significant advancement in the ability to visualize vascular anatomy and plan operations prior to the day of surgery.[14-16] The present study established CTA as a highly accurate and reliable method for identifying and mapping the perforators of the deep inferior epigastric artery, surpassing the previous modalities used for this role. It suggested the usefulness of CTA for preoperative planning of the deep inferior epigastric artery perforator flap for breast reconstruction, potentially reducing dissection and operating time and decreasing operative complications. The study's results supported the use of CTA as the gold standard for preoperative imaging of the abdominal wall vasculature before reconstructive procedures.

Building on the foundation laid by this study, subsequent research and clinical experiences have further refined the application of CTA in the preoperative planning of DIEP flaps. Enhanced imaging techniques and advanced processing software have enabled more precise mapping of the vascular territory, facilitating the identification of the optimal perforators for flap harvest.[14,17] This progress has led to increased confidence among surgeons in the reliability of CTA, resulting in more tailored and efficient surgical approaches. The integration of CTA into the standard preoperative workflow has thus augmented the planning of breast reconstruction, making it a more predictable and safe procedure.

In recent times, surgeons have continually strived to improve and augment preoperative visualization of anatomy to further improve their understanding and planning prior to surgery. Magnetic resonance angiography (MRA) emerged as a promising alternative to CTA that lacked the downside of ionizing radiation.[18,19] Furthermore, innovations such as 3D printing and virtual reality have been integrated into surgical planning, allowing for more precise and individualized reconstructions.[7,20,21] 3D printing, in particular, can create patient-specific models of the vascular anatomy, aiding surgeons in visualizing and planning complex procedures. Virtual reality, meanwhile, offers an immersive environment for surgical training and planning, enabling surgeons to rehearse and refine their techniques before actual surgery. On the horizon, artificial intelligence represents an emerging technology that could accurately automate perforator identification from imaging, further enhancing efficiency.[22]

Currently, CTA remains the gold standard for preoperative visualization of the vascular anatomy of the abdominal wall. Looking ahead, ongoing research and technological developments are expected to continue to develop new technologies and improve the process of preoperative planning of breast reconstruction.

REFERENCES

1. Masia J, Clavero JA, Larrañaga JR, et al. Multidetector-row computed tomography in the planning of abdominal perforator flaps. *J Plast Reconstr Aesthet Surg* 2006;59(6):594–599
2. Allen RJ, Treece P. Deep inferior epigastric perforator flap for breast reconstruction. *Ann Plast Surg* 1994;32(1):32–38
3. Rozen WM, Bhullar HK, Hunter-Smith D. How to assess a CTA of the abdomen to plan an autologous breast reconstruction. *Gland Surg* 2019;8(Suppl 4):S291–s296
4. Onishi K, Maruyama Y. Cutaneous and fascial vasculature around the rectus abdominis muscle: anatomic basis of abdominal fasciocutaneous flaps. *J Reconstr Microsurg* 1986;2(4):247–253
5. Taylor GI, Corlett R, Boyd JB. The extended deep inferior epigastric flap: a clinical technique. *Plast Reconstr Surg* 1983;72(6):751–765
6. Cevik J, Hunter-Smith DJ, Rozen WM. Current advances in breast reconstruction. *J Clin Med* 2022;11(12):3328
7. Cevik J, Seth I, Hunter-Smith DJ, Rozen WM. A history of innovation: tracing the evolution of imaging modalities for the preoperative planning of microsurgical breast reconstruction. *J Clin Med* 2023;12(16):Pages.
8. Rozen WM, Ashton MW, Pan WR, Taylor GI. Raising perforator flaps for breast reconstruction: the intramuscular anatomy of the deep inferior epigastric artery. *Plast Reconstr Surg* 2007;120(6):1443–1449
9. Blondeel PN, Beyens G, Verhaeghe R, et al. Doppler flowmetry in the planning of perforator flaps. *Br J Plast Surg* 1998;51(3):202–209
10. Taylor GI, Doyle M, McCarten G. The Doppler probe for planning flaps: anatomical study and clinical applications. *Br J Plast Surg* 1990;43(1):1–16
11. Yu P, Youssef A. Efficacy of the handheld Doppler in preoperative identification of the cutaneous perforators in the anterolateral thigh flap. *Plast Reconstr Surg* 2006;118(4):928–933
12. Stekelenburg CM, Sonneveld PM, Bouman MB, et al. The hand held Doppler device for the detection of perforators in reconstructive surgery: what you hear is not always what you get. *Burns* 2014;40(8):1702–1706

13. Berg WA, Chang BW, DeJong MR, Hamper UM. Color Doppler flow mapping of abdominal wall perforating arteries for transverse rectus abdominis myocutaneous flap in breast reconstruction: method and preliminary results. *Radiology* 1994;192(2):447–450

14. Cevik J, Rozen W. A Novel optimization technique of Computed Tomography Angiographic 3D-reconstructions for pre-operative planning of DIEP flaps. *JPRAS Open* 2023;3538–3541

15. Rozen WM, Ashton MW, Grinsell D, et al. Establishing the case for CT angiography in the preoperative imaging of abdominal wall perforators. *Microsurgery* 2008;28(5):306–313

16. Rozen WM, Phillips TJ, Ashton MW, Stella DL, Taylor GI. A new preoperative imaging modality for free flaps in breast reconstruction: computed tomographic angiography. *Plast Reconstr Surg* 2008;122(1):38e–40e

17. Teunis T, Heerma van Voss MR, Kon M, van Maurik JF. CT-angiography prior to DIEP flap breast reconstruction: a systematic review and meta-analysis. *Microsurgery* 2013;33(6):496–502

18. Pauchot J, Aubry S, Kastler A, et al. Preoperative imaging for deep inferior epigastric perforator flaps: a comparative study of computed tomographic angiography and magnetic resonance angiography. *Eur. J. Plast. Surg.* 2012;35(11):795–801

19. Schaverien MV, Ludman CN, Neil-Dwyer J, McCulley SJ. Contrast-enhanced magnetic resonance angiography for preoperative imaging of deep inferior epigastric artery perforator flaps: advantages and disadvantages compared with computed tomography angiography: a United Kingdom perspective. *Ann Plast Surg* 2011;67(6):671–674

20. Chae MP, Hunter-Smith DJ, Spychal RT, Rozen WM. 3D volumetric analysis for planning breast reconstructive surgery. *Breast Cancer Res Treat* 2014;146(2):457–460

21. Phan R, Chae MP, Hunter-Smith DJ, Rozen WM. Advances in perforator imaging through holographic CTA and augmented reality: a systematic review. *Australas J Plast Surg.* 2022;5(1):32–38

22. Cevik J, Seth I, Rozen WM. Transforming breast reconstruction: the pioneering role of artificial intelligence in preoperative planning. *Gland Surg* 2023;12(9):1271–1275

EXPERT COMMENTARY

Song Daijan

The study by Rozen et al. (2008) aims to evaluate the accuracy of CTA for mapping the perforators of the deep inferior epigastric artery in patients prior to autologous breast reconstruction.

The study design was a randomized controlled single-blind, prospective cohort study with 42 participants who eventually had the CTA and DIEP flaps. The primary outcome was whether CTA identified perforators successfully. The study was well designed, with clear inclusion and exclusion criteria. However, the small sample size limited the statistical power.

The results showed that CTA has very high sensitivity and positive predictive value for perforator mapping by comparing CTA findings with operative findings. There were no complications arising from the use of CTA per se; all flaps were successful. The conclusion was that CTA is accurate and safe for identifying and mapping the perforators of deep inferior epigastric artery is reasonable; however, the study is limited by the small sample size and lack of long-term follow-up data. Future studies would address these limitations.

EDITOR COMMENTARY

Plastic surgery was described by Harold Gillies (c. 1957) as the "perpetual battle of beauty versus blood supply," and this is no more evident than in the evolution of breast reconstruction. The preoperative imaging of perforators is all about trying to win this battle. During the harvest of DIEP flaps, multiple perforators from the epigastric arteries are encountered as the flap is elevated. Often it is usually choosing the "best" perforator from the many that takes up the most time and causes the most stress for the surgeon, particularly whilst they are gaining experience.

This study, a subsequent cadaveric study (Rozen WM et al., 2008) and a clinical study by Masia J et al. (2006) confirmed that CTA could identify perforators with almost 100% concordance with operative/dissection findings and high positive predictive value (PPV). This capability relied on the advent of important technological developments; spiral CT and multidetector row CT (MDCT) were crucial as standard mode CT did not have the speed or resolution to identify the relatively small perforators. I remember reading about the development of MDCT for detailed pulmonary angiography in 2002 and had suggested to our radiologists that this may be a way of identifying flap perforators, but they thought it was unlikely to be useful.

CTA imaging allows the surgeon to preoperatively select the best perforator(s) on the basis of their diameter and configuration, which potentially allows for maximization of the flap blood supply, adjustment of the flap design to properly incorporate/centralize the perforator, as well improve the ease of dissection. It has been well established by subsequent studies that CTA can lead to a statistically significant reduction in time required to harvest DIEP flaps and the overall operative time – 100 minutes per patient according to Masia J et al. (2006) though gains reported by others have generally been more modest. For reference, it takes an additional 30–45 minutes to dissect a DIEP flap compared to a free TRAM flap (Blondeel P et al., 1998). Preoperative perforator localization may be particularly useful in patients with preexisting scars, e.g., Pfannenstiel.

The crucial clinical question has been whether this would make a difference to the clinical outcomes and whilst Masia et al. (2006) reported on one fewer flap failure and partial necrosis in the CTA group, overall, the literature has not been wholly convincing on this point. In all likelihood, CTA (or MRA or CDU) should tend to improve outcomes, but the differences between them (after you standardize for surgeon skill/ experience) are likely to be so minor that it would be difficult to establish definitively with clinical studies. All flaps in this study were successful, and, like most studies, did not show significant difference in complications (Colakoglu S et al., 2022).

The CTA has become an integral part of the preoperative workup in autologous breast reconstruction in high-resource centres and predominates as a "gold standard" of sorts in the literature. There are some well-established benefits to CTA though it falls short of being regarded as "essential." The utility of CTA is well established particularly in high-resource centres; however, the routine use of CTA (or MRA) depends largely on local resources, and, even where available, there may be significant waiting times. The time-savings may be more important for the those wanting to do more than one flap a day, whilst the preoperative vascular roadmap may benefit those still learning to do DIEP flaps (Thakur I et al., 2024) or may facilitate those using innovative approaches, such as robotic-assisted DIEP harvest (Daar DA et al., 2022). The use of 3D printing and augmented reality overlays have been described as possible ways to further facilitate the dissection and save time, but they remain at a preliminary stage. The use of artificial intelligence (AI) may reduce the time needed to identify the course of perforators in scans (Mavioso C et al., 2020).

MRA is preferred by Robert Allen because it avoids the issue of radiation exposure (personal communication) and has fewer issues with nephrotoxicity and allergic/contrast reactions. Doppler ultrasound (both handheld and colour duplex) is still in relatively common use despite the criticisms/shortcomings. Mijuskovic B et al. (2019) found that if CDU was performed by experienced radiologists, then it was slightly better than CTA at locating perforators. Zinser MJ et al. (2023) revived the use of contrast-enhanced ultrasound (CEUS) that potentially improves the intramuscular detail of CDU. Recently, the use of high-frequency and ultra-high-frequency ultrasound technology that allows visualization of small vessels (<0.5 mm diameter), including the point where the perforator pierces the superficial fascia and enters the dermis, may facilitate the harvest of super-thin perforator flaps as well as lymphatic surgery.

REFERENCES

Blondeel PN, Beyens G, Verhaeghe R, Van Landuyt K, Tonnard P, Monstrey SJ, Matton G. Doppler flowmetry in the planning of perforator flaps. *Br J Plast Surg.* April 1998;51(3):202–209. doi: 10.1016/s0007-1226(98)80010-6.

Colakoglu S, Tebockhorst S, Freedman J, Douglass S, Siddikoglu D, Chong TW, Mathes DW. CT angiography prior to DIEP flap breast reconstruction: a randomized controlled trial. *J Plast Reconstr Aesthet Surg.* January 2022;75(1):45–51. doi: 10.1016/j.bjps.2021.05.050.

Daar DA, Anzai LM, Vranis NM, Schulster ML, Frey JD, Jun M, Zhao LC, Levine JP. Robotic deep inferior epigastric perforator flap harvest in breast reconstruction. *Microsurgery.* May 2022;42(4):319–325. doi: 10.1002/micr.30856.

Masia J, Clavero JA, Larrañaga JR, et al. Multidetector-row computed tomography in the planning of abdominal perforator flaps. *J Plast Reconstr Aesthet Surg.* 2006;59(6):594–599

Mavioso C, Araújo RJ, Oliveira HP, et al. Automatic detection of perforators for microsurgical reconstruction. *Breast* 2020;50:19–24.

Mijuskovic B, Tremp M, Heimer MM, Boll D, Aschwanden M, Zeindler J, Kurzeder C, Schaefer DJ, Haug MD, Kappos EA. Color Doppler ultrasound and computed tomographic angiography for perforator mapping in DIEP flap breast reconstruction revisited: a cohort study. *J Plast Reconstr Aesthet Surg.* October 2019;72(10):1632–1639. doi: 10.1016/j.bjps.2019.06.008.

Rozen WM, Palmer KP, Suami H, Pan WR, Ashton MW, Corlett RJ, Taylor GI. The DIEA branching pattern and its relationship to perforators: the importance of preoperative computed tomographic angiography for DIEA perforator flaps. *Plast Reconstr Surg.* February 2008;121(2):367–373. doi: 10.1097/01.prs.0000298313.28983.f4.

Thakur I, Shepherd H, Soliman B. The first 150 consecutive DIEP free flaps: lessons learnt and a guide to efficiency for the junior plastic surgeon. *JPRAS Open.* 5 July 2024;41:336–346. doi: 10.1016/j.jpra.2024.06.014.

Zinser MJ, Kröger N, Malter W, Schulz T, Puesken M, Mallmann P, Zirk M, Schröder K, Andree C, Seidenstuecker K, et al. Preoperative perforator mapping in DIEP flaps for breast reconstruction. The impact of new contrast-enhanced ultrasound techniques. *J Pers Med.* 2023;13:64.

CHAPTER 2

PET–CT Surveillance versus Neck Dissection in Advanced Head and Neck Cancer

Mehanna H. *N Engl J Med.* 2016

METHODS

This was a prospective, randomized, controlled trial, comparing the noninferiority of positron emission tomography–computed tomography (PET-CT)–guided surveillance performed 12 weeks after the end of CRT, with a planned neck dissection in patients with stage N2 or N3 disease. In the experimental arm patients received a neck dissection if the PET-CT showed an incomplete or equivocal response). The primary end point was overall survival.

RESULTS

From 2007 through 2012, 564 patients were recruited (282 patients in the planned surgery group and 282 patients in the surveillance group) from 37 centres in the United Kingdom. Among these patients, 17% had nodal stage N2a disease and 61% had stage N2b disease. (TNM 7 was used for staging, and while p16 was recorded, when possible, this was not mandated and no stratification on p16 status was made.) A total of 84% of the patients had oropharyngeal cancer, and 75% had tumour specimens that stained positive for the p16 protein. The median follow-up was 36 months. PET-CT–guided surveillance resulted in fewer neck dissections than did planned dissection surgery (54 vs. 221); rates of surgical complications were similar in the two groups (42% and 38%, respectively). The 2-year overall survival rate was 84.9% (95% confidence interval [CI], 80.7 to 89.1) in the surveillance group and 81.5% (95% CI, 76.9 to 86.3) in the planned surgery group. The hazard ratio for death slightly favoured PET-CT–guided surveillance and indicated noninferiority (upper boundary of the 95% CI for the hazard ratio, <1.50; $P = 0.004$). There was no significant difference between the groups with respect to p16 expression. Quality of life was similar in the two groups. PET-CT–guided surveillance, as compared with neck dissection, resulted in savings of £1,492 (approximately US$2,190) per person over the duration of the trial.

DOI: 10.1201/9781003413738-2

CONCLUSION

Survival was similar among patients who underwent PET-CT–guided surveillance and those who underwent planned neck dissection, but surveillance resulted in considerably fewer operations, and it was more cost-effective. (Funded by the National Institute for Health Research Health Technology Assessment Programme and Cancer Research UK; PET-NECK Current Controlled Trials number, ISRCTN13735240.)

EXPERT COMMENTARY

Hiro Ishii and Stuart Winter

Study Design

This was a prospective, unblinded, multicentre, randomised, controlled trial, assessing the non-inferiority of positron-emission tomography-computed tomography (PET-CT) surveillance compared to neck dissection (ND) in patients with nodal disease staged N2 or N3 following completion of chemoradiotherapy (CRT). PET-CT was performed at 12 weeks with ND performed when there was incomplete or equivocal nodal response but complete metabolic response at the primary site.

Sample Size

564 patients were centrally randomised in a 1:1 ratio, to the planned surgery group (n = 282) or to the surveillance group (n = 282). Patients were recruited from UK head and neck centres between 2007 and 2012.

Follow-Up

Patients were followed up for up to 5 years from the time of randomisation, with a median follow-up period of 36 months, with 520 patients (92%) being followed up for at least 2 years.

INCLUSION/EXCLUSION CRITERIA

Eligible patients were those who were at least 18 years of age with a histologically confirmed diagnosis of SCC of the oropharynx, hypopharynx, larynx, oral cavity or an unknown primary site in the head or neck, with a clinical and radiological (computed tomography [CT] or magnetic resonance imaging [MRI]) stage N2 or N3 nodal metastases according to TNM 7 staging. These patients had to be suitable for CRT with curative intent and could not have any contraindications to ND.

Intervention/Treatment Received

Within the surveillance group, a PET-CT was performed 12 weeks after the completion of CRT. An incomplete or equivocal response of the PET-CT was defined as intense or mild FDG uptake, with or without incomplete structural resolution of the enlarged lymph nodes. Patients who had an incomplete or equivocal response with complete response at the primary site underwent ND (modified radical or selective) within 4 weeks of the PET-CT.

Within the planned surgery group, ND was performed within 4 weeks before or 4 to 8 weeks after completion of CRT; the type of ND was left to clinical assessment by the surgeon (either modified radical or selective).

RESULTS

Overall

There were no notable differences (age, sex, tumour site, tumour and nodal stage, and p16 status) between the surveillance and the operative groups. Males dominated both groups (79.1 and 84%, respectively) and the mean age was 58 years. A total of 84% had oropharyngeal cancer. 79% (n = 446) had N2a/N2b disease. 79% of patients were tested for p16 expression; all characteristics were well matched between tested and non-tested groups. Of the 446 specimens tested for p16, 75% were p16 positive.

Overall, 221 NDs were performed in the surgery group compared to 54 in the surveillance group.

Surgical Group

Of the 282 patients, 78% underwent ND (pre- and post-CRT); of the 22% who did not go ahead with surgery, half declined surgery, and the other half were deemed inoperable either due to disease progression or due to medical fitness. A total of 57% of those that underwent surgery pre-CRT had modified radical ND, with the rest undergoing selective ND. In contrast, only 38% of those who underwent surgery post-CRT had modified radical ND.

Surveillance Group

Of the 282 patients, 96% (n = 270) underwent PET-CT at 12 weeks; there was a high level of concordance between local and central PET-CT reviewers with respect to nodal and primary site assessment, 92% and 97%, respectively.

Local PET-CT reports indicated complete response in both primary and nodal sites in 185/270 patients (69%). Complete metabolic responses in the primary site with incomplete or equivocal responses at the nodal side were seen in 47/270 patients (17%). A total of 36/47 (77%) underwent ND; the reasons for patients not undergoing surgery were listed in Table S6 in the Supplementary Appendix; 15/270 (6%) had incomplete response at the primary site, but complete response in the neck nodes and as such, did not undergo surgery. A total of 19/270 (7%) had incomplete responses at both primary and neck sites, with 12 of these patients undergoing ND.

OUTCOMES AND EFFICACY

Follow-up was for 5 years, with a median of 36 months; 520 patients (92%) were followed up for at least 2 years. Overall, 122 patients died (60 in the surveillance and 62 in the surgical group). The 2-year overall survival rate was 84.9% in the surveillance group, compared to 81.5% in the surgery group. The hazard ratio for death with surveillance compared against surgery was 0.92, which favoured the surveillance group and met the pre-specified definition of non-inferiority. This hazard ratio excluded unfavourable difference of more than 4 percentage points. The two-sided P value for the difference between the management strategies was not statistically significant (0.66). The results were similar after adjusting for treatment centre, tumour and nodal stage, primary tumour site, CRT schedules, sex and age at randomisation, as well as p16 status.

Disease specific morbidity and mortality from other causes did not differ significantly between the two groups. P16 expression positivity was highly prognostic of overall survival in both groups. There was no significant difference in overall survival in p16 positive and negative patients between the two groups.

Patterns of Relapse

The 2-year rate of locoregional control was 91.9% and 91.4% in the surveillance and surgery groups, respectively. Within the surgery group, locoregional control was 90.4% and 94.8% in those who had surgery after and before CRT, respectively.

Surgical Complications and Global Quality of Life

Complication rate following ND in the surveillance group was 42%. Within the surgery group, rates of complications and severe complications were 38% and 26%, respectively. There was no statistical difference in complication and severe complications rates between those who had surgery pre-CRT (35% and 23%) or post-CRT (39% and 20%).

There was a small difference in global health state scores on the EORTC QLQ-C30 questionnaires in favour of the surveillance group at 6 months after randomisation, but this difference disappeared by 24 months post-randomization.

Cost-Effectiveness

Over the 2-year minimum follow-up period, the surveillance group was more cost-effective than the surgical group, with cost savings of £1,492 (approximately US$2,190), with an additional 0.08 QLAYs per person.

Study Limitations

Surgical trials are notoriously difficult to undertake, and this trial is no different. The second most common reason for surgical trials not recruiting is due to patient refusal of randomisation.[1] As such, this trial had to randomise patients in a pragmatic manner to allow sufficient recruitment.

The authors reported p16 status when it was available from immunohistochemical analysis and used a cutoff at more than 70% of malignant cells, demonstrating strong diffuse nuclear and cytoplasmic staining of p16, to call that tumour p16 positive. No further assessment of HPV infection was made. There was no planned stratification based on p16 status. The American Joint Committee on Cancer's *Cancer Staging System*, 7th Edition (TNM 7) was used for the duration of the trial.

The authors did not calibrate the standard uptake values (SUVs) among various scanning systems. Therefore, it was not possible to analyse the SUVs in determining the patients' response to treatment. This is especially relevant in those with p16 negative disease with an equivocal FDG uptake in the nodal site as these patients should probably continue with a neck dissection. This highlights the importance of having clear criteria/set SUVs for interpreting equivocal PET-CT findings.

The median follow up was 36 months, with 92% meeting the minimum 2-year follow-up period. Both these time spans are relatively short for assessing long-term outcomes, so it is not possible to draw long-term conclusions based on this data. However, the long-term cost-effectiveness of using PET-CT as a tool for surveillance is being looked at in the PETNECK2 trial.[2]

Debate remains ongoing about the 3-month time point with emerging evidence that delaying the PET-CT to 4 months can avoid more neck dissections. The American National Comprehensive Cancer Network (NCCN) guidelines[3] suggest post-treatment PET-CT to be undertaken between 3 and 6 months following completion of treatment, and that PET-CT performed before 12 weeks are associated with significant false-positive rates and should be avoided in the absence of signs of recurrence or progression. In line with the NCCN guidelines, the National Institute for Health and Care Excellence (NICE) guidance[4] made recommendations that for patients completing radical CRT, PET-CT should be performed 3 to 6 months following completion of treatment.

STUDY IMPACT

This study has demonstrated that in those patients being treated with CRT, a post-treatment PET-CT can safely avoid a planned neck dissection if there is complete structural and metabolic response in the tumour. This has resulted in a reduced number of operations, fewer complications, and short-term improved quality of life. These findings also support the concept of patient-tailored treatment using PET-CT as a means of assessing their response to CRT.

Crucially, in a system such as the National Health Service, it is important to consider the cost-effectiveness of each intervention, and the authors have demonstrated that PET-CT follow-up was more cost effective than planned surgical intervention by £1,492 per patient over the duration of the trial.

This study served as the basis of the updated NICE guidance: "Cancer of the Upper Aerodigestive Tract: Assessment and Management in People Aged 16 and Over," initially published in 2016. Then, in 2018,[4] these guidelines were revised and the recommendation on using PET-CT to inform the decision about surgery following completion of radical CRT were added. The 2018 recommendations are as follows:

- Offer PET-CT to guide the management for patients treated with radical CRT who have an oropharyngeal primary cancer site **and** 2 or more positive nodes in the neck, all of which are less than 6 cm across.
- To consider PET-CT to guide management in patients who have been treated with radical CRT who have:
  - an oropharyngeal primary site with 1 positive node in the neck that is less than 6 cm across **or**
  - an oropharyngeal primary site with 1 or more positive nodes larger than 6 cm across in the neck **or**
  - a hypopharyngeal or laryngeal primary site with 1 or more positive nodes in the neck.
- For patients who have completed CRT, perform a PET-CT 3–6 months after completion of treatment.
- Do not offer neck dissection to patients who have no abnormal FDG uptake or residual soft tissue masses on post-treatment PET-CT.

REFERENCES

1. Kaur G, Hutchison I, Mehanna H, Williamson P, Shaw R, Smith CT. Barriers to recruitment for surgical trials in head and neck oncology: a survey of trial investigators. *BMJ Open*. 2013;3(4):2625. doi:10.1136/BMJOPEN-2013-002625.
2. PETNECK2 Home | PETNECK2. Accessed 8 March 2024. https://www.petneck2.com/.
3. NCCN guidelines version 3.2024 Head and neck cancers. Published 2024. https://www.nccn.org/professionals/physician_gls/pdf/head-and-neck.pdf.
4. Cancer of the upper aerodigestive tract: assessment and management in people aged 16 and over. 2018. https://www.nice.org.uk/guidance/ng36.

EDITOR COMMENTARY

This trial builds on previous retrospective and observational data. The only way to solve the controversy between those advocating for systematic ND and those supporting a response-guided indication for ND was to test with a randomised trial. This study found that there were fewer NDs, fewer complications, and better quality of life in the surveillance group. As a bonus, there was also a cost saving.

Some argue that a particular shortcoming of this study is that the rates of residual pathologically positive nodes at neck dissection is not stated. This would have been useful in theory but less so in practice when there is no reliable way of knowing if this represents viable disease.

It would be very important to know if this can be extrapolated to patients with non-HPV related HNSCC – the 12-week cutoff would probably need to be adjusted as this cohort tends to have a slower but better response rate. This is reflected in the "3–6 months" suggested by NICE. The study seems most focused for N2 oropharyngeal cancer, with only 3% N3 disease and similarly low rates of hypopharyngeal (5%) and laryngeal (6%) cancers.

CHAPTER 3

A Systematic Review: Current Trends and Take Rates of Cultured Epithelial Autografts in the Treatment of Patients with Burn Injuries

Lo CH, Chong E, Akbarzadeh S, Brown WA, Cleland H.
Wound Repair Regen. 2019;27:693–701

METHODS

A structured literature search was performed in Ovid MEDLINE from 1946 and Ovid EMBASE from 1974 till present. All published peer-reviewed randomized or non-randomized clinical studies, cohort studies, prospective or retrospective series involving human application of cultured epithelial autografts in the setting of burn injury were included.

RESULTS

From 7,267 studies initially identified, 77 studies were included in the analysis. A total of 96% (74/77) of these series had a sample size of less than 100 patients. In 76.6% (59/77) of publications, average burn treatment exceeded 40% total body surface area. Overall, cultured epithelial autograft take rates reported in the literature were inconsistent and varied significantly from 0% to 100%. There was a recent trend for co-application of cultured grafts with autologous skin grafts, achieving relatively high and consistent take rates of 73%–96%. Results from cultured epithelial autograft application remained unpredictable.

CONCLUSION

This technology remains an adjunct or biological dressing and not an alternative to conventional split skin graft. However, it has contributed to wound closure and it has been life-saving in selected circumstances. Skin tissue engineering should continue as the clinical need for skin replacement is foreseeable into the future.

DOI: 10.1201/9781003413738-3

STUDY REGISTRATION

The review was conducted according to the PRISMA statement for reporting systematic reviews and prospectively registered in PROSPERO (registration number CRD42018089599).

AUTHOR COMMENTARY

Wen Shien Tai and Cheng Hean Lo

The following excerpt from Genesis 2:21-22 has been regarded as the oldest written reference to tissue engineering:

> And the Lord God caused a deep sleep to fall on Adam, and he slept; and He took one of his ribs, and closed up the flesh in its place. Then the rib which the Lord God had taken from man He [a]made into a woman, and He brought her to the man.

There were many studies of the epidermis in culture from the 1890s to the 1950s, and these were reviewed by Matoltsy.[1] In 1974, Howard Green learned about embryogenesis from study of cultivated murine teratomas and had no intention of studying therapy with cultured cells or the treatment of human burns.[2] With his graduate student, James Rheinwald, Green noted that teratoma cell cultivation gave rise to interesting colonies of epithelial appearance against a background of fibroblasts. Almost simultaneously, in the field of skin tissue engineering, John Burke and Ioannis Yannas were collaborating in studies in both the laboratory and on humans to generate a tissue-engineered skin substitute using collagen matrix to support the growth of dermal fibroblasts.[3,4] Their work resulted in Integra™, a dermal regeneration template still commercially available and used today. At the same time, Eugene Bell was developing living human skin equivalents consisting of fibroblasts cast in collagen lattices and seeded with epidermal cells.[3,5]

Propagation and culture of human keratinocytes was explored as the answer to limited donor site and autograft availability in patients with massive burn injuries.[6] In 1977, clinical use of cultured epithelium in burn patients was first presented at the Ninth Annual Meeting of the American Burn Association.[7] By 1979, techniques of in vitro cultivation of epidermal cells were further advanced, producing epithelial sheets suitable for grafting and highlighting the possibility of using autologous culture-grown epithelium to treat epidermal defects.[8,9]

This systematic review published in 2019 summarized the current state of play regarding clinical application of cultured epithelial autografts (CEA) in patients with massive burn injuries.[10] A literature search of major databases identified 7,267 studies, from which 77 studies were included in the study. All published, peer-reviewed, randomized or non-randomized clinical studies, cohort studies, prospective or retrospective series were included in the analysis. CEA had been used to treat patients for almost 50 years and was demonstrated to be potentially life-saving. However, CEA was also unreliable, with take rates quoted ranging from 0% to 100%. The more recent trend of combining CEA with autologous skin grafts seemed to improve take rates to 73%–96%, but determining the exact contributions of CEA versus autologous skin grafts to wound healing remains difficult.

Wound infection is the most common cause of CEA failure.[11–14] On poorly granulated or severely infected chronic wounds, and areas subject to contamination with fecal matter or sputum, grafted epithelium has a poor chance of success and often disappeared within 2–3 days.[15,16] CEA is highly vulnerable to bacterial proteases and cytotoxins during the first weeks of maturation and attachment.[15] Proteases are capable of completely digesting cultured epithelium, which is much more sensitive to proteolytic activity than split autografts.[11,17]

Wounds covered with only cultured epithelium display poor skin function and continued wound contraction.[18] The absence of dermis causes a greater degree of secondary wound contraction and skin fragility.[19] Areas of transplanted cultured epidermis where skin feels soft with no tendency toward scar contracture are attributed to the presence of residual dermis or dermal components in the wound bed.[16] It is long recognized that CEA may provide early wound closure, but, alone, it does not provide adequate long-term burn wound coverage and the risk of contracture formation is high.[18]

The production of CEA is expensive, and cost remains a limiting factor.[15,20] As numbers of major burn patients are low, for financial, organizational, and workforce reasons, culture laboratories of burn units are often organized for research and not for CEA production.[15] Staff then sporadically deviate from original assignments for the benefit of patients. This setup potentially leads to poorer quality grafts, quality control, staff expertise, and, eventually, poor laboratory credibility and closure.[15] Furthermore, the cost-benefit ratio may not compare favorably with other graft expansion techniques, such as widely meshed autografting with allograft overlay.[21]

The ideal skin substitute or human skin equivalent matches natural or uninjured skin, restoring form (cosmesis) and function.[22,23] It should restore function by restoring nerve, vascular plexus and adnexa (gland, follicles), and both dermis and epidermis to avoid wound contraction and scarring.[23,24] There have been many attempts to design the ideal composite skin substitute.[5,25,26] Overall, human clinical application of composite skin substitutes has been limited and disappointing, with few patients treated, usually as case reports or small clinical series.[27]

Boyce et al. is the only group to have treated and reported on large clinical series using a composite skin substitute with barrier function at time of grafting and an architecture that mimics normal skin, with a defined epidermis, dermis, and basement membrane.[22,28,29] They developed their skin substitute using separate, parallel cultures of autologous epidermal keratinocytes and dermal fibroblasts inoculated onto a biopolymer substrate composed of bovine skin collagen and chondroitin-6-sulfate (GAG). According to Steven Boyce (personal communication, March 2019), their group has treated more than 150 patients with their engineered skin substitute, making it the largest clinical experience with cultured composite substitute and burn wound closure. The results achieved were promising.

More recently, Meuli et al. published their experience with the treatment of 10 children (1 with acute burn injury, 9 had elective surgery) with bovine collagen type 1 hydrogel composite (denovoSkin TM and Zurich Skin, CUTISS Inc.) and reported a median graft take of 78% 3 weeks after surgery.[30] From 10 wounds treated, 7 were partial thickness in depth. In further separate reports, the same skin substitute was used to treat a 5-year-old child with 95% total body surface area (TBSA) burns with excellent engraftment rates of 80%–90% and a 4-day-old neonate with 40% TBSA burns.[31,32] A phase II clinical trial involving this composite skin is nearing completion and a phase III clinical trial is currently under preparation.[33]

Another promising approach is the application of stem cell-based therapy involving self-renewal and differentiation of stem cells.[34] Replication of "sister" stem cells and replacement of lost cells is potentially unlimited, thereby maintaining the constant number of aging somatic cells.[34] Healing and wound closure are potentially accelerated, and wound contraction and scar formation prevented.[34,35] Natesan et al. isolated stem cells from the adipose layer of discarded burned skin obtained during debridement of burn eschar.[36] Adipose-derived stromal cells (ASCs) isolated from debrided burned skin had similar morphological appearances to that of ASCs isolated from adipose tissue obtained from abdominoplasty procedures.[36] There was no significant difference in the cell proliferation rate of ASCs derived from these two sources.[36] These ASCs were successfully incorporated into a PEGylated fibrin-collagen-ASC bilayer hydrogel and used to treat full-thickness excision wounds in mice, leading to less wound contraction, improved dermal matrix deposition and epithelial margin progression.[36] This approach has significant therapeutic potential for wound healing in patients with massive burn injury.

To date, the full potential for skin substitutes has not yet been realized as none has yet been duplicated in vitro with all structures and function of native human skin.[5,22,23] The search for the ideal composite skin substitute continues.

REFERENCES

1. Matoltsy AG. Epidermal cells in culture. *Int Rev Cytol.* 1960;10:315–351.
2. Green H. The birth of therapy with cultured cells. *Bioessays* 2008;30(9):897–903.
3. Vacanti CA. The history of tissue engineering. *J Cell Mol Med.* 2006;10(3):569–576.
4. Burke JF, Yannas IV, Quinby WC, Jr, Bondoc CC, Jung WK. Successful use of a physiologically acceptable artificial skin in the treatment of extensive burn injury. *Ann Surg.* 1981;194(4):413–428.
5. Bell E, Ehrlich HP, Sher S, Merrill C, Sarber R, Hull B, et al. Development and use of a living skin equivalent. *Plast Reconstr Surg.* 1981;67(3):386–392.
6. Compton CC. Current concepts in pediatric burn care: the biology of cultured epithelial autografts: an eight-year study in pediatric burn patients. *Eur J Pediatr Surg.* 1992;2(4):216–222.
7. Igel H BC, Klein R et al. Clinical application of in vitro cultured skin as autografts. In: *Ninth Annual Meeting of the American Burn Association.* 1977. https://doi.org/10.1016/S0022-3468(05)80266-0.
8. Compton CC, Gill JM, Bradford DA, Regauer S, Gallico GG, O'Connor NE. Skin regenerated from cultured epithelial autografts on full-thickness burn wounds from 6 days to 5 years after grafting. A light, electron microscopic and immunohistochemical study. *Lab Invest.* 1989;60(5):600–612.

9. Green H, Kehinde O, Thomas J. Growth of cultured human epidermal cells into multiple epithelia suitable for grafting. *Proc Natl Acad Sci USA*. 1979;76(11):5665–5668.

10. Lo CH, Chong E, Akbarzadeh S, Brown WA, Cleland H. A systematic review: Current trends and take rates of cultured epithelial autografts in the treatment of patients with burn injuries. *Wound Repair Regen*. 2019;27(6):693–701.

11. Teepe RG, Kreis RW, Koebrugge EJ, Kempenaar JA, Vloemans AF, Hermans RP, et al. The use of cultured autologous epidermis in the treatment of extensive burn wounds. *J Trauma* 1990;30(3):269–275.

12. O'Connor NE, Mulliken JB, Banks-Schlegel S, Kehinde O, Green H. Grafting of burns with cultured epithelium prepared from autologous epidermal cells. *Lancet* 1981;1(8211):75–78.

13. Lo CH, Akbarzadeh S, McLean C, Ives A, Paul E, Brown WA, et al. Wound healing after cultured epithelial autografting in patients with massive burn injury: a cohort study. *J Plast Reconstr Aesthet Surg*. 2019;72(3):427–437.

14. Hernon CA, Dawson RA, Freedlander E, Short R, Haddow DB, Brotherston M, et al. Clinical experience using cultured epithelial autografts leads to an alternative methodology for transferring skin cells from the laboratory to the patient. *Regen Med*. 2006;1(6):809–821.

15. Guilbaud J. Problems created by the use of cultured epithelia. *Ann Medit Burns Club*. 1993;VI(2):1–4.

16. Kumagai N, Nishina H, Tanabe H, Hosaka T, Ishida H, Ogino Y. Clinical application of autologous cultured epithelia for the treatment of burn wounds and burn scars. *Plast Reconstr Surg*. 1988;82(1):99–110.

17. Eldad A, Burt A, Clarke JA, Gusterson B. Cultured epithelium as a skin substitute. *Burns Incl Therm Inj*. 1987;13(3):173–180.

18. Desai MH, Mlakar JM, McCauley RL, Abdullah KM, Rutan RL, Waymack JP, et al. Lack of long-term durability of cultured keratinocyte burn-wound coverage: a case report. *J Burn Care Rehabil*. 1991;12(6):540–545.

19. Donati L, Magliacani G, Bormioli M, Signorini M, Preis FW. Clinical experiences with keratinocyte grafts. *Burns* 1992;18 Suppl 1:S19–S26.

20. Still JM, Jr., Orlet HK, Law EJ. Use of cultured epidermal autografts in the treatment of large burns. *Burns* 1994;20(6):539–541.

21. Heimbach D, Luterman A, Burke J, Cram A, Herndon D, Hunt J, et al. Artificial dermis for major burns. A multi-center randomized clinical trial. *Ann Surg*. 1988;208(3):313–320.

22. Boyce ST, Warden GD. Principles and practices for treatment of cutaneous wounds with cultured skin substitutes. *Am J Surg*. 2002;183(4):445–456.

23. Boyce ST. Cultured skin substitutes: a review. *Tissue Eng*. 1996;2(4):255–266.

24. MacEwan MR, MacEwan S, Kovacs TR, Batts J. What makes the optimal wound healing material? A review of current science and introduction of a synthetic nanofabricated wound care scaffold. *Cureus* 2017;9(10):e1736.

25. Boyce ST. Skin substitutes from cultured cells and collagen-GAG polymers. *Med Biol Eng Comput*. 1998;36(6):791–800.

26. Boyce ST, Simpson PS, Rieman MT, Warner PM, Yakuboff KP, Bailey JK, et al. Randomized, paired-site comparison of autologous engineered skin substitutes and split-thickness skin graft for closure of extensive, full-thickness burns. *J Burn Care Res*. 2017;38(2):61–70.

27. Compton CC, Hickerson W, Nadire K, Press W. Acceleration of skin regeneration from cultured epithelial autografts by transplantation to homograft dermis. *J Burn Care Rehabil*. 1993;14(6):653–662.

28. Boyce ST, Kagan RJ, Greenhalgh DG, Warner P, Yakuboff KP, Palmieri T, et al. Cultured skin substitutes reduce requirements for harvesting of skin autograft for closure of excised, full-thickness burns. *J Trauma*. 2006;60(4):821–829.

29. Boyce S, Michel S, Reichert U, Shroot B, Schmidt R. Reconstructed skin from cultured human keratinocytes and fibroblasts on a collagen-glycosaminoglycan biopolymer substrate. *Skin Pharmacol*. 1990;3(2):136–143.

30. Meuli M, Hartmann-Fritsch F, Huging M, Marino D, Saglini M, Hynes S, et al. A cultured autologous dermo-epidermal skin substitute for full-thickness skin defects: a phase I, open, prospective clinical trial in children. *Plast Reconstr Surg*. 2019;144(1):188–198.

31. Moiemen NS, Schiestl C, Hartmann-Fritsch F, Neuhaus K, Reichmann E, Low A, et al. First time compassionate use of laboratory engineered autologous Zurich skin in a massively burned child. *Burns Open*. 2021;5:113–117.

32. Schiestl C, Zamparelli M, Meuli M, Hartmann-Fritsch F, Cavaliere A, Neuhaus K, *et al.* Life threatening non-accidental burns, pandemic dependent telemedicine, and successful use of cultured Zurich Skin in a neonate: a case report. *Burns Open.* 2023;7:28–32.
33. CUTISS. Clinical development program. [cited 2024 29 May]. Available from: https://cutiss.swiss/clinical-problem-scars/.
34. Nourian Dehkordi A, Mirahmadi Babaheydari F, Chehelgerdi M, Raeisi Dehkordi S. Skin tissue engineering: wound healing based on stem-cell-based therapeutic strategies. *Stem Cell Res Ther.* 2019;10(1):111.
35. Dash BC, Xu Z, Lin L, Koo A, Ndon S, Berthiaume F, *et al.* Stem cells and engineered scaffolds for regenerative wound healing. *Bioengineering (Basel)* 2018;5(1):23
36. Natesan S, Zamora DO, Wrice NL, Baer DG, Christy RJ. Bilayer hydrogel with autologous stem cells derived from debrided human burn skin for improved skin regeneration. *J Burn Care Res.* 2013;34(1):18–30.

EDITOR COMMENTARY

The systematic review includes 77 studies; most have small sample sizes. The commentary by Professor Lo provides an excellent update on this difficult and often confusing topic.

Cultured epithelium as pioneered by Rheinwald and Green is one of the few options for wound closure in massive burn injuries when the usual strategies of meshing/Meek grafting and reharvesting are unable to meet the needs. There are, however, significant practical barriers to the wider use of CEA, including the expertise/ facilities needed, the lag time involved, and the lack of a consistently reliable delivery system.

Over the decades, it has been difficult to scale up production of cultured skin substitutes beyond the research laboratory. Production of layered cells as a sheet remains a challenge and many choose to spray preconfluent cells. Interest in commercialization peaked in the 1990s with Epicel, though there has been a (re)surgence more recently in Asia with JACE, Keraheal, and Holoderm. The review shows a wide range of practices, reflecting the variable facilities/products available. The results remain largely unpredictable.

CEA is best applied to flat areas, avoiding joints, bony prominences, and the areas around orifices. CEA has also been applied to graft donor sites to accelerate healing. Wound colonization is probably one of the most difficult adverse factors to "control"; large acute burn wounds are prone to colonization/infection whilst antiseptics, such as chlorhexidine, and antibiotics, such as norfloxacin, are cytotoxic. The best current practice that yields consistent reproducible results probably involves using CEA with autologous graft (Meek or widely meshed, with or without cadaveric skin cover) over a vascularized dermal substitute, e.g., BTM/Nevelia/Integra, though it is then difficult to quantify the contribution of the CEA to the overall healing. Experience with newer commercial products from Japan and South Korea would be particularly informative. Holoderm was approved in 2002 and is covered by insurance (Korean industrial accident compensation insurance); it has supposedly saved over 850 lives, but there is very little written about it in the literature.

CHAPTER 4

Vacuum-Assisted Closure: State of Clinic Art

Argenta LC, Morykwas MJ, Marks MW, DeFranzo AJ, Molnar JA, David LR.
Plast Reconstr Surg. June 2006;117(7 Suppl):127S–142S

EXPERT COMMENTARY

Chenyu Huang

Study Design/Objective

This wide-ranging review was published in 2006. It describes the authors' first published case (also the first case in the world) of negative-pressure wound therapy (NPWT) (also known as vacuum-assisted closure, VAC) in 1997, how this seminal technology advanced in the next decade, and how its great efficacy meant it could be used to close many different types of wounds. Other advantages, namely, its simplicity and cost-effectiveness, were also highlighted. In addition, the rare complications of this technique were summarized.

Follow-Up

The effectiveness and safety of NPWT is discussed for clinical applications.

RESULTS

Argenta et al. mentioned several key technological advances that led to the widespread uptake of NPWT: the track device, which permits the vacuum pump to modulate pressure based on the needs of the treated area, large units that can remove several liters of fluid, and devices that irrigate contaminated wounds by continuously instilling fluids during NPWT. The addition of alarms that warn of bleeding, excessive output, or seal loss also increased confidence in these devices. In addition, the foam interface used together with NPWT device was refined: by 2006, polyurethane black foam, polyvinylalcohol (PVA) white foam, and silver-coated sponges became available. Argenta et al. reported that while NPWT was initially used to close chronic wounds, it was subsequently employed for many other clinical applications, including closing acute wounds, full- and partial-thickness abdominal wall defects, enterocutaneous fistulas, perineal/urological/gynecological wounds, traumatic extremity/orthopedic wounds, and degloving injuries. It also effectively treated sternal infection/mediastinitis and

DOI: 10.1201/9781003413738-4

diabetic-foot disease, and it facilitated split- or full-thickness skin grafting, grafting over bone, and fibrous ingrowth and colonization of synthetic matrices. In 2006, its utility in grafted burn wounds was still being assessed. The complications of NPWT were rare but included toxic shock syndrome (particularly when the wounds contained foreign bodies), granulation around detached sponge pieces, and excessive bleeding, particularly when the NPWT device was placed near major vessels. Argenta et al. discouraged the use of NPWT without safety alarms or with large reservoirs and condemned the use of NPWT with wall suction.

STUDY LIMITATIONS

N/A

Relevant Studies

After publication of the review, NPWT was subsequently found to be effective in several other clinical settings, including healing of pharyngocutaneous fistulae post-laryngectomy surgery[1] and nonoperative management of scleroderma ulcers.[2] Endoscopic application of NPWT can also treat perforated duodenal ulcers that have formed abscesses.[3] Moreover, NPWT can serve as adjuvant wound therapy after surgical management of axillary hidradenitis suppurativa,[4] colon perforation,[5] and perineal laceration.[6] In addition, NPWT has been used prophylactically to reduce wound complications after limb-sparing resection of pediatric primary bone sarcoma[7] and to prevent overall/deep surgical site infections after cardiac surgery.[8]

STUDY IMPACTS

A number of technical advances that could promote and broaden the clinical applications of NPWT have been proposed. They include using cheaper, more readily available interface materials (loofah sponge)[9] or employing mechanically powered devices rather than the classic electrically powered devices,[10] and single-use NPWT with canisters that collect excess wound fluids[11] or without canisters (this approach relies on evaporation of the fluids from the dressing).[12] Personal/home-use NPWT systems have also been developed and have been shown to be effective. For example, portable incisional NPWT effectively reduces the incidence of local wound complications after post-bariatric brachioplasty.[13] Such personal/home-use applications have been particularly advanced by employing an electrical feedback system that maintains optimal levels of negative pressure[14] and by improving device portability. Studies also show that different treatment parameters can affect NPWT efficacy, including the magnitude of applied pressure,[15] cycling parameters,[16] and instillation of topical wound solutions (e.g., antiseptics) and allowing them to dwell for specific times. The latter approach has been shown to decrease the time to wound closure by reducing the bacterial bioburden and promoting granulation-tissue formation.[17] NPWT can also be combined with regenerative medicine or pharmaceuticals to improve healing. For example, when mesenchymal stem cells were placed in full-thickness wounds in rats, covered with an acellular dermal matrix and subjected to NPWT, the matrix demonstrated much greater neovascularization than when NPWT and/or stem cells were not used.[18] Moreover, NPWT followed by basic fibroblast growth factor (bFGF) spray therapy eliminated partial necrosis of a distal sural flap used for calcaneal osteomyelitis.[19] In addition, NPWT not only effectively secures meshed split-thickness skin grafts that are used to treat full-thickness burn wounds, but also this effect is enhanced by first spraying the grafts with autologous skin-cell suspensions.[20] Similarly, use of NPWT after placing a platelet-rich fibrin gel into bone-exposed wounds accelerates wound healing in rats.[21] Finally, continuous intra-soft tissue or intramedullary antibiotic perfusion of antimicrobial agents during NPWT effectively prevents further infections in hard to heal ulcers.[22]

The advent of smart technology and artificial intelligence is likely to lead to new generations of NPWT. This is exemplified by a study on the effect of NPWT on abdominal-compartment syndrome in pigs. Six pressure sensors of a microcontroller-based multichannel pressure-sensor system were placed in the abdominal cavity and covered by a special foam that prevented their direct contact with the bowel wall. The intra-abdominal pressure was measured at the six locations during minus 50, 100, and 150 mmHg NPWT. This showed that NPWT at 100 mmHg demonstrated the best results and induced negative pressure in even the deep layers of the peritoneal cavity, thereby effectively decompressing the cavity.[23] Similarly, optical sensors utilizing the principle of dynamic fluorescence quenching were used to measure the oxygen levels in the foam interface of a NPWT device. That analysis showed that the foam oxygen levels dropped by as much as 22.8% and this reduction correlated inversely with the applied vacuum. This suggested that excessive vacuum could lead to oxygen deprivation in the underlying wound tissue.[24] Such technologies could be used to improve NPWT efficacy and applications in the future.

Research into cellular mechanotransduction may also lead to novel NPWT applications. Mechanotransduction involves cells sensing external mechanical forces that are then transduced into biochemical signals that alter cellular gene expression and behavior.[25,26] Therapies that achieve beneficial clinical effects by inducing cellular mechanotransduction are known as mechanotherapies. In 2013, we defined mechanotherapies as "therapeutic interventions that reduce and reverse injury to damaged tissues or promote the homeostasis of healthy tissues by mechanical means at the molecular, cellular, or tissue level."[27] Examples of mechanotherapies include using positive mechanical forces to expand soft tissues, e.g., via breast-reconstruction expander implants. Several mechanotherapies are also commonly used to promote wound healing, including using tension-reducing surgical approaches and postoperative silicone sheets to limit destabilizing stretch/abrasion forces on wounds. These approaches promote timely cutaneous wound healing and prevent hypertrophic scarring. Hyperbaric oxygen and shock-wave therapy are also classical wound-healing mechanotherapies. NPWT is also a wound-healing mechanotherapy because its mechanical force (negative pressure) not only draws the wound edges together and stabilizes the wound by removing excess fluid, but it also induces microdeformation at the foam-wound surface interface that stretches wound-bed cells. This stretching activates mechanotransduction pathways that promote beneficial cellular activities, such as proliferation, differentiation, migration, angiogenesis, neurogenesis, and granulation-tissue formation.[28] At present, the molecular mechanisms that underlie NPWT-induced mechanotransduction (and mechanotransduction in general) are poorly understood. Nonetheless, research into various NPWT indications has revealed the involvement of several molecules and pathways. For example, NPWT attenuates local inflammation in porcine acute wounds by downregulating multiple pro-inflammatory cytokines (IL-8, TGF-β1, and TNF-α).[29] This inflammation-reducing activity may also involve the Th17 cytokine IL-17, whose local expression in acute wounds in rats is increased by NPWT: the IL-17 inhibitor secukinumab completely abolishes the beneficial effects of NPWT on acute-wound healing in rats.[30] The anti-inflammatory effect of NPWT may also promote diabetic foot-ulcer healing: NPWT in this setting is associated with local downregulation of pro-inflammatory cytokine-producing signaling pathways (MAPK/JNK)[31] and reduced expression of the pro-inflammatory pattern-recognition receptor NOD1.[32] NPWT may also facilitate diabetic foot-ulcer healing by promoting angiogenesis (as shown by elevated VEGF levels) and extracellular matrix production/remodeling (as shown by elevated TGF-β1 and TIMP-1 expression and reduced IL-1β, TNF-α, MMP-1, and MMP-9 expression).[33] Moreover, NPWT can improve open fracture healing potentially by promoting MAPK-mediated osteogenic differentiation and proliferation of muscle-derived stem cells.[34] We believe that further research into these and other mechanobiological mechanisms will help to improve the efficacy and safety of NPWT and further broaden its applications.

REFERENCES

1. Malik MFMA, Azman M, and Baki MM. Negative pressure wound therapy in pharyngocutaneous fistula. *Cureus.* 2024;16(5):e60457.
2. Patel RM and Nagle DJ. Nonoperative management of scleroderma of the hand with tadalafil and subatmospheric pressure wound therapy: case report. *J Hand Surg.* 2012;37(4):803–806.
3. Ciuntu BM, Tanevski A, Buescu DO, Lutenco V, Mihailov R, Ciuntu MS, Zuzu MM, Vintila D, Zabara M, Trofin A, Cadar R, Nastase A, Ursulescu CL, and Lupascu CD. Endoscopic vacuum-assisted closure (E-VAC) in septic shock from perforated duodenal ulcers with abscess formations. *J Clin Med.* 2024;13(2):470.
4. Vinnicombe Z, Singh GV, Spiers J, Pouncey AL, McEvoy H, and Lancaster K. Comparison of negative pressure wound therapy with or without a split-thickness skin graft in the surgical management of axillary *Hidradenitis suppurativa*: a retrospective cohort study. *Plast Surg (Oakv).* 2024;32(2):314–320.
5. Lin CY and Pu TW. Colon perforation with severe peritonitis caused by erotic toy insertion and treated using vacuum-assisted closure: a case report. *World J Clin Cases.* 2024;12(18):3548–3554.
6. Mitsusada K, Dote H, Irabu S, and Atsumi T. Perineal laceration treated with negative pressure wound therapy following colostomy. *Trauma Case Rep.* 2024:52:101059.
7. Cuthbert C, Zaghloul T, Bhatia S, Mothi SS, Davis E, Heavens HG, Bishop MW, Talbot LJ, Neel MD, and Abdelhafeez AH. Use of vacuum-assisted closure to reduce the likelihood of wound complications after limb-sparing resection of pediatric primary bone sarcomas of the femur. *J Pediatr Surg.* 2024;59(9):1735–1739.
8. Fiocco A, Dini M, Lorenzoni G, Gregori D, Colli A, and Besola L. The prophylactic use of negative-pressure wound therapy after cardiac surgery: a meta-analysis. *J Hosp Infect.* 2024;148:95–104.
9. Tuncel U, Turan A, Markoc F, Erkorkmaz U, Elmas C, and Kostakoglu N. Loofah sponge as an interface dressing material in negative pressure wound therapy: results of an in vivo study. *Ostomy Wound Manage.* 2014;60(3):37–45.
10. Armstrong DG, Marston WA, Reyzelman AM, and Kirsner RS. Comparative effectiveness of mechanically and electrically powered negative pressure wound therapy devices: a multicenter randomized controlled trial. *Wound Repair Regen.* 2012;20(3):332–341.

11. Orlov A and Gefen A. The potential of a canister-based single-use negative-pressure wound therapy system delivering a greater and continuous absolute pressure level to facilitate better surgical wound care. *Int Wound J.* 2022;19(6):1471–1493.

12. Orlov A and Gefen A. Effective negative pressure wound therapy for open wounds: The importance of consistent pressure delivery. *Int Wound J.* 2023;20(2):328–344.

13. Facchin F, Pagani A, Marchica P, Pandis L, Scarpa C, Brambullo T, Bassetto F, and Vindigni V. The role of portable incisional negative pressure wound therapy (piNPWT) in reducing local complications of post-bariatricbrachioplasty: a case-control sstudy. *Aesthetic Plast Surg.* 2021;45(4):1653–1659.

14. Mullins RF, Wilson J, Hassan Z, Homsombath B, Craft-Coffman B, Paglinawan R, Cregan I, and Fagan S. The role of personal-use negative pressure wound therapy with enhanced functionality in achieving wound-related treatment goals: a small prospective study. *Wounds.* 2023;35(3):53–58.

15. Timmers MS, Cessie SL, Banwell P, and Jukema GN. The effects of varying degrees of pressure delivered by negative-pressure wound therapy on skin perfusion. *Ann Plast Surg.* 2005;55(6):665–671.

16. Dastouri P, Helm DL, Scherer SS, Pietramaggiori G, Younan G, and Orgill DP. Waveform modulation of negative-pressure wound therapy in the murine model. *Plast Reconstr Surg.* 2011;127(4):1460–1466.

17. Diehm YF, Fischer S, Wirth GA, Haug V, Orgill DP, Momeni A, Horch RE, Lehner B, Kneser U, and Hirche C. Management of acute and traumatic wounds with negative-pressure wound therapy with instillation and dwell Time. *Plast Reconstr Surg.* 2021;147(1S-1):43S–53S.

18. Sahin I, Ozturk S, Deveci M, Ural AU, Onguru O, and Isik S. Experimental assessment of the neo-vascularisation of acellular dermal matrix in the wound bed pretreated with mesenchymal stem cell under subatmospheric pressure. *J Plast Reconstr Aesthet Surg.* 2014;67(1):107–114.

19. Mikami T, Kaida E, Yabuki Y, Kitamura S, Kokubo K, and Maegawa J. Negative pressure wound therapy followed by basic fibroblast growth factor spray as a recovery technique in partial necrosis of distally based sural flap for calcaneal osteomyelitis: a case report. *J Foot Ankle Surg.* 2018;57(4):816–820.

20. Carney BC, Johnson LS, Shupp JW, and Travis TE. Initial experience combining negative pressure wound therapy with autologous skin cell suspension and meshed autografts. *J Burn Care Res.* 2021;42(4):633–641.

21. Zhang H, Wang S, Lei C, Li G, and Wang B. Experimental study of negative pressure wound therapy combined with platelet-rich fibrin for bone-exposed wounds. *Regen Med.* 2022;17(1):23–35.

22. Kitano D, Sakurai A, Kuwazuru K, Kitagawa H, Taniguchi T, and Takahara S. Intra-soft tissue and intramedullary antibiotic perfusion in combination with negative pressure wound therapy. *J Wound Care.* 2023;32(Sup11):S14–S23.

23. Csiszkó A, Balog K, Godó ZA, Juhász G, Pető K, Deák A, Berhés M, Németh N, Bodnár Z, and Szentkereszty Z. Pressure distribution during negative pressure wound therapy of experimental abdominal compartment syndrome in a porcine model. *Sensors (Basel).* 2018;18(3):897.

24. Biermann N, Geissler EK, Brix E, Schiltz D, Prantl L, Kehrer A, and Taeger CD. Oxygen levels during negative pressure wound therapy. *J Tissue Viability.* 2019;28(4):223–226.

25. Ingber DE. Tensegrity-based mechanosensing from macro to micro. *Prog Biophys Mol Biol.* 2008;97(2–3):163–179.

26. Ingber DE. Mechanobiology and diseases of mechanotransduction. *Ann Med.* 2003;35(8):564–577.

27. Huang C, Holfeld J, Schaden W, Orgill D, and Ogawa R. Mechanotherapy: revisiting physical therapy and recruiting mechanobiology for a new era in medicine. *Trends Mol Med.* 2013;19(9):555–564.

28. Huang C, Leavitt T, Bayer LR, and Orgill DP. Effect of negative pressure wound therapy on wound healing. *Curr Probl Surg.* 2014;51(7):301–331.

29. Norbury K and Kieswetter K. Vacuum-assisted closure therapy attenuates the inflammatory response in a porcine acute wound healing model. *Wounds.* 2007;19(4):97–106.

30. Xiao S, Wang W, Zhao C, Ren P, Dong L, Zhang H, Ma F, Li X, and Bian Y. A new mechanism in negative pressure wound therapy: interleukin-17 alters chromatin accessibility profiling. *Am J Physiol Cell Physiol.* 2024;327(1):C193–C204.

31. Wang T, Li X, Fan L, Chen B, Liu J, Tao Y, and Wang X. Negative pressure wound therapy promoted wound healing by suppressing inflammation via down-regulating MAPK-JNK signaling pathway in diabetic foot patients. *Diabetes Res Clin Pract.* 2019:150:81–89.

32. Wang T, Li X, Fan L, Chen B, Liu J, Tao Y, and Wang X. Negative pressure wound therapy promoted wound healing by suppressing inflammation via down-regulating MAPK-JNK signaling pathway in diabetic foot patients. *Diabetes Res Clin Pract.* 2019 Apr;150:81–89. doi:10.1016/j.diabres.2019.02.024. Epub 2019 Feb 27. PMID: 30825563.

33. Karam RA, Rezk NA, Rahman TMA, and Saeed MA. Effect of negative pressure wound therapy on molecular markers in diabetic foot ulcers. *Gene.* 2018:667:56–61.
34. Liu H, Zheng X, Chen L, Jian C, Hu X, Zhao Y, Li Z, and Yu A. Negative pressure wound therapy promotes muscle-derived stem cell osteogenic differentiation through MAPK pathway. *J Cell Mol Med.* 2018;22(1):511–520.

EDITOR COMMENTARY

A pedant's note: Negative pressure per se does not actually exist; a vacuum is a pressure below atmospheric. What "negative pressure" refers to is the way gases follow the pressure gradient.

NPWT has fundamentally changed wound care over the past few decades, applied as an alternative or adjunct to the "conventional" options of the reconstructive ladder. The original paper described experience with the safe and effective use of NPWT in a large number of varied wounds but lacks true control or experimental groups; each indication often includes a small number of cases, and the results were largely qualitative.

Despite hundreds of papers published and accumulated experience of thousands of physicians, the advice of clinical guidelines, including NICE UK, has been quite variable, and endorsements have generally been slow in coming. For example, it took until 2013 for NPWT to be "considered" for the open abdomen, whilst, in 2015, there was the first support of the use of NPWT by NICE in diabetic foot ulcers after surgical debridement on "advice of the multidisciplinary foot care service." Similarly, in 2019 single-use NPWT (in the form of PICO) was recognized to provide potentially better outcomes in patients at high risk of SSI, i.e., high BMI, DM, renal insufficiency, and smoking. Its use in complex open fractures was supported in 2022 after some modifications following the UK WOLLF trial (Costa ML et al., 2018). Use increased significantly during the COVID-19 pandemic as a way of managing wounds with the minimum of dressing changes and reducing hospital admissions.

This paper is a comprehensive review on the theories explaining the actions of NPWT and the then current clinical indications. In particular, there is the intriguing finding (of Labanaris AP et al., 2009) of an increase in lymphatic density at wound edges after NPWT seen in wound debridement samples.

Also, in the context of all the ligitation associated with the 'ownership' of NPWT, it would be remiss not to mention that Soviet surgeon Nail Bagautdinov described the use of negative pressure with foam dressings to treat wounds sustained during the Soviet-Afghanistan War in 1986. Ironically, a patent (or "inventor's certificate" in the Soviet Union) was declined because it was thought to be too similar to the Bier Cup from the 1890s. As it turned out, there were actually several other instances of possible "prior art," particularly from Europe. However, this particular work by a surgeon in Kazan City, Russia, was enough for KCI to lose its lawsuit with BlueSky and Smith and Nephew, which meant that, in addition to KCI, Wake Forest and also Argenta and Morykwas could not lay claim to NPWT. Bagautdinov (1980) was paid US$350 an hour for his time by Smith and Nephew; he immigrated to the United States in 1995 and currently works as an emergency physician in New York.

In her master's thesis in 2007, Danielle Zurovcik (2015) described a prototype for a hand-powered NPWT "bellows" pump, and this heralded a number of "economical" designs that would be potentially useful for NPWT in the developing world.

REFERENCES

Bagautdinov NA. Variant of External Vacuum Aspiration in the Treatment of Purulent Diseases of Soft Tissue. *In Current Problems of Modern Clinical Surgery: Interdepartmental Collection*, ed. V.Ye. Volkov et al. Cheboksary: Chuvashia State University, 1986:94–96.

Costa ML, Achten J, Bruce J, Tutton E, Petrou S, Lamb SE, Parsons NR, UK WOLLF Collaboration. Effect of negative pressure wound therapy vs standard wound management on 12-month disability among adults with severe open fracture of the lower limb: the WOLLF randomized clinical trial. *JAMA*. 12 June 2018;319(22):2280–2288. doi: 10.1001/jama.2018.6452.

Labanaris AP, Polykandriotis E, Horch RE. The effect of vacuum-assisted closure on lymph vessels in chronic wounds. *J Plast Reconstr Aesthet Surg*. August 2009;62(8):1068–1075. doi: 10.1016/j.bjps.2008.01.006.

Zurovcik DR, Mody GN, Riviello R, Slocum A. Simplified negative pressure wound therapy device for application in low-resource settings. *J Orthop Trauma*. October 2015;29 Suppl 10(10):S33–S36.

CHAPTER 5

Fibular Osteoseptocutaneous Flap: Anatomic Study and Clinical Application

Wei FC, Chen HC, Chuang CC, Noordhoff MS. *Plast Reconstr Surg.* 1986 Aug;78(2):191–200. doi: 10.1097/00006534-198608000-00008 PMID: 3523559

From anatomic studies of 20 cadaver legs and 15 clinical cases, it has been possible to demonstrate adequate circulation to the skin of the lateral aspect of the lower leg from the septocutaneous branches of the peroneal artery alone. This finding has allowed the development of a new concept and technique to elevate the fibula as an osteoseptocutaneous flap for reconstruction, which provides the following advantages:

1. Elevation of the fibular osteoseptocutaneous unit is easy and fast.
2. The cutaneous flap of the fibular osteoseptocutaneous unit can slide almost freely while attached to the paper-thin posterior crural septum without being tethered by a bulky muscle cuff, facilitating the setting of the fibular osteocutaneous flap when the bone and skin are widely separated.
3. Intraoperatively, in a situation in which it is necessary to change from originally selected recipient vessels to ones more suitable, the thin posterior crural septum can be folded around the fibula, allowing more flexibility in choice of recipient vessels.
4. The fibular osteoseptocutaneous flap meets the criteria outlined for composite tissue reconstruction of defects of the extremities.

This fibular osteoseptocutaneous flap was used in 15 clinical cases without any significant complications.

AUTHOR COMMENTARY

Curtis Hanba and Fu-Chan Wei

Introduction

This commentary reviews the landmark paper "Fibular osteoseptocutaneous flap: Anatomic study and clinical application" originally published in 1986. Still applicable in current practice, this technique helped to foster a new paradigm for both long bone and jaw reconstruction. Technical pearls are shared, and updated practice patterns are discussed.

DOI: 10.1201/9781003413738-5

The fibula and iliac crest were introduced in the early to mid-1970s as donor sites for vascularized bone flaps with the fibula primarily used for long bone reconstruction and the iliac crest commonly applied for jaw reconstruction.[1-3] In that era, when necessary, the fibula was harvested as a compound osteocutaneous or osteomyocutaneous flap with a relatively poor understanding of the vascular supply to the soft tissue of the lower lateral leg. This led to unreliable outcomes and challenges with soft tissue design. In 1986, Wei et al.'s anatomical study detailed the blood supply of the skin of the lateral aspect of the leg from septocutaneous branches of the peroneal vessels.[4] This finding allowed the fibula to be harvested as a more reliable "osteoseptocutaneous flap," which greatly expanded its clinical application in treating not only compound long bone defects but also could be used in mandible and maxillary reconstruction.[4]

The landmark article has demonstrated an impactful contribution to the field of reconstructive microsurgery as evidenced by an impressive citation index. The technique is likely to continue as a mainstay of vascularized bone transfer for many years to come.

STUDY DESIGN AND RESULTS

The authors dissected the cutaneous blood supply of the lower lateral leg in 20 cadavers and reported their experience treating 15 patients. During the anatomic component of the study, septocutaneous vessels were identified in the posterior crural septum between the peroneus and soleus muscles and followed toward their origin. Musculocutaneous vessels that penetrated a cuff of flexor hallucis longus (FHL), posterior tibialis (PT), or soleus were ligated. Methylene blue was injected into the origin of the peroneal artery and photographs documented the cutaneous perfusion patterns of the dissected specimens. The results identified an average of 4 to 7 cutaneous vessels per side, with an average of 1 to 4 of them being strictly septocutaneous, which were mostly located along the posterior border of the fibula at the middle and lower third of the leg. Authors reported a reliable skin paddle of 22 to 25 cm by 10 to 14 cm.[4] In clinical practice, an average of 12 cm of bone was utilized although typically 20–26 cm of vascularized bone can reliably be harvested from a standard adult sized fibula.[5,6]

ADVANCES IN TECHNIQUE

Prior to this article, two significant barriers prevented the widespread use of the fibula free flap. First, postoperative monitoring was challenging in cases without a cutaneous component, and, second, the inadequate knowledge about blood supply to the skin of the lower leg hindered the reliable incorporation of soft tissue into the flap's design. Chen and Yan's description of the fibula osteocutaneous flap in 1983 required resection of a large portion of the soleus and prioritized musculocutaneous perforating vessels to supply the lower lateral leg's cutaneous tissue.[7] The drawback of this technique was that the posterior crural septum was left behind, and a significant soft tissue bulk needed to be included for skin flap harvest. Both of these technical disadvantages limited the rotation of the soft tissue and thus the overall utility of the fibula osteocutaneous flap.

HARVEST TECHNIQUE

A tourniquet is placed on the midthigh and inflated to 350 mmHg.[4,8] An elliptical incision is centered over the posterior crural septum. Although a majority of septal vessels are identified in the middle and the lower 1/3 of the leg, the senior author designs his skin flap to include the entire potential area supplied by the cutaneous vessels thus allowing selection of the most convenient cutaneous supply during harvest. The incision is carried through the subcutaneous tissue above the deep fascia. Along the anterior incision, the peroneal tendons are identified, and the deep fascia is entered 1 cm posterior to the tendon to avoid its denudation and for better take of skin grafts if required. Subfascial dissection continues posteriorly to identify the intermuscular septum and septocutaneous vessels. Posteriorly, branches of the sural nerve are preserved, as are the lesser saphenous veins. The septocutaneous vessels are traced proximally, most commonly to the peroneal artery, near the posterior aspect of the fibula. Next, the lateral compartment musculature, including the peroneus longus and brevis and anterior compartment, including extensor digitorum longus, and extensor hallucis are dissected from the fibula. A thin muscular cuff is left on the bone to support the periosteal blood supply. The anterior tibial neurovascular bundle is identified and preserved. Next, bony cuts are designed with preservation of the proximal and distal 6 cm of bone to maintain joint stability. Once the osteotomies are done, the fibula bone can be mobilized to expose the interosseous membrane (IOM). After division of the IOM, the fibula is further released to allow rotation with traction by bone clamps at both divided ends; thus, the distal runoff of the peroneal vessels is exposed and followed, superiorly releasing the FHL and PT. It is currently the practice of the senior author to preserve the nerve to the FHL when possible and to divide distal runoff of the peroneal artery in a location that allows perfusion of the most distal end of the skin flap while maintaining muscular branches to the residual FHL to preserve its blood supply, which may reduce the incidence of great toe contracture. In a separate study from the senior author, postoperative MRI demonstrated viable FHL if the blood supply is protected during the procedure, although this data remains unpublished (Lin et al., "Fate of the Flexor Hallucis Longus Muscle at the Donor Site after Fibula FLap Harvest: Assessing muscle Viability Using Novel MRI Techniques – A Cohort Study"). Next, the tourniquet is released, and blood flow is re-established for 20 minutes prior to division of the vascular pedicle of the flap.

FOLLOW-UP AND CONTROVERSIES

In the original article, only one of the 15 patients reported mild numbness of the dorsal foot without major donor site complications.[4] Sensory alterations related to the osteoseptocutaneous flap harvest can be the result of manipulation of the sural nerve or deep peroneal nerve.[9] Generally these disturbances are mild, and often the sural nerve can be used as a nerve graft source when sensory reconstruction is necessary.[10] In this clinical series, one of the patients had a history of congenital pseudoarthosis, and the remaining cases were trauma-related reconstructions. In the case of the 4½-year-old patient with pseudoarthrosis, sacrifice of the posterior tibial artery and peroneal artery together as a unit was needed as there was no cutaneous supply from the peroneal system. Sacrifice of 2 of the 3 blood vessels supplying the foot is generally considered high risk and often an awareness of this risk preoperatively would lead surgeons to seek alternative donor sites.[9] In fact, in the senior author's personal experience of over 950 fibula-free flaps, vascular compromise to the foot has not been encountered. It is the senior author's practice to request preoperative CT angiography of the lower extremity when either the pedis dorsalis or the posterior tibial artery are abnormal during preoperative clinical assessment or in the setting of prior trauma of the lower extremity.[11] Primary closure of the donor site without tension is feasible only if a less than 3.5 cm wide skin paddle is taken with the vascularized fibula.[4] An overly tight closure can compromise blood flow to the foot or lower leg musculature mimicking a Volkmann's ischemic contracture.[12,13]

STUDY IMPACT

The fibula osteoseptocutaneous flap has become a workhorse bone flap with a multitude of applications largely because of the reliability of circulation in the skin paddle. Furthermore, the freely movable septocutaneous vessels in the posterior crural septum allowed simultaneous reconstruction of an adjacent coverage defect. Although segmental jaw defect reconstruction with fibula was first introduced by Hidalgo in 1989, it was the pioneering work of this 1986 study in lower extremity reconstruction which dramatically expanded the capacity of the fibula to replace the iliac crest and other vascularized bony flaps as the primary choice.[14] In 1994, Wei reported a series of 27 patients who underwent segmental mandibular reconstruction, noting a 96.3% bone flap survival rate without cutaneous compromise in any of the cases.[15] As noted, release of the posterior crural septum allows extra rotational freedom in the event that an originally planned recipient vessel is deemed unsatisfactory intraoperatively and alternate recipient vessels are needed, which is not an uncommon scenario in patients with previously treated head and neck pathology.[16] This study, among others, firmly supported the reliability of the fibula osteoseptocutaneous flap and its legacy is maintained to this day.

REFERENCES

1. Taylor, G. I., Townsend, P., & Corlett, R. (1979). Superiority of the deep circumflex iliac vessels as the supply for free groin flaps. Clinical work. *Plastic and Reconstructive Surgery*, 64(6), 745–759. https://doi.org/10.1097/00006534-197912000-00001.
2. Taylor, G. I., Townsend, P., & Corlett, R. (1979). Superiority of the deep circumflex iliac vessels as the supply for free groin flaps. *Plastic and Reconstructive Surgery*, 64(5), 595–604.
3. Taylor, G. I., Miller, G. D., & Ham, F. J. (1975). The free vascularized bone graft. A clinical extension of microvascular techniques. *Plastic and Reconstructive Surgery*, 55(5), 533–544. https://doi.org/10.1097/00006534-197505000-00002.
4. Wei, F. C., Chen, H. C., Chuang, C. C., & Noordhoff, M. S. (1986). Fibular osteoseptocutaneous flap: anatomic study and clinical application. *Plastic and Reconstructive Surgery*, 78(2), 191–200. https://doi.org/10.1097/00006534-198608000-00008.
5. Taylor G. I. (1983). The current status of free vascularized bone grafts. *Clinics in Plastic Surgery*, 10(1), 185–209.
6. Weiland, A. J., Moore, J. R., & Daniel, R. K. (1983). Vascularized bone autografts. Experience with 41 cases. *Clinical Orthopaedics and Related Research*, (174), 87–95.

7. Chen, Z. W., & Yan, W. (1983). The study and clinical application of the osteocutaneous flap of fibula. *Microsurgery, 4*(1), 11–16. https://doi.org/10.1002/micr.1920040107.

8. Al Deek, N. F., Kao, H. K., & Wei, F. C. (2018). The fibula osteoseptocutaneous flap: concise review, goal-oriented surgical technique, and tips and tricks. *Plastic and Reconstructive Surgery, 142*(6), 913e–923e. https://doi.org/10.1097/PRS.0000000000005065.

9. Lezak, B., Massel, D. H., & Varacallo, M. (2024). Peroneal nerve injury. In *StatPearls*. StatPearls Publishing.

10. Hanba, C., Lin, T. C., & Wei, F. C. (5 August 2024). The fibula osteoseptocutaneous flap - evolution in concepts, techniques and technologies during mandibular reconstruction: a review. *International Journal of Surgery*. https://doi.org/10.1097/JS9.0000000000001972.

11. Lutz, B. S., Wei, F. C., Ng, S. H., Chen, I. H., & Chen, S. H. (1999). Routine donor leg angiography before vascularized free fibula transplantation is not necessary: a prospective study in 120 clinical cases. *Plastic and Reconstructive Surgery, 103*(1), 121–127. https://doi.org/10.1097/00006534-199901000-00019.

12. Linderson, A., Dimovska, E. O. F., & Rodriguez-Lorenzo, A. (2022). Donor site ischemic events following fibula flap harvest in head and neck reconstruction: a case report and perioperative management strategies. *International Microsurgery Journal,6*(1), 1. https://doi.org/10.24983/scitemed.imj.2022.00159.

13. Santi, M. D., & Botte, M. J. (1995). Volkmann's ischemic contracture of the foot and ankle: evaluation and treatment of established deformity. *Foot & Ankle International, 16*(6), 368–377. https://doi.org/10.1177/107110079501600610.

14. Hidalgo D. A. (1989). Fibula free flap: a new method of mandible reconstruction. *Plastic and Reconstructive Surgery, 84*(1), 71–79.

15. Wei, F. C., Seah, C. S., Tsai, Y. C., Liu, S. J., & Tsai, M. S. (1994). Fibula osteoseptocutaneous flap for reconstruction of composite mandibular defects. *Plastic and Reconstructive Surgery, 93*(2), 294–306.

16. Prince, A. D. P., Broderick, M. T., Neal, M. E. H., & Spector, M. E. (August 2020). Head and neck reconstruction in the vessel depleted neck. *Frontiers of Oral and Maxillofacial Medicine, 2*, 13. https://doi.org/10.21037/fomm-20-38.

EDITOR COMMENTARY

For a long time, microsurgical bony mandibular reconstruction had been regarded as a particularly challenging surgery with few options. In 1982, Ian Taylor described his method of mandibular reconstruction using free composite iliac bone "grafts" with microvascular techniques (i.e., flaps) with a success rate of 87% – one flap failed due to arterial thrombosis (1982). Although use of the iliac bone has declined in recent decades, it remains the preferred option in several centers – virtual surgical planning, bone-shaping with templates and techniques to increase pedicle length have increased its versatility. Meticulous re-suturing of the abdominal muscles may reduce the incidence of herniae, one of the main donor site concerns.

As Wei F.C. (1994) stated, David Hidalgo (1989) was the first to use fibula flaps for segmental mandibular defects. It provided a long length of fibular bone with a robust periosteal blood supply that permits multiple osteotomies and a pedicle with sizable blood vessels that are straightforward to anastomose. However, he encountered significant problems with the skin paddle when it was harvested with the fibula (4 cases). The skin paddle was thus deemed unreliable and was often excised. This contrasts with the findings in this study by Wei F.C. et al. that demonstrated that a reliable fibular skin paddle could be harvested by basing it on septocutaneous supply from the peroneal artery. The retrospective study describes use of the flap for long bone reconstructions, after having been defined in cadaveric dissection. Inclusion and exclusion criteria are not mentioned. Three cases were discussed in the paper; however, the study lacks details of the outcomes, including any complications and there was no long-term follow-up.

In a subsequent 1994 article, Wei et al. presented their findings on a total of 27 cases of composite mandibular reconstruction. A success rate of 96.3% was reported with no cases of loss of skin paddle (partial or total) and a 100% success rate of primary healing at the osteotomy sites. In 1995, Hidalgo confirmed the reliability of the flap and skin island in a retrospective series with 60 patients (1995).

Although these are all retrospective case series with short follow-up and inherent limitations as such, the collective experience has allowed the fibula osteoseptocutaneous flap to become the standard of care for reconstruction of segmental jaw defects.

REFERENCES

Hidalgo DA. Fibula free flap: a new method of mandible reconstruction. *Plast Reconstr Surg.* 1989;84(1):71–79.

Hidalgo DA, Rekow A. A review of 60 consecutive fibula free flap mandible reconstructions. *Plast Reconstr Surg.* 1995;96:585–596, discussion 597–602.

Taylor GI. Reconstruction of the mandible with free composite iliac bone grafts. *Ann Plast Surg.* November 1982;9(5):361–376.

Wei FC, *et al.* Fibula osteoseptocutaneous flap for reconstruction of composite mandibular defects. *Plast Reconstr Surg.* 1994;93(2):294–306.

CHAPTER 6

Early Microsurgical Reconstruction of Complex Trauma of the Extremities

Godina M. *Plast Reconstr Surg.* 1986;78(3):285–292
doi: 10.1097/00006534-198609000-00001

MATERIAL AND METHOD

They were divided into three groups for the purpose of review. Group 1 underwent free-flap transfer within 72 hours of the injury, group 2 between 72 hours and 3 months of the injury, and group 3 between 3 months and 12.6 years, with a mean of 3.4 years.

RESULT AND CONCLUSION

The results were analyzed with respect to flap failure, infection, bone-healing time, length of hospital stay, and number of operative procedures. The flap failure rate was 0.75% in group 1, 12% in group 2, and 9.5% in group 3 (p less than 0.0005 early versus delayed; p less than 0.0025 early versus late). Postoperative infection occurred in 1.5% of group 1, 17.5% of group 2, and 6% of group 3. Bone-healing time was 6.8 months in group 1, 12.3 months in group 2, and 29 months in group 3. The average length of total hospital stay was 27 days for group 1, 130 days for group 2, and 256 days for group 3. The number of operations averaged 1.3 for group 1, 4.1 for group 2, and 7.8 for group 3.

EXPERT COMMENTARY

Joon Pio Hong

Lower extremity reconstruction, particularly in the setting of trauma, remains one of the most challenging tasks for the plastic and reconstructive surgeon.[1, 2] Relevant factors to consider include bony restoration, dead space obliteration, infection debridement, flap choice, and timing. Marko Godina in his landmark paper in 1986 established the principle of early flap coverage for reconstruction of traumatic lower extremity injuries to minimize oedema, fibrosis, and infection while optimizing outcomes.[3] This paper remains a landmark paper in the field of lower extremity reconstruction due to the impact it has made to the overall principles in the approach to the problem.

His large series of over 500 patients demonstrated lower rates of flap failure and postoperative infection in the early surgery group compared with patients who had flaps

DOI: 10.1201/9781003413738-6

after 72 hours, making this an essential guideline for decades after this work. In this work, early coverage of complex lower extremity trauma both improved flap success rate and decreased the rate of long-term infection, showing that only 1% of patients with lower extremity trauma developed infections when they were acutely debrided, washed out, and reconstructed with a free tissue transfer within 72 hours of injury.[4] This subgroup of patients also enjoyed a 0.75% flap failure rate, which grew substantially to between 9% and 12% in patients who were reconstructed after the 72-hour mark. The implications of this finding were substantial and the concept of the "emergency free flap" was born.[4]

Of course, one can debate whether this concept is still valid today as the wider user of negative pressure wound therapy has changed the way some complex wounds are managed. In addition, the introduction of high-level supermicrosurgery using small perforators as potential recipients may allow surgeons to avoid major vessels that may have become scarred during the prolonged wound preparation phase, which would increase the chance of complications.[5–8] One must also consider the fact that trauma patients are often initially seen in hospitals where reconstruction is not readily offered, and, thus, by the time the patient reaches a higher level center, the "golden time" has already passed. However, it seems that they can still have reasonably good outcomes by adjusting their management; thus, the debate on whether or not the timing of reconstruction is *that* critical may be a valid one. Nevertheless, one can still agree that reconstruction in an acute setting still provides many benefits compared to the delayed setting.

In addition to his work on timing of reconstructive surgery, one must understand the overall thinking of Godina. Marko's legacy lives on in the care of our patients today as a standard for the management of lower extremity trauma. His work on the concepts of end-to-side anastomosis is still widely respected.[9] His lasting contributions continue with the first clinical uses of the latissimus dorsi free muscle flap, free lateral arm flap, and saphenous neurovascular flap, as well as advocating the use of arterial autografts in microvascular surgery.[10–12] These concepts all tie in together with the concept of optimal timing.

I strongly believe that this concept of timing remains a golden principle for now, and this paper remains a landmark paper in the field of lower extremity reconstruction. In addition to these critical concepts, one must be aware of new concepts, such as the orthoplastic approach, and other innovations that will provide the best possible outcome in modern-day reconstruction for the lower extremity.

REFERENCES

1. Hong JP, Hallock GG. Our premise for lower extremity reconstruction. *J Reconstr Microsurg.* 2021;37(1):1.
2. Suh HS, Lee JS, Hong JP. Consideration in lower extremity reconstruction following oncologic surgery: patient selection, surgical techniques, and outcomes. *J Surg Oncol.* 2016;113(8):955–961.

3. Godina M. Early microsurgical reconstruction of complex trauma of the extremities. *Plast Reconstr Surg.* 1986;78(3):285–292.

4. Colen DL, Colen LB, Levin LS, Kovach SJ. Godina's Principles in the twenty-first century and the evolution of lower extremity trauma reconstruction. *J Reconstr Microsurg.* 2018;34(8):563–571.

5. Hong JP, Koshima I. Using perforators as recipient vessels (supermicrosurgery) for free flap reconstruction of the knee region. *Ann Plast Surg.* 2010;64(3):291–293.

6. Hong JP, Park CJ, Suh HP. Importance of vascularity and selecting the recipient vessels of lower extremity reconstruction. *J Reconstr Microsurg.* 2021;37(1):83–88.

7. Kim KN, Hong JP, Park SW, Kim SW, Yoon CS. Overcoming the obstacles of the ilizarov device in extremity reconstruction: usefulness of the perforator as the recipient vessel. *J Reconstr Microsurg.* 2015;31(6):420–425.

8. Power HA, Cho J, Kwon JG, Abdelfattah U, Pak CJ, Suh HP, *et al.* Are perforators reliable as recipient arteries in lower extremity reconstruction? Analysis of 423 free perforator flaps. *Plast Reconstr Surg.* 2022;149(3):750–760.

9. Godina M. Preferential use of end-to-side arterial anastomoses in free flap transfers. *Plast Reconstr Surg.* 1979;64(5):673–682.

10. Godina M. Arterial autografts in microvascular surgery. *Plast Reconstr Surg.* 1986;78(3):293–294.

11. Godina M. The tailored latissimus dorsi free flap. *Plast Reconstr Surg.* 1987;80(2):304–306.

12. Arnez ZM, Kersnic M, Smith RW, Godina M. Free lateral arm osteocutaneous neurosensory flap for thumb reconstruction. *J Hand Surg Br.* 1991;16(4):395–399.

EXPERT COMMENTARY

Odhran Shelley

Marko Godina's paper entitled "Early microsurgical reconstruction following complex trauma of the extremities" is one of the most important in plastic surgery.[1] It combines concepts of tissue management, debridement, and complex reconstruction. It fuses astute observation and exceptional skill applied to treat challenging problems. It considers the impact of timing following injury and appraises outcomes such as rates of infection, number of anaesthesias, length of hospital stay, and function in ways reconstructive outcomes had not been considered before. It is a timeless classic with results that remain difficult to match today.

STUDY DESIGN

This paper is a case control study of 532 patients with post-traumatic defects of the extremities who underwent free flap reconstruction by a single microsurgical service. Patients were divided into three groups for the purpose of the review. The first group had an early free flap performed within 72 hours from injury. The second (group 2) had delayed reconstruction with a free flap performed at a timepoint between 72 hours and 3 months; and the third (group 3) had a late reconstruction with a free flap performed more than 3 months following the injury. The groups were evaluated by the criteria of free-flap failure, post-reconstruction infections, time to achieve bone healing, total hospitalization time, and number of anaesthetics. Bone healing time was evaluated by clinical weight- or load-bearing ability. Hospitalization included all time spent in hospital.

FOLLOW-UP

Follow-up was performed in two centres supported by the service, the microsurgical centre in Ljubljana (470 cases) and Kuwait (62) cases. The exact range of follow-up is not stated, but the average time to bone healing ranged from 6.8 months in the early group to 29 months in the delayed group. This implies that there was a significant follow-up time in all groups studied.

INCLUSION/EXCLUSION CRITERIA

All patients who underwent microsurgical reconstruction of the extremities under the auspices of the Microsurgical Service of the University Department of Plastic Surgery and Burns in Ljubljana between 1976 and 1983. Of those, 470 were performed in Ljubljana, Slovenia and 62 in Kuwait. No exclusion criteria are listed.

RESULTS

Godina's paper links outcomes with experience and relates a 26% failure rate in the first 100 free flaps, which took an average of 7.2 hours to perform, and 4% in the last 100 free flaps, which took, on average, 4.7 hours to perform.

Each outcome measured favoured early free-flap reconstruction. There were 134 patients in the early group (25.2%) with 1 failure (0.75%), 2 postoperative infections (1.5%), average time to bone healing 6.8 months, 27 days average hospitalization, and 1.3 anaesthesias performed. The delayed group had 167 patients (31.4%) with 20 failures (12%), 29 postoperative infections (17.5%), average time to bone healing 12.3 months, 130 days average hospitalization, and 4.1 anaesthesias performed. The late group had 231 patients (43.4%) with 22 failures (9.5%), 14 postoperative infections (6%), average time to bone healing 29 months, 256 days average hospitalization, and 7.8 anaesthesias performed.

STUDY LIMITATIONS

The paper itself was not submitted by the author but posthumously by a close friend and colleague, Graham Lister (of 'The Hand'). As such, certain details are lacking. It is not clear how much information was collected prospectively, although there was considerable detail included. It is unstated but expected that most of the extremity reconstructions were of the lower limb, and it would have been very interesting to have a subgroup analysis to determine differences in outcome between upper and lower extremities. While the paper states that it was carried out at two sites, there is no mention of the proportion of early, delayed, and late reconstructions performed at each site, but it states that there was no difference in outcomes between sites. There was no universally applied system to describe injury severity at the time, and now we recognise differences in severity accorded by the Gustilo and Anderson,[2] Byrd and Spicer,[3] and MESS scores.[4] The author states that in their early group, they applied topical antiseptic, and that in their experience the wound remained clean; now we would certainly wish to know whether there was microbiological surveillance and whether any antibiotics were used perioperatively and, if so, which and for how long. Certain questions were not considered in the paper, such as whether there were differences in outcomes between muscle and fasciocutaneous free tissue transfer.

It would also be useful to know whether any salvage surgeries were performed following failure, whether these were successful, and what the limb amputations rates were in those cases with both successful and unsuccessful reconstruction. Lastly, the paper states that microsurgeon availability was never a problem, but the paper itself raises the very important question of what constitutes a microsurgeon . In the first 100 free flaps performed, itself a not inconsiderable number, the author reports a 26% free flap failure rate. In the last 100 cases performed the failure rate was 4%. Obviously, the author's own experience helped to shape our understanding of the timing of surgery following injury, but it also indirectly introduces the question: What defines a competent microsurgeon? With the answer being someone with not only the combination of knowledge and skill but also an ability to understand the individuals particular needs and treat accordingly.

RELEVANT STUDIES

While the essence of the paper is the impact and benefit of early definitive closure with free tissue transfer within 72 hours, much more is unsaid in the paper but which contribute to it. These include Godina's aggressive "anatomical" debridement, as is clearly seen in the case illustrated in the paper itself. He advocates that a thorough debridement needs to be done in a bloodless field, under tourniquet control. This ensures that all devitalised and contaminated tissue is adequately removed. But bone debridement needs to be less radical in early reconstruction. This has been further defined by Arnez and Khan with the concept of preservation of longitudinal structures where possible.[5] Godina had previously advocated the benefits of end-to-side anastomosis (ETS)[6] – potential vessel spasm will tend to cause an end-to-side anastomosis to open, whereas an end-to-end anastomosis will close, are expanded in the paper to relate that end-to-end anastomoses can be safely performed within the early period. This follows commentary from Rollin Daniel, when Godina had first advocated ETS anastomoses, to urge caution particularly in single-vessel limbs.[7]

Godina's paper used the concept of "zone of injury," which guides the selection of the appropriate vessels in limb reconstruction. Godina also developed a posterior approach to the posterior tibial vessels when the patient was positioned on their side.[8] This allowed simultaneous debridement of the wound, preparation of the vessels, and raising of the free flap. This efficiency allowed his team to reduce their operative time significantly from 7.2 hours to 4.7 hours in this paper. His other great contributions to reconstructive surgery, which included ectopic reimplantation[9] and arterial grafts,[10] likely also played roles in the success of his limb salvage programme.

The impact of timing and early reconstruction has been further studied, and Godina's observation revalidated by many independent studies and metanalysis,[11–16] as well as showing cost-effectiveness.[16] Recently, the Nationwide Readmission Database (2014– 2019) was reviewed by Habarth-Morales, who identified 1,030 patients who underwent free flap reconstruction after lower extremity trauma.[11] They report that the lowest rate of complications was indeed in the early group < 72 hours. They also noted that although there is increased risk of complications > 10 days following the injury compared to < 72 hours, that there is no difference in outcomes when reconstruction is performed < 10 days. This reinforces the principle of early reconstruction being more favourable, while extending the window for "early" reconstruction to 10 days.

Godina's paper relates that timing depends mainly on the organisation of the services and needs a strong team encompassing both orthopaedic surgeons and microsurgeons. Lack of such collaboration results in huge variance in care and impacts outcomes to the present day, as the recent INTELLECT study reports.[17]

STUDY IMPACTS

Based on the results in this paper, Godina could strongly advocate for early reconstruction within 72 hours of injury following extremity trauma. He showed that not only was early reconstruction safe, but also it was associated with the fewest anaesthetics, least failures, shortest hospital stay, fewest infections, and lowest rates of non-union compared to any later time point. His observations of inflammation and infection in the delayed phase allowed him to postulate that these changes were drivers of poor outcome, which resolved to a degree by 3 months following injury. Free tissue transfer is now an important tool in the reconstructive surgeon's armamentarium. This paper highlights the importance of assessment of the vessels and need for thorough debridement, and it includes observations on the surgeons own learning curve, providing a roadmap to guide the management of complex injuries. Multiple studies continue to show a difference with better outcomes with early versus delayed reconstruction of the lower limb emphasising the enduring truth of Godina's observations.[11–16]

As such, this is one of the greatest papers in plastic surgery, which provided the evidence to change clinical practice thereafter, and it remains the cornerstone paper which underpins many national policies and international practice on the management of complex lower limb trauma.

It also summarised the extensive experience of a skilled microsurgeon and team which provided 24/7 service in two different health systems. The principles in the paper are built on a number of Godina's unique contributions to the literature, which continue to influence care and provide insight to the present day. Given that major lower limb trauma has become less frequent, these insights are unlikely to be gained by any practitioner today.

Godina's paper also reflects on the need to work in collaboration with anaesthetic colleagues regarding optimising the patient and measures to keep the wound clean with topical antiseptics. He also eschews the use of topical antibiotics on the wound itself, showing good antibiotic stewardship.

He also discusses surgical failure and relates that the sole flap failure observed in the early period was related to poor surgical planning. He introduces the need for the surgeon to understand that the injured limb undergoes a dynamic inflammatory process, with necrotic tissue, infection, and fibrosis providing increased barriers to successful reconstruction with delayed reconstruction resulting in poorer outcomes.

As such, this paper is incredibly important in the context of reconstructive surgery. His observations and adaptations also inspire surgeons to be more ergonomic, manage patients holistically, and consider their outcomes and reasons for failure.

One of the final reasons this is an exceptional paper relates to the timing and circumstance of its publication. Marko Godina had visited Canniesburn Plastic Surgery unit in Glasgow, where he became a good friend with the erudite and acclaimed Graham Lister. Godina changed the lives of many with major trauma, but, unfortunately, he lost his own life in a road traffic accident. The observations for the paper were found, after his death, on his desk, and they were collated by Lister and submitted on his behalf. Listers comment says it all: Godina's observations "represent an aspect of his unique personality. The first is his untiring energy, the second his simple logic, and the third his innovative approach to unsolved problems." May his paper continue to be an inspiration to us all.

REFERENCES

1. Godina M. Early microsurgical reconstruction of complex trauma of the extremities. *Plast Reconstr Surg.* September 1986;78(3):285–292.
2. Gustilo RB, Anderson JT. Prevention of infection in the treatment of one thousand and twenty-five open fractures of long bones: retrospective and prospective analyses. *J Bone Joint Surg Am.* June 1976;58(4):453–458.
3. Byrd HS, Spicer TE, Cierney G 3rd. Management of open tibial fractures. *Plast Reconstr Surg.* November 1985;76(5):719–730.
4. Durham RM, Mistry BM, Mazuski JE, Shapiro M, Jacobs D. Outcome and utility of scoring systems in the management of the mangled extremity. *Am J Surg.* November 1996;172(5):569–573.
5. Arnez ZM, Tyler MP, Khan U. Describing severe limb trauma. *Br J Plast Surg.* June 1999;52(4):280–285.
6. Godina M. Preferential use of end-to-side arterial anastomoses in free flap transfers. *Plast Reconstr Surg.* November 1979;64(5):673–682.
7. Daniel RK. Preferential use of end-to-side arterial anastomoses in free flap transfers. *Plast Reconstr Surg.* June 1980;65(6):849.
8. Godina M, Arnez ZM, Lister GD. Preferential use of the posterior approach to blood vessels of the lower leg in microvascular surgery. *Plast Reconstr Surg.* August 1991;88(2):287–291.
9. Godina M, Bajec J, Baraga A. Salvage of the mutilated upper extremity with temporary ectopic implantation of the undamaged part. *Plast Reconstr Surg.* September 1986;78(3):295–299.

10. Godina M. Arterial autografts in microvascular surgery. *Plast Reconstr Surg.* September 1986;78(3):293–294.
11. Habarth-Morales TE, Davis HD, Rios-Diaz AJ, Broach RB, Serletti JM, Azoury SC, Levin LS, Kovach SJ 3rd, Rhemtulla IA. The Godina Principle in the 21st Century: Free Flap Timing after Isolated Lower Extremity Trauma in a Retrospective National Cohort. *J Reconstr Microsurg.* 2025 Jul;41(6):469–477. doi:10.1055/a-2404-7634. Epub 2024 Aug 27. PMID: 39191415.
12. Brown C, Ash M, Menon A, Knaus W, Hernandez-Irizarry R, Ghareeb P. Incidence and risk factors for secondary surgery and amputation after lower extremity limb salvage. *Ann Plast Surg.* 2025 Jan 1;94(1): 75–78. doi:10.1097/SAP.0000000000004125. Epub 2024 Oct 18. PMID: 39477226.
13. Le ELH, McNamara CT, Constantine RS, Greyson MA, Iorio ML. The continued impact of Godina's Principles: outcomes of flap coverage as a function of time after definitive fixation of open lower extremity fractures. *J Reconstr Microsurg.* October 2024;40(8):648–656.
14. Lee ZH, Stranix JT, Rifkin WJ, Daar DA, Anzai L, Ceradini DJ, Thanik V, Saadeh PB, Levine JP. Timing of microsurgical reconstruction in lower extremity trauma: an update of the godina paradigm. *Plast Reconstr Surg.* September 2019;144(3):759–767.
15. Verheul E, Berner JE, Oflazoglu K, Troisi L, Arnež Z, Ortega-Briones A, Nanchahal J, Rakhorst H. Development of guidelines for the management of patients with open fractures: the potential cost-savings of international collaboration. *J Plast Reconstr Aesthet Surg.* January 2022;75(1):439–488.
16. Lee ZH, Stranix JT, Levine JP. The optimal timing of traumatic lower extremity reconstruction: current consensus. *Clin Plast Surg.* April 2021;48(2):259–266.
17. Haykal S, Roy M, Patel A. Meta-analysis of timing for microsurgical free-flap reconstruction for lower limb injury: evaluation of the Godina principles. *J Reconstr Microsurg.* May 2018;34(4):277–292.
18. BernerJE, Chan JKK, Gardiner MD, Navia A, Tejos R, Ortiz-Llorens M, Ortega- Briones A, Rakhorst HA, Nanchahal J, Jain A, INTELLECT Collaborative. International Lower Limb Collaborative (INTELLECT) study: a multicentre, international retrospective audit of lower extremity open fractures. *Br J Surg.* 16 August 2022;109(9):792–795.

EDITOR COMMENTARY

This was one of the first papers that provided evidence for the benefits of early reconstruction of complex extremity trauma. Prior to its publication, microvascular reconstructions were usually performed in a delayed or "late" manner for various injuries, often after local or regional soft tissue reconstructions had failed. As microsurgery spread, plastic surgeons came to be involved earlier, but even then these subacute wounds would often be colonised with bacteria and had a burden of necrotic tissue. In 1976, after the development of a microsurgery service at the University of Ljubljana Hospital, Dr. Marko Godina instituted a change in policy to facilitate early (i.e., within 72 hours) free tissue transfer reconstruction of large traumatic soft tissue extremity wounds in concert with orthopaedic surgeons. Godina visited Canniesburn well before Odhran Shelley or myself were there. He was known to be a speedy surgeon; the joke being that it was due to his craving for cigarettes.

The clinical outcome results come from this period after 1976 through to 1983, and they were published posthumously on his behalf in 1986. They clearly demonstrated improved outcomes in the early reconstruction group, which prompted a paradigm shift in the treatment of complex lower limb trauma. However, there have also been significant changes in reconstructive surgery since Godina's time – maturation of microsurgery as a discipline with increased surgeon skill/experience, new local perforator flaps, the development of negative pressure wound therapy, and the availability of effective skin substitutes. These have actually led to a reduction in the use of free flaps for lower limb trauma. Thus, whilst the "emergency free flap" does not seem to be mandatory, an early reconstruction is still preferable.

Although it had inherent limitations being a retrospective single institution study with limited data analysis and also lacked meaningful measures of functional outcomes (except for weight bearing), the study triggered a change in philosophy and practice in lower limb trauma.

CHAPTER 7

The Search for the Ideal Thin Skin Flap: Superficial Circumflex Iliac Artery Perforator Flap – A Review of 210 Cases

Terence LH Goh, Sung Woo Park, Jae Young Cho, Jong Woo Choi, Joon Pio Hong
Plast Reconstr Surg. 2015 Feb;135(2):592–601 doi: 10.1097/PRS.0000000000000951

AUTHOR COMMENTARY

Joon Pio Hong

The groin flap, supplied by the superficial circumflex iliac artery, was one of the first free flaps to be used successfully in reconstruction. This flap was first described as a pedicle flap by McGregor and Jackson and then introduced as a free flap by Daniel and Taylor.[1,2] The groin donor site is well concealed, provides a moderate amount of thin skin, and has a reasonably good color match with the face. Despite these benefits, it did not gain common popularity as a workhorse flap: as it was raised subfascially, it could be bulky especially in obese patients and be difficult to inset; the pedicle anatomy was variable in its course; the venae commitantes were often too small; and donor site lymphorrhea and wound dehiscence were problems.[3–7] It was not till Koshima et al. revisited the groin flap and modified it as a skin flap elevated above the deep fascia based on the superficial circumflex iliac artery (SCIA) perforator that the groin region as a free flap received appropriate recognition.[8] The SCIP flap was able to overcome some disadvantages, such as bulkiness and variable arterial anatomy, by using the free style free flap approach in harvesting.[8–12] However, even with these evolved techniques and concepts, the SCIP flap was still challenging to use due to the short pedicle and small vessel calibre, and it still had the problems of relative bulkiness, especially in obese patients, and donor site morbidity such as lymphorrhea. Further modifications were made where Hong et al. harvested the flap on the superficial fascia, making the flap even thinner (super-thin flaps) while avoiding injuries to the lymphatic system, which would be located in the deep fat below the superficial fascia, thus minimizing lymphorrhea.[13–18] Further studies clarified the contributions of the superficial (medial) branch and deep (lateral) branches of SCIA as well as the venous outflow, which helped to achieve better design, vascular supply, harvest multiple components, and appreciation of the limits of the flap.[16,19–23] Although both medial and lateral branches arise from the SCIA, it can be seen as two different flaps based on each perforating branch as it provides very distinctive and unique characteristics. It was this pivotal information included in the paper, that added clarity to the groin flap and facilitated the progression to the thin SCIP flap.

DOI: 10.1201/9781003413738-7

The medial branch, depending on the type of perforator, either takes an axial pathway underneath the dermis or directly anchors to the dermis, and the surgeon can design accordingly the dimension of the flap.[18,19] The lateral branch is usually an axial pattern perforator, allowing larger dimensions as well as the inclusion of the iliac bone as a chimeric flap.[23] Using the ultrasound to map the pathway of the perforators adds accuracy and allows prediction of the dimensions of the SCIP flap.[24–26] Based on this approach, the authors have elevated flaps as large as 12 × 36 cm. Furthermore, one can design the flap laterally to harvest a longer pedicle, overcoming one of the pitfalls for this flap.[27,28]

Although the SCIP, which is the evolved form of groin flap, is steadily gaining popularity, the learning curve remains steep.[29] To maximize the advantages of the SCIP flap, one must understand the anatomy and the relative characteristics of the two perforators, the medial and lateral branches, from the SCIA. In defect reconstruction, the SCIP flap offers the advantages of being a thin flap, able to be harvested as a composite flap, and a large skin dimension while having a well-hidden donor site scar. Thus, this paper deserves to be recognized as a landmark paper, being an evolved extension of the groin flap.

REFERENCES

1. McGregor IA, Jackson IT. The groin flap. *Br J Plast Surg.* 1972;25(1):3–16.
2. Daniel RK, Taylor GI. Distant transfer of an island flap by microvascular anastomoses. A clinical technique. *Plast Reconstr Surg.* 1973;52(2):111–117.
3. Calderon W, Chang N, Mathes SJ. Comparison of the effect of bacterial inoculation in musculocutaneous and fasciocutaneous flaps. *Plast Reconstr Surg.* 1986;77(5):785–794.
4. Jeng SF. Free composite groin flap and vascularized external oblique aponeurosis for traumatic avulsion injuries of the foot. *J Trauma.* 1993;35(1):71–74.
5. Iwaya T, Harii K, Yamada A. Microvascular free flaps for the treatment of avulsion injuries of the feet in children. *J Trauma.* 1982;22(1):15–19.
6. Cooper TM, Lewis N, Baldwin MA. Free groin flap revisited. *Plast Reconstr Surg.* 1999;103(3):918–924.
7. Garrett JC, Buncke HJ, Brownstein ML. Free groin-flap transfer for skin defects associated with orthopaedic problems of the lower extremity. *J Bone Joint Surg Am.* 1978;60(8):1055–1058.
8. Koshima I, Nanba Y, Tsutsui T, Takahashi Y, Urushibara K, Inagawa K, *et al.* Superficial circumflex iliac artery perforator flap for reconstruction of limb defects. *Plast Reconstr Surg.* 2004;113(1):233–240.
9. Hsu WM, Chao WN, Yang C, Fang CL, Huang KF, Lin YS, *et al.* Evolution of the free groin flap: the superficial circumflex iliac artery perforator flap. *Plast Reconstr Surg.* 2007;119(5):1491–1498.
10. Wei FC, Mardini S. Free-style free flaps. *Plast Reconstr Surg.* 2004;114(4):910–916.
11. Chang CC, Wong CH, Wei FC. Free-style free flap. *Injury.* 2008;39 Suppl 3:S57–S61.
12. Berner JE, Nikkhah D, Zhao J, Prousskaia E, Teo TC. The versatility of the superficial circumflex iliac artery perforator flap: a single surgeon's 16-year experience for limb reconstruction and a systematic review. *J Reconstr Microsurg.* 2020;36(2):93–103.
13. Hong JP, Koshima I. Using perforators as recipient vessels (supermicrosurgery) for free flap reconstruction of the knee region. *Ann Plast Surg.* 2010;64(3):291–293.
14. Hong JP. The use of supermicrosurgery in lower extremity reconstruction: the next step in evolution. *Plast Reconstr Surg.* 2009;123(1):230–235.
15. Choi DH, Goh T, Cho JY, Hong JP. Thin superficial circumflex iliac artery perforator flap and supermicrosurgery technique for face reconstruction. *J Craniofac Surg.* 2014;25(6):2130–2133.

16. Goh TL, Park SW, Cho JY, Choi JW, Hong JP. The search for the ideal thin skin flap: superficial circumflex iliac artery perforator flap: a review of 210 cases. *Plast Reconstr Surg.* 2015;135(2):592–601.
17. Hong JP, Sun SH, Ben-Nakhi M. Modified superficial circumflex iliac artery perforator flap and supermicrosurgery technique for lower extremity reconstruction: a new approach for moderate-sized defects. *Ann Plast Surg.* 2013;71(4):380–383.
18. Suh YC, Hong JP, Suh HP. Elevation technique for medial branch based superficial circumflex Iliac artery perforator flap. *Handchir Mikrochir Plast Chir.* 2018;50(4):256–258.
19. Suh HS, Jeong HH, Choi DH, Hong JP. Study of the medial superficial perforator of the superficial circumflex iliac artery perforator flap using computed tomographic angiography and surgical anatomy in 142 patients. *Plast Reconstr Surg.* 2017;139(3):738–748.
20. Yoshimatsu H, Steinbacher J, Meng S, Hamscha UM, Weninger WJ, Tinhofer IE, *et al.* Superficial circumflex iliac artery perforator flap: an anatomical study of the correlation of the superficial and the deep branches of the artery and evaluation of perfusion from the deep branch to the sartorius muscle and the iliac bone. *Plast Reconstr Surg.* 2019;143(2):589–602.
21. Yoshimatsu H, Iida T, Yamamoto T, Hayashi A. Superficial circumflex iliac artery-based iliac bone flap transfer for reconstruction of bony defects. *J Reconstr Microsurg.* 2018;34(9):719–728.
22. Yoshimatsu H, Yamamoto T, Hayashi A, Fuse Y, Karakawa R, Iida T, *et al.* Use of the transverse branch of the superficial circumflex iliac artery as a landmark facilitating identification and dissection of the deep branch of the superficial circumflex iliac artery for free flap pedicle: anatomical study and clinical applications. *Microsurgery.* 2019;39(8):721–729.
23. Yoshimatsu H, Yamamoto T, Iida T. Deep branch of the superficial circumflex iliac artery for backup. *J Plast Reconstr Aesthet Surg.* 2015;68(10):1478–1479.
24. Cho MJ, Kwon JG, Pak CJ, Suh HP, Hong JP. The role of duplex ultrasound in microsurgical reconstruction: review and technical considerations. *J Reconstr Microsurg.* 2020;36(7):514–521.
25. Hong JP. The color duplex ultrasound: the reconstructive surgeon's stethoscope. *J Reconstr Microsurg.* 2022;38(3):169.
26. Hong JP, Kim HB, Park CJ, Suh HP. Using duplex ultrasound for recipient vessel selection. *J Reconstr Microsurg.* 2022;38(3):200–205.
27. Kim HB, Min JC, Pak CJ, Hong JPJ, Suh HP. Maximizing the versatility of thin flap from the groin area as a workhorse flap: the selective use of Superficial Circumflex Iliac Artery Perforator (SCIP) Free Flap and Superficial Inferior Epigastric Artery (SIEA) free flap with precise preoperative planning. *J Reconstr Microsurg.* 2023;39(2):148–155.
28. Kwon JG, Pereira N, Tonaree W, Brown E, Hong JP, Suh HP. Long pedicled superficial circumflex iliac artery flap based on a medial superficial branch. *Plast Reconstr Surg.* 2021;148(4):615e–619e.
29. Altiparmak M, Cha HG, Hong JP, Suh HP. Superficial circumflex iliac artery perforator flap as a workhorse flap: systematic review and meta-analysis. *J Reconstr Microsurg.* 2020;36(8):600–605.

CHAPTER 8

Geometric Considerations in the Design of Rotation Flaps in the Scalp and Forehead Region

Ahuja RB. *Plast Reconstr Surg.* 1988 Jun;81(6):900–906
doi: 10.1097/00006534-198806000-1 PMID: 3375351

EXPERT COMMENTARY

R.B. Ahuja and Pallab Chatterjee

The use of local flaps for the closure of full-thickness defects is a fundamental technique in plastic surgery that follows the principle of replacing like-with-like tissue.[1] Among the numerous and innovative techniques described, transposition flaps and rotation flaps can be regarded as the very basic foundation techniques on which the other local flaps are based. The standard rotation flap and transposition flaps are commonly taught and illustrated in the mainstream plastic surgery texts and journal publications.[2,3] Ahuja elucidated his concept of the modified rotation flap in 1988 with the above paper,[4] and with the follow up in 1989.[5] A local flap template (LFT) was proposed for triangulated defects which incorporated the principles of both classical rotation and transposition flaps. This technique was demonstrated to be particularly useful in closing large scalp and forehead defects. The scalp is an anatomical area which has relatively inextensible skin covering the three-dimensional area of the head which places limits on the design of local flaps for defects exceeding 2 cm width if a skin graft is to be avoided for optimal cosmetic results. The LFT design can be effectively employed for the primary coverage of scalp defects as large as 6–7 cm, without needing skin grafting of the secondary donor site. This geometric design was further explained by studying the mechanics of movements of this flap in its several variations.[5]

It is important to have an optimal rotation flap design for scalp defects as there are no perforator flaps in this region. The LFT (or modified rotation flap) had its genesis in the recognition that there were two possible local flap designs for triangulated defects (classical rotation and classical transposition), each rotating about a different pivot point around the triangulated defect. While a transposition flap moves the skin adjacent to the defect, the rotation flap moves skin diametrically opposite the defect. A transposition flap leaves a donor defect because the arc of rotation is incomplete. The modified rotation flap template completes this arc of rotation for a transposition flap, an important concept in enhancing the mechanics of the movement of the leading edge of the flap, as explained in the 1989 paper.[5]

DOI: 10.1201/9781003413738-8

However, the modified template flap was slow to find acceptance by plastic surgeons as it challenged established beliefs and the claims seemed unbelievable. It was accepted that the triangulated defect could be considered as a sector within an imaginary circle of surrounding skin tissue in a classical rotation design, wherein the local tissue is moved from an area diametrically opposite to the defect to obtain closure. However, in this modified rotation flap concept, the triangulated defect is placed such within the imaginary circle that the flap is designed from an area adjacent to the defect, as in a transposition flap, albeit with a larger rotational arc. A classical rotation flap will always require a longer incision (and thus a larger flap) to cover a comparable defect than a rotation template design. In the scalp and forehead region, very large flaps are required with the classical design and this requirement is exaggerated by the three-dimensional anatomy of the region. Such large incisions can compromise the cosmetic result. Even a well-designed classical rotation flap in the scalp region may require a back cut, which may produce a secondary defect that cannot be closed primarily. In some situations, the back cut may even jeopardize the blood supply of the flap.

Critical to the template design is the placement of the geometric pivot point. This is done as in a classical transposition flap, but with a caveat that the triangulated defect should be an isosceles triangle with the pivot point placed at a distance slightly more than the maximum width of the triangulated defect (Figure 8.1a, CP slightly more than AB). Several designs are possible with the template design to accommodate the anatomical

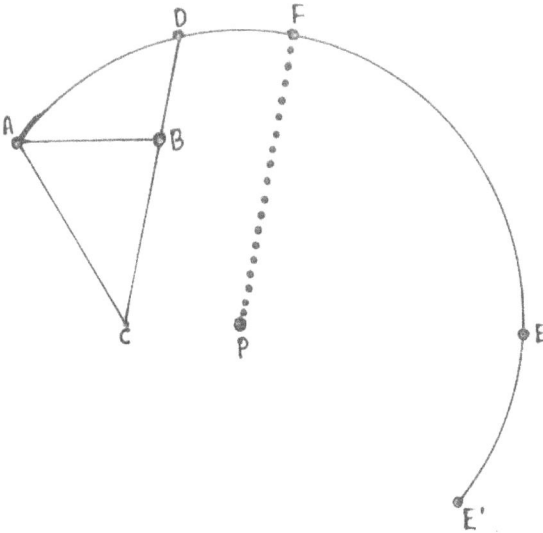

Figure 8.1a.   Rotation template flap design. The defect is triangulated (ABC) as an isosceles triangle with angle C not exceeding 30 degrees. Pivot point P is selected with CP slightly more than AB and parallel to it. With pivot point P as centre and AP as radius, a semicircle ADE' is drawn. CDE is the local flap template and CE is the base of the template. Depending on the extent of recruitment along DE', the flap will be predominantly transposition till F, rotation equals transposition till E (most often adequate) and predominantly rotation if recruited till E'.

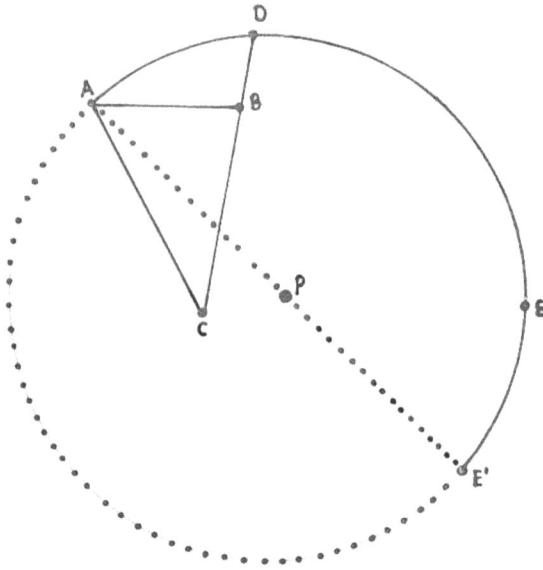

Figure 8.1b. The local flap template (LFT) concept. The selection of geometric pivot point P closer to AB causes the triangulated defect to be placed strategically within an imaginary circle of surrounding skin tissue and not as a sector of that circle, as in a classical rotation flap design. This placement eases the flap movement into the defect. The segment E to E' is only employed, in a cut as you go manner, as and when required. This does not compromise the flap blood supply as it is a design reserve and not a 'back cut.'

limitations in the scalp region. For example, the pivot point can be moved closer to the apex of the defect and extending the arc of rotation flap, in a "cut as you go" manner to ease the tension of this design compromise, without affecting the blood supply of the flap (Figure 8.1b). This flexibility in the design of the flap makes the flap truly appealing as it is facilitating flap movement without being a "back cut." Triangulated defects between 6 and 7 cm width can be easily closed by designing flaps on this principle on either side of the defect.[4,5] This was never possible in the classical rotation flap design and only small defects could be closed primarily. The ability to use the template design on both sides of the triangulated defect lends versatility to the technique.

The small area of tissue at the leading edge of the template design that represents a "discardable area" in the template design, just as in a classical transposition flap, is sacrificed only minimally on a *need-to* basis after closure of other areas of the flap.

With time, the use of the modified rotation flap gained wider acceptance. Leedy et al. mentioned this as a method for reconstruction of small to moderate scalp defects in an excellent review in 2005.[6] It has also been accepted as a recommendation for use in post-burn alopecia in *Total Burn Care* (5th Edition) when the affected surface area is mild to moderate.[7] When plastic surgeons use this technique for the first time in anatomically challenging areas, such as the forehead and scalp, they are often struck by its simplicity and geometric precision in obtaining the primary closure of moderately large defects. Understanding the elegant combination of transposition and rotation movements afforded by modified rotation flap enables one to close large defects in the inextensible scalp and forehead area. This versatile technique will continue to bail plastic surgeons out of a sticky situation with its ability to use design reserve in a "cut as you go" approach.

REFERENCES

1. Gillies H, Millard Jr DR. *The Principles & Art of Plastic Surgery*. London: Butterworth & Co Ltd; 1957.
2. McGregor AD, McGregor IA. *Fundamental Techniques of Plastic Surgery*, 10th ed. Edinburgh: Churchill Livingstone; 2000.
3. Jankauskas S, Cohen IK, Grabb WC. Basic techniques of plastic surgery. In: Smith JW, Aston SJ, editors. *Grabb & Smith's Plastic Surgery*. Boston, MA: Little, Brown & Company; 1991 [chapter 1].
4. Ahuja RB. Geometric considerations in the design of rotation flaps in the scalp and forehead region. *Plast Reconstr Surg*. 1988 Jun;81(6):900–906. doi: 10.1097/00006534-198806000-00012.
5. Ahuja RB. Mechanics of movement for rotation flaps and a local flap template. *Plast Reconstr Surg*. 1989 Apr;83(4):733–737. doi: 10.1097/00006534-198904000-00024.
6. Leedy JE, Janis JE, Rohrich RJ. Reconstruction of acquired scalp defects: an algorithmic approach. *Plast Reconstr Surg*. 2005 Sep 15;116(4):54e–72e. doi: 10.1097/01.prs.0000179188.25019.6c.
7. Rajeev B. Ahuja, Pallab Chatterjee. 51 - management of postburn alopecia. In: Herndon DN, editor. *Total Burn Care*, 5th ed. Elsevier; 2018:555–561.e1. https://doi.org/10.1016/B978-0-323-47661-4.00051-4.

EXPERT COMMENTARY

Karen Vuong and Cheng Hean Lo

In this publication, Ahuja described the modified rotation flap and its application in closure of scalp and forehead defects.[1] The step-by-step approach and adherence to the mathematical design provided precision and geometrical advantage. The modified rotation flap incorporated elements of both rotation and transposition flaps. Similar to previous authors, the leading edge of the rotation flap was made longer to enable reach and reliable closure of the defect.[2] The anatomic limitations, convexity, and inextensibility of the skin in the scalp and forehead regions were recognized as challenges which curtail flexibility in flap design.[1] However, with multiple well-illustrated diagrams and case examples, Ahuja demonstrated the advantages and reliability of the modified rotation flap in these regions. Through his experience, Ahuja provided reassurance that if it is geometrically possible to design this flap in the scalp and forehead, then primary closure will always be obtained. The exactness of the geometric design of this flap provided confidence in primary closure. A forehead donor defect up to 6.5 cm in width following forehead flap rhinoplasty was closed primarily.[1]

Numerous modifications exist and opinions vary with regards to the ideal design of a rotation flap.[3] The standard rotation flap is still the most widely described and used. The "divine rotation flap" design is based on concepts of divine proportion and Fibonacci sequence, concepts previously employed in studies of aesthetics and theories regarding facial beauty.[2,4,5] However, it is relatively difficult to apply, involving convoluted mathematical calculations and geometrical measurements. It also leads to relatively high tension at wound closure.[3] Ahuja's MRF is well described and reasonably straightforward to learn for the young surgeon.[1,6] It has been applied successfully in unforgiving regions, including forehead and scalp. The standard and modified rotation flap designs have similar scar burdens; however, the modified rotation flap results in higher closing tension despite being a bigger flap with higher surface area.[3] Wound closure with excessive tension may lead to impaired vascularity, flap necrosis, and wound dehiscence or breakdown.[3]

Ultimately, the aim in flap design is to close a particular defect in the most simple, efficient, and aesthetic manner.[3] Modifications may be necessary to respect anatomical or donor site boundaries or to camouflage scars in the most aesthetic manner (an example being pretrichial incisions). Application of further techniques (such as galeal scoring and back cuts) may also be called upon when complexity of the task at hand exceeds expectations. Herein lies the art of plastic surgery.

REFERENCES

1. Ahuja RB. Geometric considerations in the design of rotation flaps in the scalp and forehead region. *Plast Reconstr Surg.* 1988;81(6):900–906.
2. Jackson IT. *Local Flaps in Head and Neck Reconstruction.* St. Louis: Mosby; 1985.
3. Lo CH, Kimble FW. The ideal rotation flap: an experimental study. *J Plast Reconstr Aesthet Surg.* 2008;61(7):754–759.
4. Sandhir RK. Divine rotation flap. *Ann Plast Surg.* 1997;38(2):194–195.
5. Ricketts RM. Divine proportion in facial esthetics. *Clin Plast Surg.* 1982;9(4):401–422.
6. Ahuja RB. Mechanics of movement for rotation flaps and a local flap template. *Plast Reconstr Surg.* 1989;83(4):733–737.

EDITOR COMMENTARY

Rotation flaps can be difficult to get right and is something that younger surgeons may struggle with. The conventional or classical rotation flap triangulate the defect to become a sector of a large rotation flap with a length to base ratio of 2:1; the length of the arc along the circle has been said to be ideally 4× the width of the defect (base of the triangle). This design has some geometric issues – first, there will be tension at the opposite point and, second, flaps shorten with rotation. These shortcomings become less significant when a large enough flap is designed in tissue that has lax/spare/stretchable skin to compensate; otherwise, a back cut will be needed. The back cut moves the functional pivot nearer the defect and is effective, but it potentially threatens the blood supply and some regard it as "bad planning." A Burow's triangle will equalize the incision lengths but does little to reduce tension. More undermining around a rotation flap does not significantly decrease wound tension.

Dr. Ahuja looked at the geometry and adjusted the pattern so that it was more logical and less reliant on having lax tissues. The triangulated defect is pivoted inwards on the circumference away from the flap to combine elements of transposition and rotation. A triangle of skin is discarded in between the base of the triangle and the arc of the circle; some may argue that this is the equivalent of the Burow's triangle as above to compensate for unequal lengths. There is a comprehensive commentary by Lo C.H. (2008).

REFERENCE

Lo CH, Kimble FW. The ideal rotation flap: an experimental study. *J Plast Reconstr Aesthet Surg.* 2008 Jul;61(7):754–759. doi: 10.1016/j.bjps.2007.12.032.

CHAPTER 9

Deep Inferior Epigastric Perforator Flap for Breast Reconstruction

Allen RJ, Treece P. *Ann Plast Surg.* 1994 Jan;32(1):32–38
doi: 10.1097/00000637-199401000-00007 PMID: 8141534

.

AUTHOR COMMENTARY

Robert J. Allen Sr.

The genesis of the DIEP Flap for breast reconstruction began in the 1980s during my NYU Fellowship in Microsurgery. Bill Shaw's technique for breast reconstruction with the superior gluteal free flap expanded the field of reconstructive microsurgery and, upon returning to New Orleans, I performed 10 breast reconstructions with the gluteal flap before abandoning this method due to the difficulty associated with the short pedicle.

Hans Holmstrom published "The Free Abdominoplasty flap and Its Use in Breast Reconstruction" in 1979. This was a rectus abdominus musculocutaneous free flap. In 1982, Carl Hartrampf introduced the transverse island abdominal flap (TIAF), renamed the TRAM flap in his honor. This non-microsurgical procedure appealed to most plastic surgeons worldwide, but, over time, the significant donor site morbidity became obvious.

As a microsurgeon, I investigated ways to transfer the "free abdominoplasty flap" without muscle sacrifice. I investigated the superficial vascular system first by injecting abdominoplasty specimens with methylene blue and radio-opaque dye. In June 1989, I performed the first superficial inferior epigastric artery (SIEA) flap for breast reconstruction at the Charity Hospital in New Orleans. Of 7 SIEA breast reconstructions, 3 flaps failed due to technical mistakes. A paper on it was submitted for publication but was rejected. Besides an unacceptable failure rate, one reviewer stated that with the TRAM flap no other flap from the abdomen was needed. Another reviewer suggested doing another 100 cases without a failure and resubmitting the paper; we have recently resubmitted a paper with over 400 SIEA breast reconstructions since 1989 with greater than 97% success rate. At the time, due to the variability of the SIEA anatomy including no artery in some cases, my investigation turned to the deep inferior epigastric artery (DIEA) perforators. Injection studies were done on a dominant perforator of abdominoplasty specimens. The vascular territory was superomedial as opposed to the SIEA being inferolateral, illustrating the complimentary nature of these vascular systems.

DOI: 10.1201/9781003413738-9

Just before my first clinical case, I read an article in the *Annals of Plastic Surgery* by Koshima I et al. on "Free Thin Paraumbilical Perforator-Based Flaps." His article cited an earlier article of his from 1989, "Inferior Epigastric Artery Skin Flaps" in the *British Journal of Plastic Surgery*. I realized then that perforator skin flaps were evolving independently around the world.

I performed the first deep inferior epigastric perforator (DIEP) flap at the Charity Hospital in New Orleans in August 1992. The patient had a unilateral modified radical mastectomy defect with contralateral mammary hypertrophy with a reduction planned at the second stage. A hemiabdomen was used leaving the other hemiabdomen as backup. The patient liked her DIEP flap so much, she requested and received a contralateral prophylactic skin-sparing mastectomy with DIEP flap reconstruction at the second stage.

This DIEP flap for breast reconstruction paper was submitted to the *Annals of Plastic Surgery* in November 1992 and published in January 1994. A 3-minute presentation was given at the 1993 ASPRS meeting in New Orleans; I was surprised there was no immediate feedback on my presentation. Just after my talk I caught a presentation by Claudio Angrigiani on the "The Latissimus Flap without Muscle," demonstrating that perforator flaps were also being performed in Argentina. A plastic surgery resident from Belgium, Phillip Blondeel, heard my talk and took the DIEP back to his program in Europe. I first met Phillip in 1995 at the ISRM meeting in Singapore where he had a poster presentation on DIEP flap for breast reconstruction. I also met Isao Koshima at that meeting. We three became close friends from then on. Phillip came to New Orleans for an extended visit to learn about our work with perforator flaps. We co-founded the International Course on Perforator Flaps, which was held annually for over 20 years.

My publication "10-Year Retrospective Review of 758 DIEP Flaps for Breast Reconstruction" in *PRS* (Apr 2004), won the 2005 James Barrett Brown Award for best publication in plastic surgery. This award increased wider acceptance for, and contributed to, the DIEP flap becoming known as the gold standard in breast reconstruction.

CTA imaging in 2004 and MRA imaging in 2006 for preoperative perforator mapping has made the DIEP technique easier and quicker. In 2019, we began incorporating a surgical delay procedure in selected patients, increasing the vascular territory and simplifying the flap dissection on transfer. More recently, we have reduced the time between delay to transfer to 24 hours with good outcomes.

Innovations are continuously occurring, resulting in better outcomes. DIEP augmentation mammoplasty is increasingly pushing into the field of aesthetic surgery. It has been over 32 years since the first DIEP breast reconstruction, and I continue to perform more DIEP flaps every year than any other flap.

REFERENCES

Angrigiani C, Grilli D, Siebert J. Latissimus dorsi musculocutaneous flap without muscle. *Plast Reconstr Surg.* 1995 Dec;96(7):1608–1614. doi: 10.1097/00006534-199512000-00014.

Gill PS, Hunt JP, Guerra AB, Dellacroce FJ, Sullivan SK, Boraski J, Metzinger SE, Dupin CL, Allen RJ. A 10-year retrospective review of 758 DIEP flaps for breast reconstruction. *Plast Reconstr Surg.* 2004 Apr 1;113(4):1153–1160. doi: 10.1097/01.prs.0000110328.47206.50.

Koshima I, Moriguchi T, Soeda S, Tanaka H, Umeda N. Free thin paraumbilical perforator-based flaps. *Ann Plast Surg.* 1992 Jul;29(1):12–17. doi: 10.1097/00000637-199207000-00004.

Koshima I, Soeda S. Inferior epigastric artery skin flaps without rectus abdominis muscle. *Br J Plast Surg.* 1989 Nov;42(6):645–648. doi: 10.1016/0007-1226(89)90075-1.

EXPERT COMMENTARY

Whitney Chow

Dr. Robert Allen's work on the deep inferior epigastric perforator (DIEP) flap, published in the *Annals of Plastic Surgery* in 1994, represents a significant evolution in autologous tissue-based breast reconstructive surgery. His work focused on using the DIEP flap for breast reconstruction; his technique preserved abdominal muscle integrity, thereby reducing the potential for complications often associated with the traditional transverse rectus abdominis myocutaneous (TRAM) flap, such as abdominal weakness, hernia, and bulging. His pioneering work set a new standard to maximize aesthetic and functional outcomes in breast reconstruction patients. To date, this remains the gold standard operation performed worldwide for microsurgery autologous breast reconstruction.

In 1982, Hartrampf introduced the pedicled TRAM flap. However, this technique had significant drawbacks, including the risk of abdominal hernia, partial flap necrosis, and unsatisfactory aesthetic outcomes. In 1989, further advancements were made by Koshima and Soeda, who described the paraumbilical perforator-based flap, allowing harvest of lower abdominal tissue for a variety of non-breast defects without sacrificing the rectus abdominis muscle. This concept was refined and popularized in the field of breast reconstruction by Robert Allen in 1994.

KEY MESSAGE FROM ALLEN'S PAPER

Allen's anatomical studies in his landmark paper demonstrated reliable infraumbilical perforators within a 7 cm radius of the umbilicus. These perforators pass through the rectus muscle to supply the subcutaneous fat and skin. The vascular territories supplied by these perforators were visualized through contrast studies. By meticulously dissecting the course of these perforators, it was possible to isolate the DIEP pedicle without needing to harvest any rectus muscle. This advancement in technique allows patients to achieve natural breast reconstruction with reduced risk of abdominal weakness, enhancing quality of life and functional outcomes following mastectomy.

KEY EVOLUTIONS SINCE ALLEN'S WORK

Over the past decades, the DIEP flap operation has continued to transform and improve, with advances in preoperative imaging/planning, refinement in flap dissection, evolving microsurgical technique, improvement of flap-shaping, and postoperative Enhanced Recovery After Surgery (ERAS) protocols.

PREOPERATIVE IMAGING/PLANNING

Major advancements came with the use of computed tomography angiography (CTA) and magnetic resonance angiography (MRA) to map the location, course, and calibre of perforating vessels. This helps surgeons to meticulously plan surgical steps and select vessels to optimize flap perfusion, ultimately reducing operation time (Rozen et al., 2019). CTA has become the primary imaging tool for preoperative planning due to its accessibility, reproducible results, and affordability. Studies have demonstrated its sensitivity and specificity in detecting perforators as high as 100% (Chae et al., 2015). MRA offers advantages such as no radiation exposure, a safer allergy profile with contrast agents, and a clearer definition of the intramuscular course of perforators. However, MRA imaging has a higher average cost, requires a longer breathhold time and thus is more susceptible to artifacts, and incompatibility with certain patient devices.

REFINEMENT IN FLAP DISSECTION

The superficial inferior epigastric artery (SIEA) flap is an alternative option for autologous breast reconstruction. One of its advantages over the DIEP flap is that its blood supply is derived from the superficial system, eliminating the need for pedicle dissection within the muscle layer. This approach preserves the abdominal muscles integrity, resulting in less postoperative pain and a quicker recovery compared to the DIEP flap. However, the SIEA is anatomically variable and less reliable, making it unsuitable for all cases (Park et al., 2016).

MINIMALLY INVASIVE DISSECTION WITH ROBOTIC TECHNIQUE

Traditional DIEP flap surgery typically requires a large fascial incision to allow separation of the pedicle from the rectus muscle, which can contribute to postoperative pain and a higher risk of abdominal bulges and hernias despite not harvesting muscle. However, a new and innovative approach utilizing minimally invasive robotic techniques reduces the fascial incision to just 2–3 cm. This allows for the dissection of perforators from the intraperitoneal cavity (Bishop and Selber, 2021) and has been associated with less postoperative pain, shorter hospital stays, and improved overall recovery. However, it presents technical challenges that require surgical expertise and expensive equipment, and there is a learning curve associated with this technique. Additionally, the smaller fascial incision may result in longer operative times and limited access if complications arise intraoperatively. This approach is suitable only for selected cases, specifically those with one or two perforators located closely together and with a short intramuscular course.

MICROSURGICAL TECHNIQUE – VENOUS COUPLER

Traditionally, vessel anastomosis was performed by hand-sewing with monofilament microsutures under magnification. The use of a venous coupler for venous anastomosis in microsurgical breast reconstruction is now well established in clinical practice (Jandali et al., 2010). This reliable device features interlocking rings containing 12 metal pins that come together to achieve a patent microvascular anastomosis. The coupling device has been shown to be a safe and effective method for venous anastomosis, reducing flap ischemic time, managing vessel size discrepancies, and minimizing complications associated with microvascular anastomosis compared to standard suture techniques (Fitzgerald O'Connor et al., 2016).

FLAP SHAPING – STACKED FLAP/BIPEDICLE FLAP

Tailoring abdominal flaps to enhance breast contour and symmetry is particularly important when a significant volume is required from a small abdomen. Stacked and bipedicle flaps are both reliable and reproducible options. Various techniques for shaping abdominal tissue to achieve optimal aesthetic outcomes have been reported by Patel et al. (2016). These flap-shaping techniques, including folding, dividing, and coning, can be used in combination to create a flap design that best matches the contralateral breast, resulting in a safe, natural, and durable aesthetic outcome.

POSTOPERATIVE ENHANCED RECOVERY

Recent advances in the ERAS protocols for microsurgery breast reconstruction have significantly improved postoperative recovery times and overall patient outcomes (Pierzchajlo et al., 2023). Enhancements in anaesthesia, surgical techniques, postoperative pain management, and early mobilization allow patients undergoing DIEP flap surgery to experience better pain management, resulting in shorter hospital stays. The ERAS protocol encourages reduced use of opioid-based analgesics and incorporates intraoperative regional blocks using local anaesthetics, such as liposomal bupivacaine. Additionally, improved patient education and support facilitate the safe early discharge of patients after surgery.

CONCLUSION

Dr. Robert Allen's 1994 paper on the DIEP flap marked a milestone in microsurgical breast reconstruction, showcasing how innovation can significantly enhance patient outcomes through continuous advancements, refined techniques, and pushing the boundaries of microsurgery. Today, the DIEP flap remains the gold standard in autologous breast reconstruction, known for its high success rates and high patient satisfaction.

REFERENCES

Bishop S, Selber J. Minimally invasive robotic breast reconstruction surgery. *Gland Surg.* 2021 Jan;10(1):469–478.

Chae MP, Hunter-Smith DJ, Rozen WM. Comparative analysis of fluorescent angiography, computed tomographic angiography and magnetic reasonance angiography for planning autologous breast reconstruction. *Gland Surg.* 2015;4:164–178.

Fitzgerald O'Connor E, Rozen WM, Chowdhry M, Patel NG, Chow WTH, Griffiths M, Ramakrishnan VV. The microvascular anastomotic coupler for venous anastomoses in free flap breast reconstruction improves outcomes. *Gland Surg.* 2016 Apr;5(2):88–92.

Jandali S, Wu L, Vega S, Kovach S, Serletti J. 1000 consecutive venous anastomoses using the microvascular anastomotic coupler in breast reconstruction. *Plast Reconstr Surg.* 2010 Mar;125(3):792–798.

Park JE, Shenaq DS, Silva AK, Mhlaba JM, Song DH. Breast reconstruction with SIEA flaps: a single Institution Experience with 145 free flaps. *Plast Reconstr Surg.* 2016 Jun;137(6):1682–1689.

Patel NG, Rozen WM, Chow WTH, Chowdhry M, Fitzgerald O'Connor E, Sharma H, Griffiths M, Ramakrishnan VV. Stacked and bipedicle abdominal free flaps for breast reconstruction: considerations for shaping. *Glad Surg.* 2016 Apr;5(2):115–121.

Pierzchajlo N, Zibitt M, Hinson C, Stokes J, Neil ZD, Pierzchajilo G, Gendreau J, Buchanan P. Enhanced recovery after surgery pathways for deep inferior epigastric perforator flap breast reconstruction: a systemic review and meta-analysis. *J Plast Reconstr Aesthet Surg.* 2023 Dec;87:259–272.

Rozen WM, Bhullar HK, Hunter-Smith D. How to assess a CTA of the abdomen to plan an autologous breast reconstruction. *Gland Surg.* 2019 Oct;8(Suppl 4):S291–S296.

EDITOR COMMENTARY

The abdomen is in many ways an ideal donor site for breast reconstruction; the tissue is reasonably well matched and there is often some excess tissue in the lower abdomen. Hartrampf (1982) used the superior epigastric pedicle whilst a paper by Holmstrom in 1979 described a "free abdominoplasty flap" performed by Hamilton and Fogdestam 3 years before the pedicled flap. Donor site morbidity was the most significant issue; there was a risk of ventral hernia or muscle weakness.

There were attempts to reduce the morbidity with muscle-sparing TRAM techniques. Koshima I et al. (1989, 1992) had described the use of perforator-based flaps from the abdomen without muscle for non-breast reconstruction. To come up with the free deep inferior epigastric perforator (DIEP), Allen RJ dissected injected cadavers and injected abdominoplasty specimens to delineate the vascular patterns. He used Doppler ultrasound to evaluate the abdominal perforators in 120 patients and found that each patient had at least 2 perforators in the abdominoplasty region, within a 7 cm radius of the umbilicus. The authors then embarked on 15 breast reconstructions using the DIEP flap where the blood vessels supplying the skin are first found by dissection above the muscle fascia and then followed in a retrograde fashion through the muscle to the source vessel without sacrifice of muscle or fascia. Most cases in this series were delayed reconstruction; with immediate reconstruction, the 4th intercostal nerves were preserved where feasible and then co-apted to the flap nerves. The thoracodorsal arteries were used as the recipient vessel in this series before the use of the IMA/V became popular. The DIEP has become what most regard as the gold standard for breast reconstruction.

This paper was a well-designed study with both experimental and clinical evidence. However, it was a retrospective study without a control group and follow up was limited to 6–24 months postoperatively, which may not have been enough time for all donor site issues to become apparent. However, many subsequent studies have followed to provide confirmation of the efficacy and advantages of the DIEP compared to the TRAM (Blondeel et al., 1998).

REFERENCES

Blondeel PN, Morris SF, Hallock GG, *et al.* The versatility of the deep inferior epigastric perforator flap: a prospective study of 100 consecutive patients. *Plast Reconstr Surg.* 1998;102(6):1788–1796.

Hamilton R, Fogdestam I. Australia's contribution to the free abdominoplasty flap in breast reconstruction. *AJOPS.* 2019;2(2):8–12. doi:10.34239/ajops.v2n2.185.

CHAPTER 10

Osseointegrated Titanium Implants: Requirements for Ensuring a Long-Lasting, Direct Bone-to-Implant Anchorage in Man

Albrektsson T, Brånemark PI, Hansson HA, Lindström J.
Acta Orthop Scand. 1981;52(2):155–170

EXPERT COMMENTARY

Michael Leung

Osseointegration is a technique that allows direct bone-to-implant anchorage without the use of cement. It was invented by Professor P.I. Brånemark from the University of Gothenburg, Sweden. Initially pioneered in the 1960s for dental applications, it has since been extended to other craniofacial applications, particularly in the attachment of prostheses and dental rehabilitation following head and neck tumour resection. Another revolutionary application is the attachment of prostheses in cases of short above-knee and above-elbow amputations, especially when conventional prostheses cannot be used due to various soft tissue and bony problems.

This landmark paper by T. Albrektsson and P.I. Brånemark, though conducted in the early stages of the development of osseointegration, is one of the classic studies that delves into the ultrastructure of the bone-implant interface. Professor Brånemark discovered the concept of osseointegration while studying microcirculation in rabbit tibia using a titanium camera, which proved difficult to remove, leading to his ground-breaking insights.

Osseointegration is defined as the "direct anchorage of an implant by the formation of bony tissue around the implant without the formation of fibrous tissue at the bone-implant interface." In this paper, the authors investigated the bone-implant interface using X-ray, scanning electron microscopy (SEM), transmission electron microscopy (TEM), and histology. To my knowledge, no other study since then has examined this interface in such detail.

The surface of the titanium implant becomes instantaneously coated with an oxide layer, preventing direct exposure of metal or metal compounds to surrounding tissues. This oxide layer, composed of TiO, TiO_2, Ti_2O_3, and Ti_3O_4, apparently reduces the risk of

DOI: 10.1201/9781003413738-10

infection. The stable oxide coating, about 100 Å thick, prevents direct contact between bone and metal.

Using SEM, the authors demonstrated that the cells adjacent to the implant are of normal shape and size. The actual border area between the cell and the implant consisted of ground substance composed of glycoproteins. There were no white cells or other types of inflammatory cells infiltrating the border area of the soft tissues. The thick collagenous fibrils of the bone split into thin filaments, which embedded in the amorphous or granular material formed by proteoglycans, thus establishing a layer directly covering the titanium oxide. The anchorage mechanism of the collagen filaments appeared to be similar to the attachment of Sharpey's fibres to bone, i.e., gluing by the amorphous coating formed by the ground substance.

In the discussion section, the authors outlined the prerequisites for osseointegration:

1. *Implant material*: Non-alloyed titanium is the only metal shown to establish direct bone-to-implant contact.
2. *Implant design*: Cylindrical threaded implants create maximal contact between bone and implant.
3. *Implant finish*: The importance of this parameter is difficult to evaluate.
4. *Status of the bone*: Healthy bone tissue is essential for proper osseointegration, with potential corticalisation of cancellous bone around the implant. Bone grafting may be required.
5. *Surgical technique*: Adherence to the principles of "minimal tissue violence" is crucial, with constant cooling important during slow surgical insertion of the implant.
6. *Implant loading conditions*: The implant should heal in situ without loading for 3–4 months.

Since the publication of this article in 1981, osseointegration has become the mainstay of dental restoration and plays an increasing role in head and neck reconstruction post-tumour resection. Its applications in craniofacial reconstruction include:

1. Attachment of facial prostheses (e.g., eye, nose, ear) and occasionally large facial prostheses.
2. Bone-anchored hearing aids.
3. Dental rehabilitation post-maxillary and mandibular reconstruction.

In hand reconstructive surgery, it is commonly used for attaching thumb, finger, and occasionally hemi-hand prostheses. It was also used in finger joint replacements (e.g., MP and PIP joint replacements in rheumatoid arthritis patients), but osseointegrated joint replacements are no longer used due to issues with silicone joint fractures.

Osseointegration use is rapidly expanding for upper and lower limb prosthesis attachment in amputation cases. In upper limb amputation, it is mainly used for patients with short above-elbow amputation stumps, applicable in both acute and chronic settings. Osseointegration, combined with targeted muscle reinnervation (TMR), has revolutionized upper limb amputee rehabilitation.

In lower limb amputation cases, osseointegration has given patients with short above-knee amputation stumps a realistic chance of walking and is also used in below-knee amputations under special circumstances. However, its widespread (over)use in some centres over the past decade may be detrimental to patients due to potential complications. Therefore, I believe osseointegration should be reserved for patients unable to wear a conventional limb prosthesis, as it carries inherent surgical risks, particularly regarding soft tissue and implant infections.

The main challenge in osseointegration is soft tissue management. The goal is to aim to have the tissue around the implant as thin and immobile as possible. This is usually not an issue in dental osseointegration, where gum tissue is inherently immobile and saliva production helps maintain cleanliness. For craniofacial prosthesis attachments, such as ears, noses, and eyes, the surrounding/overlying tissue must often be thinned down with dermal thinning or replaced with split skin grafts. This issue is particularly significant in lower limb amputation cases due to the thickness of the tissue and the need for tissue redundancy in various postures.

The Brånemark system typically involves two stages: the first stage is the insertion of the fixture, and the second stage, performed 3–4 months later, involves attaching the abutment to the fixture via a surgical stoma. The two-stage procedure allows for more opportunities for soft tissue thinning and manipulation to optimise the cutaneous opening. However, some centres propose a single-stage osseointegration procedure (Prof. Al Muderis) to shorten the rehabilitation period, though its efficacy remains under debate.

The most common complication of osseointegration is soft tissue infection, ranging from superficial soft tissue infections to deep bone infections. Deep bone infections can lead to osteomyelitis and may necessitate further shortening. Literature reports complication rates of up to 30%–40%, though deep bone infections are rare.

Another significant drawback is the cost of the implant and abutment. The implant costs approximately 50,000 AUD, and the abutment costs around 20,000 AUD, not including hospital inpatient costs, surgical fees, and rehabilitation expenses.

In conclusion, osseointegration is a valuable reconstructive tool with widespread applications but carries significant risks and complications. Its use should be judicious and limited to major reconstructive centres with specific expertise and multiple specialties available. Each case should be discussed in a multidisciplinary team (MDT) setting, including various surgical specialties, rehabilitation consultants, anaplastologists, psychologists, and perioperative pain management teams. The operation is best performed as a conjoint procedure, e.g., plastic and orthopaedic surgeons working together in limb amputation cases, and close cooperation among all disciplines is vital to its success.

EDITOR COMMENTARY

The concept of a direct-to-bone anchor without using cement was novel, so novel in fact, its existence was doubted for a long time despite published work from this team. This paper underpins what started in the Gothenburg clinic in 1965 and then became generally known as Brånemark implants. A total of 2,895 implants were placed in the maxilla and mandible whilst a minority (124) were used in the temporal, tibial, and iliac bones. The pattern of anchorage of collagen to the titanium was compared to Sharpey's fibres connecting tendons to bone. In the pioneering experiments by Leventhal GS (1951), titanium screws that were placed into rat femurs were so difficult to remove after 16 weeks that the femur fractured in one case. In 1952 Brånemark had used a titanium chamber to study blood flow in rabbit bone but found the implant could not be removed due to "osseointegration." Brånemark spent decades trying to convince others.

A delicate meticulous technique required for "minimal tissue violence" is crucial to successful osteointegration. Osseointegration has become crucial to modern dental rehabilitation – the first dental implants were placed into a patient, Gosta Larsson, in 1965 to support an obturators for his cleft palate and mandibular deformities; Gosta also had a BAHA in 1990. All the implants were still in place when he died in 2006. Limb prostheses using osseointegration are often more comfortable and consume less energy, but patients need careful selection.

As an aside, there are those who believe the more appropriate term should be "osteointegration" (Siegel, 1999) to fit in with the more common terms for bony things, e.g., "osteosarcoma," "osteogenesis." However, as Watts et al. (2000) points out "integrate" is derived from Latin, as is "osseo" whereas "osteo" is Greek (like "sarx" for sarcoma).

REFERENCES

Leventhal GS. Titanium, a metal for surgery. *J Bone Joint Surg Am*. 1951 Apr;33–A(2):473–4. PMID: 14824196.

Siegel MA. Osseointegration? *Oral Surg Oral Med Oral Pathol Oral Radiol Endod*. 1999 Aug;88(2):113. doi: 10.1016/s1079-2104(99)70101-0.

Watts TL. Osseointegration is Latin. *Oral Surg Oral Med Oral Pathol Oral Radiol Endod*. 2000 May;89(5):532. doi: 10.1067/moe.2000.106694.

CHAPTER 11

The Keystone Design Perforator Island Flap in Reconstructive Surgery

Behan FC. *ANZ J Surg*. 2003 Mar;73(3):112–120
doi: 10.1046/j.1445-2197.2003.02638.x PMID: 12608972

We have coined the term "keystone design perforator island flap" (KDPIF) because of its curvilinear-shaped trapezoidal design borrowed from architectural terminology. It is essentially elliptical in shape with its long axis adjacent to the long axis of the defect. The flap is based on randomly located vascular perforators. The wound is closed directly, the mid-line area is the line of maximum tension, and by V-Y advancement of each end of the flap, the 'islanded' flap fills the defect. This allows the secondary defect on the opposite side to be closed, exploiting the mobility of the adjacent surrounding tissue. The importance of blunt dissection is emphasized in raising these perforator island flaps as it preserves the vascular integrity of the musculocutaneous and fasciocutaneous perforators together with venous and neural connections. The keystone flap minimizes the need for skin grafting in the majority of cases and produces excellent aesthetic results. Four types of flaps are described: Type I (direct closure), Type II (with or without grafting), Type III (employs a double-island flap technique), and Type IV (involves rotation and advancement with or without grafting). The patient is almost pain free in the postoperative phase. Early mobilization is possible, allowing this technique to be used in short-stay patients.

RESULTS

In a series of 300 patients with flaps situated over the extremities and trunk and facial region, primary wound healing was achieved in 99.6% with one out of 300 developing partial necrosis of the flap.

CONCLUSION

The technique described in the present article offers a simple and effective method of wound closure in situations that would otherwise have required complex flap closure or skin grafting, particularly for melanoma.

EXPERT COMMENTARY

Nicola Fleming and Cheng Hean Lo

As a research fellow at the Royal College of Surgeons in London, FC Behan carried out cadaveric injection studies and demonstrated that the integument is supplied by a system of axial vessels with their random communications or "linkage vessels."[1] The term "angiotome" was devised to refer to any area of integument supplied by an axial vessel. In 1973, Behan and Wilson first presented the angiotome concept at the Second Congress of the European Section of the International Confederation of Plastic and Reconstructive Surgery (Madrid, Spain).[1,2] In 1975, they further elaborated on the angiotome concept at the Sixth International Congress of Plastic and Reconstructive Surgery (Paris, France).[3] It was observed that each angiotome may be safely raised as a flap or extended by random communications or linkage vessels with an adjacent angiotome.[1]

In 1987, Taylor and Palmer introduced the in vitro concept of angiosome to define composite three-dimensional units or blocks of tissue supplied by named source arteries.[4] In 1994, Morrison noted: "Taylor chose the word angiosome to describe the three-dimensional linkage in both the horizontal and vertical dimensions. Several years before this, Behan had by injection studies demonstrated and described the linkage of one axial pattern vascular territory with another and coined the term angiotome to complement the well understood territory of the dermatome."[5] The angiotome concept was the foundation upon which the keystone island flap was built.

In 2003, the keystone island flap concept (or keystone design perforator island flap) was first published.[2] This personal series of 300 cases explained the origins and naming of the keystone island flap, followed by a detailed description of flap design and surgical technique, including flap elevation and defect closure. Keystone island flaps were classified as Types I–IV based on extent of dissection, requirement for division of deep fascia (Type IIA), and need for split-skin grafting of the secondary defect (Type IIB). Double keystone flaps (type III) were raised to exploit maximum laxity of surrounding tissues and subfascial flap undermining (Type IV) up to 50% allowed safe mobilization and coverage of complex defects. This series was highlighted by the safe and extensive application of the technique in many areas of the body with a flap necrosis rate less than 1%. The sympathectomy effect was proposed as the physiological explanation for his regular observations of "red dot sign" and "vascular flare" not seen with other local fasciocutaneous flap techniques. Patients experienced excellent healing, minimal pain, minimal oedema and superior aesthetics, which were noted as key advantages of this technique.

In 2012, Behan et al. comprehensively described the clinical application of the keystone island flap by anatomical regions.[6] This book also demonstrated the successful application of this reconstructive technique in different settings, including head and neck surgery, melanoma surgery, trauma surgery, and even reconstruction of irradiated wounds.

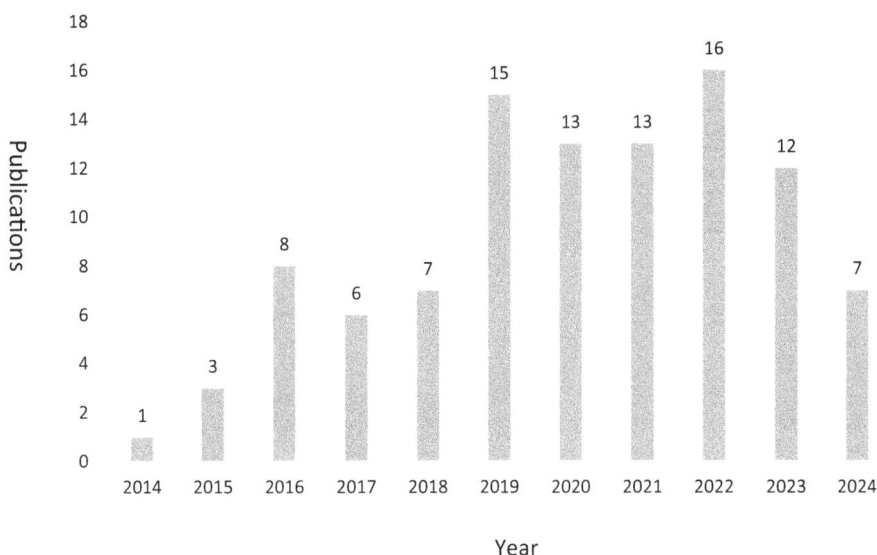

Figure 11.1   Increasing number of publications involving keystone island flaps over the last 10 years (January 2014–May 2024).

A review of literature from January 2014 to May 2024 (English-language publications only, key terms "keystone" or "key stone" and "flap") identified 100 publications (69 case series, 24 case reports, 7 comparative studies) originating from 27 different countries (Figure 11.1). From these publications, 39 described reconstruction of trunk defects, 26 involved extremities, 15 involved the head and neck region, and 20 involved a combination of anatomical regions. Clinical applications were further expanded to include conditions such as myelomeningocoele, burns, breast cancer, pilonidal sinus, hidradenitis suppurativa, and chronic pressure sores.[7–14] Low complication rates and relatively short operative duration times compared to other reconstructive options, such as the microvascular free flap, were consistently reported.[15] Healing times and limb mobility were significantly improved with use of the keystone island flap compared to split-thickness skin grafts.[7,16]

Application of the keystone island flap continues to grow.

REFERENCES

1. Behan FC, Wilson JSP. The Vascular Basis of Laterally Based Forehead Island Flaps and their Clinical Applications, *Transactions of the Second Congress of the European Section of the International Confederation of Plastic and Reconstructive Surgery.* Madrid, Spain; 1973:3–26.
2. Behan FC. The keystone design perforator island flap in reconstructive surgery. *ANZ J Surg.* 2003;73(3):112–120.
3. Behan FC, Wilson JSP. Marchac D, Hueston JT, editors. The principle of the angiotome: a system of linked axial pattern flaps. In: Marchac D, Hueston JT, editors. *Transactions of the Sixth International Congress of Plastic and Reconstructive Surgery.* Paris, France; August 1975:6–11, 24–29.

4. Taylor GI, Palmer JH. The vascular territories (angiosomes) of the body: experimental study and clinical applications. *Br J Plast Surg.* 1987;40(2):113–141.
5. Morrison WA. Fasciocutaneous flaps in lower limb reconstruction. *Aust N Z J Surg.* 1994;64(3):145–146.
6. Behan FC, Findlay M, Lo CH. *The Keystone Perforator Island Flap Concept.* New South Wales, Australia: Elsevier Australia; 2012.
7. Darrach H, Kokosis G, Bridgham K, Stone JP, Lange JR, Sacks JM. Comparison of keystone flaps and skin grafts for oncologic reconstruction: a retrospective review. *J Surg Oncol.* 2019;119(7):843–849.
8. Virag TH, Kadar IA, Matei IR, Georgescu AV. Surgical management of hidradenitis suppurativa with keystone perforator island flap. *Injury* 2020;51 Suppl 4:S41–S47.
9. Byun IH, Kim CW, Park TH. The modified keystone flap for pressure ulcers: a modification of the keystone flap with rotation and advancement. *Ann Plast Surg.* 2019;82(3):299–303.
10. Kim HB, Lim SY, Yoon CS, Kim KN. Reconstruction of bilateral inferomedial gluteal defects after resection of hidradenitis suppurativa with symmetrical keystone flaps designed parallel to relaxed skin-tension lines: a case report. *Medicine (Baltimore)* 2020;99(14):e19779.
11. Park HS, Morrison E, Lo C, Leong J. An application of keystone perforator island flap for closure of lumbosacral myelomeningocele defects. *Ann Plast Surg.* 2016;77(3):332–336.
12. Rini IS, Gunardi AJ, Yashinta, Kevin J, Marsaulina RP, Aryandono T, *et al.* Quality of life in palliative post-mastectomy reconstruction: keystone versus rotational flap. *Plast Reconstr Surg Glob Open.* 2021;9(3):e3457.
13. Calisir A, Ece I. Comparison of the Keystone flap and the Limberg flap technique in the surgical treatment of pilonidal sinus disease. *Updates Surg.* 2021;73(6):2341–2346.
14. Gupta S, Chittoria RK, Chavan V, Aggarwal A, Reddy CL, Mohan PB, *et al.* Keystone flap for postburn finger flexion contracture release. *J Cutan Aesthet Surg.* 2021;14(1):125–128.
15. Huang J, Yu N, Long X, Wang X. A systematic review of the keystone design perforator island flap in lower extremity defects. *Medicine (Baltimore)* 2017;96(21):e6842.
16. Potet P, De Bonnecaze G, Chabrillac E, Dupret-Bories A, Vergez S, Chaput B. Closure of radial forearm free flap donor site: a comparative study between keystone flap and skin graft. *Head Neck.* 2020;42(2):217–223.

EDITOR COMMENTARY

The author presented his experience with 300 keystone design perforator island flaps (KDPIF) over 7 years with only one partial necrosis. It seemed like a completely new concept – a novel flap pattern without being overly concerned over which vessels supplied it. The paper contained a great deal of compelling information to support the concept and its clinical use but uptake was relatively slow to reach a wider audience, perhaps due to being in a lower impact journal.

We had the pleasure of hosting Felix in our unit for several weeks not that long after the publication of the paper. With Professor Behan on hand to guide us through several cases and explain points of discussion, we got to grips with it quickly. He thought the robust vascularity was related to the dermatomes. He emphasized that there could be considerable tension during closure, but that this was spread out by the VY closure of the ends and by using substantial sutures around the periphery. He particularly espoused the "red dot sign" as a favourable feature. It could be used even in irradiated tissue. Tissue deformation studies (Pelissier et al., 2007a,b) gave some interesting insight in how the tissues move.

The keystone has wide applications. It is a very useful technique to use in the extremities particularly for wider excision of leg melanoma. We used the keystone flap in a series of cases to close "tight" ALT donor sites (presented at WRSM 2009), which obviated the need for grafting and provided more aesthetic outcomes.

Some have used preoperative localization using handheld Doppler devices or duplex Doppler ultrasound to look for perforators that can be incorporated into the design; it can offer some "reassurance" but is generally unnecessary.

REFERENCES

Pelissier P, Santoul M, Pinsolle V, Casoli V, Behan F. The keystone design perforator island flap. Part I: anatomic study. *J Plast Reconstr Aesthet Surg.* 2007a;60(8):883–887. doi: 10.1016/j.bjps.2007.01.072.
Pelissier P, Gardet H, Pinsolle V, Santoul M, Behan FC. The keystone design perforator island flap. Part II: clinical applications. *J Plast Reconstr Aesthet Surg.* 2007b;60(8):888–891. doi: 10.1016/j.bjps.2007.03.023.

CHAPTER 12

Experience with a Synthetic Bilayer Biodegradable Temporising Matrix in Significant Burn Injury

John E. Greenwood, Bradley J. Schmitt, Marcus J.D. Wagstaff. *Burns Open. 2018;* 2:17–34

AUTHOR COMMENTARY

Marcus J.D. Wagstaff

Introduction

The Biodegradable Temporising Matrix (BTM, PolyNovo Biomaterials Pty Ltd, Melbourne, Aus) was devised to be a novel dermal substitute. Comprising of a 2 mm-thick biodegradable, biocompatible polyurethane (NovoSorb) open-cell foam scaffold bonded to an overlying non-biodegradable seal, it was intended to allow tissue ingress (fibroblasts, collagen, capillaries) into the pores of the foam, with the seal preventing tissue evaporative water loss (TEWL) and disrupting coalescence of granulation tissue across its surface that would cause wound contraction. In concept, this physiological closure would enable temporising of a large burn wound, affording time to allow donor sites and superficial burns to reepithelialise, for the patient to recover from the multi-system insult of their burn injury, and, in theory, for (composite) skin to be cultured before further skin graft harvest. During this time, it would deliver a new, vascularised layer of tissue to replace the missing dermis, improve scarring, and reduce wound contraction. In addition, in contrast to biological dermal substitutes, its synthetic composition was designed to resist digestion by colonising bacteria.

This paper reported on the first use of BTM as a dermal substitute in patients with significant burn injury. The translation of preclinical research to clinical use had been comprehensively published,[1–4] resulting in several iterations towards the final BTM device. Small-scale clinical trials testing safety and efficacy had been performed, starting with a short-term implantation model of a 3 cm thick unsealed NovoSorb foam used as a negative pressure wound therapy interface for 3 days at a time in decubitus ulcers.[5] No adverse reactions were noted, so the trials progressed to a long-term implantation model using the proposed sealed 2 mm dermal substitute. The model chosen was free flap donor site reconstruction as these wounds are complex, with muscle and tendon in their base, but clean, surgically controlled, predictable, and a precedent of successful use had been published in the literature using the Integra biological dermal

DOI: 10.1201/9781003413738-12

regeneration template.[6] The first 10 patients revealed problems with secondary infection of subseal collections and the removal of the seal was piecemeal, making it frustrating and time-consuming.[7] The seal and bond were then optimised in a further pig trial, and a second cohort of 10 patients were recruited for free flap donor site reconstruction with the optimised BTM, with hand-cut fenestrations in the seal to allow fluid egress.[8,9] This time delamination of the seal was more straightforward, and no secondary infections were observed. Based on this result, it was decided to proceed with a single-arm prospective cohort study in significant burn injury.

METHODS

Ethics committee approval was obtained, and the trial registered with the Australian and New Zealand clinical trials registry (ANZCTR). As a single-arm study, no comparison with standard of care or other dermal substitute was planned. The recruited numbers and power required to show significant differences in safety or efficacy in this field would need to be high, mandating a multi-centred approach. Therefore, a small sample of five patients was recruited. Inclusion criteria included patients between 18 and 70 years of age, with burns of which between 20% and 50% total body surface area (TBSA) were full thickness. This percentage was considered a severe enough burn injury, with the anticipated physiological compromise, to test the device but excluding experimenting on an extremely vulnerable patient with more extensive and deep burn wounds.

Demographic data recorded included age/sex of the patient; mechanism of burn injury; %TBSA, including full-thickness component; %TBSA receiving BTM and anatomical site; time for integration, and hospital length of stay.

Adverse events were documented, and their relation to the device was attributed when present.

Outcomes reported were %TBSA BTM removed (with the reason for removal). As a marker of clinically significant skin graft loss, the %TBSA of repeat graft application was also reported. Scar assessment was performed at 12 months using the Patient Observer Scar Assessment Scale by a senior physiotherapist.

ADVERSE EVENTS

The results and discussion of these 5 patients, on review, were prescient to so many of the qualities of BTM that have led to its global adoption and sustained use. A total of 2.5% TBSA BTM was removed from patient 1's shoulders and upper right thigh on day 4 post-implantation due to lack of adherence and faecal contamination, respectively. Given our experience that BTM takes approximately one week to adhere, in our current practice, we would probably resecure the BTM and wait for adherence to occur. When faecal contamination occurred, we prepared for the possibility of removing large amounts of BTM in the days to come. However, we were surprised that localised excision and antimicrobial administration were all that was required to control the spread of infection across the matrix and wound. For patient 3, infection of BTM and surrounding primary skin graft on the upper abdomen with *Stenotrophomonas maltophilia* led to extensive skin graft loss and the neighbouring BTM was removed. With patient 5, however, we observed widespread *Pseudomonas aeruginosa* infection under BTM on both arms at day 7 post-implantation. We discovered that serial drainage over several days via incisions in the seal, along with antimicrobial administration, enabled the entire device to persist in the presence of infection and continue to integrate.

Patient 4 experienced bleeding under the BTM. He had been anticoagulated with therapeutic-dose heparin to enable dialysis. As the haematomas appeared, the affected areas of BTM were removed at the bedside in the intensive care unit (ICU), the clots removed, haemostasis achieved with bipolar cautery, the wound cleaned, and the BTM replaced, which integrated. With patient 1, the seal remained intact and bonded to the matrix for up to 7 weeks when the final grafts were applied to the thighs. We have since learned that the seal will stay bonded to the matrix for much longer than this and that widespread spontaneous delamination, allowing the granulation to coalesce on the surface and cause wound contraction, does not tend to occur.

OUTCOMES

Aside from the safety and efficacy of BTM as a temporising dermal substitute in significant burns, there were some further significant findings. The study revealed that BTM could integrate over deep structures such as bone and tendon. Patient 4 had 21% TBSA full-thickness burns over his right flank and upper limb, necessitating removal of the superficial muscle group of the forearm, revealing the deeper neurovascular structures, exposing the medial epicondyle and at the flank two exposed ribs, all devoid of periosteum. His entire right axilla was also burned. Initially, BTM did not take over the bone, so the cortices were drilled after which the BTM then integrated. This successful cover of complex structures and bone has now led to further applications in bone and tendon cover, such as lower limb and hand trauma and scalp reconstruction over calvarium.[10–12] His total axillary reconstruction with BTM afforded him a full range of shoulder movement to extremes of abduction, without secondary release of contracture being necessary.

Patient 5 had BTM applied to the entire back and was nursed supine on an air-fluidised mattress. Our experience with other biological dermal substitutes in this scenario was that infection and loss of the product were likely. However, with this patient and with subsequent experience, we have found the back to be an excellent recipient site for BTM, and that compression through recumbence is advantageous to achieve integration. Across all subjects <2% of the 122% TBSA of BTM applied underwent repeat skin grafting secondary to loss.

In patients 1–3 it was recorded that the mesh pattern was less discernible and skin tissue quality was softer, more robust, and mobile with a superior cosmetic quality compared to areas treated by skin graft alone. Patient 3, who had dark skin, reported that there was no pigment loss in the BTM-mesh grafted areas, compared to the primary grafted sites (without BTM), which had patches of pigment loss. Attempts to qualify this using POSAS scores were incomplete, as two patients did not attend follow-up, and the scores were not compared to the areas of primary grafting. In retrospect, little meaningful information can be derived from this.

CONCLUSION

This paper pioneered the use of BTM in burns, and, through data collection, photographic documentation and problem-solving, it also uncovered many of the nuances and strengths that now routinely inform its use in hostile environments. It has since been used successfully, as initially proposed, to temporise the burn wound as the first stage prior to reconstruction with laboratory-cultured autologous composite skin in extremely large TBSA burn patients.[13–15]

There are now over 280 peer-reviewed articles published on BTM. It is stable for long periods without delamination, it reliably supports the take of skin graft when integrated, it can persist after drainage of infection or haematoma, and it can integrate to cover exposed bone and tendon. The quality of the thickness and appearance of the reconstruction, irrespective of integration time, is superior to split skin graft alone. All these qualities have broadened its indications for use in reconstruction in trauma, post-cancer excision, necrotising fasciitis, spina bifida, hidradenitis suppurativa, and diabetic foot ulcer reconstruction.[16–20]

REFERENCES

1. Li A, Dearman BL, Crompton KE, Moore TG, Greenwood JE. Evaluation of a novel biodegradable polymer for the generation of a dermal matrix. *J Burn Care Res.* 2009 Jul-Aug;30(4):717–728. doi: 10.1097/BCR.0b013e3181abffca.
2. Greenwood JE, Dearman BL. Split skin graft application over an integrating, biodegradable temporizing polymer matrix: immediate and delayed. *J Burn Care Res.* 2012 Jan–Feb;33(1):7–19. doi: 10.1097/BCR.0b013e3182372be9.
3. Greenwood JE, Dearman BL. Comparison of a sealed, polymer foam biodegradable temporising matrix against Integra® dermal regeneration template in a porcine wound model. *J Burn Care Res.* 2012 Jan–Feb;33(1):163–173. doi: 10.1097/BCR.0b013e318233fac1.
4. Dearman BL, Stefani K, Li A, Greenwood JE. "Take" of a polymer-based autologous cultured composite "skin" on an integrated temporising dermal matrix: proof of concept. *J Burn Care Res.* 2013 Jan–Feb;34(1):151–160. doi: 10.1097/BCR.0b013e31828089f9.
5. Wagstaff MJD, Driver S, Coghlan P, Greenwood JE. A randomised, controlled trial of negative pressure wound therapy via a biodegradable polyurethane foam in the management of decubitus ulceration. *Wound Repair Regen.* 2014;22(2):205–211.
6. Murray RC, Gordin EA, Saigal K, Leventhal D, Krein H, Heffelfinger RN. Reconstruction of the radial forearm free flap donor site using integra artificial dermis. *Microsurgery.* 2011 Feb;31(2):104–108. doi: 10.1002/micr.20833.
7. Wagstaff MJD, Schmitt BJ, Coghlan P, Finkemeyer JP, Caplash Y, Greenwood JE. A biodegradable polyurethane dermal matrix in reconstruction of free flap donor sites: a pilot study. *ePlasty* 2015 Apr 24;15:e13.

8. Dearman BL, Li A, Greenwood JE. Optimisation of a polyurethane dermal matrix and experience with a polymer-based cultured composite skin. *J Burn Care Res.* 2014 Sep–Oct;35(5):437–448. doi: 10.1097/BCR.0000000000000061.

9. Wagstaff MJD, Schmitt BJ, Caplash Y, Greenwood JE. Free flap donor site reconstruction: a prospective case series using an optimized polyurethane biodegradable temporizing matrix. *ePlasty.* 2015 Jun 26;15:e27.

10. Damkat-Thomas L, Greenwood JE, Wagstaff MJD. A synthetic biodegradable temporising matrix in degloving lower extremity trauma reconstruction: a case report. *Plast Reconstr Surg Glob Open.* 2019 Apr 2;7(4):e2110. doi: 10.1097/GOX.0000000000002110.

11. Greenwood JE, Wagstaff MJ, Rooke M, Caplash Y. Reconstruction of extensive calvarial exposure after major burn injury in 2 stages using a biodegradable polyurethane matrix. *Eplasty.* 2016 May 9;16:e17.

12. Concannon E, Damkat-Thomas L, Rose E, Coghlan P, Solanki N, Wagstaff M. Use of a synthetic dermal matrix for reconstruction of 55 patients with non-graftable wounds and management of complications. *J Burn Care Res.* 2023 Jan 31:irad012. doi: 10.1093/jbcr/irad012.

13. Greenwood JE, Damkat-Thomas L, Schmitt B, Dearman B. Successful proof of the 'two-stage strategy' for major burn wound repair. *Burns Open.* 2020 4:121–131. doi: 10.1016/j.burnso.2020.06.003.

14. Dearman BL and Greenwood JE. Long-term follow-up of a major burn treated using a composite cultured skin: case report. *Burns Open.* 2022;6(4):156–163. doi: 10.1016/j.burnso.2022.07.002.

15. Schiestl C, Meuli M, Vojvodic M, Pontiggia L, Neuhaus D, Brotschi B, *et al.* Expanding into the future: combining a novel dermal template with distinct variants of autologous cultured skin substitutes in massive burns. *Burns Open.* 2021;5:145–153. doi: 10.1016/j.burnso.2021.06.002.

16. Wagstaff, M. J. D., Salna, I. M., Caplash, Y., & Greenwood, J. E. Biodegradable temporising matrix (BTM) for the reconstruction of defects following serial debridement for necrotising fasciitis: a case series. *Burns Open.* 2019;3(1):12–30.

17. Tapking C, Thomas BF, Hundeshagen G, Haug VFM, Gazyakan E, Bliesener B, Bigdeli AK, Kneser U, Vollbach FH. NovoSorb® Biodegradable Temporising Matrix (BTM): What we learned from the first 300 consecutive cases. *J Plast Reconstr Aesthet Surg.* 2024 May;92:190–197. doi: 10.1016/j.bjps.2024.02.065.

18. Hasham S, O'Boyle C, Alexander S. Use of 'stacked' dermal template: biodegradable temporising matrix to close a large myelomeningocele defect in a newborn. *Scars Burn Heal.* 2024 Sep 2;10:20595131241270220. doi: 10.1177/20595131241270220.

19. Kuang B, Pena G, Cowled P, Fitridge R, Greenwood J, Wagstaff M, Dawson J. Use of Biodegradable Temporising Matrix (BTM) in the reconstruction of diabetic foot wounds: a pilot study. *Scars Burn Heal.* 2022 Sep 21;8:20595131221122272. doi: 10.1177/20595131221122272.

20. Guerriero FP, Clark RA, Miller M, Delaney CL. Overcoming barriers to wound healing in a neuropathic and neuro-ischaemic diabetic foot cohort using a novel bilayer biodegradable synthetic matrix. *Biomedicines.* 2023; 11(3):721. doi: 10.3390/biomedicines11030721.

EXPERT COMMENTARY

Nelson Low

Study Design

This study is a prospective, pilot clinical trial conducted at the Royal Adelaide Hospital. The research aimed to evaluate the effectiveness of the NovoSorb Biodegradable Temporising Matrix (BTM) in managing significant full-thickness burns, covering between 20% and 50% of the Total Body Surface Area (TBSA). Five adult subjects were included, each presenting with severe burns requiring immediate or early burn excision followed by BTM implantation. The follow-up period extended to at least 12 months post-treatment, assessing scar outcomes and integration of the BTM.

RESULTS AND FOLLOW-UP

The follow-up period involved regular clinical assessments and photographic documentation to monitor the integration of the BTM and the outcomes of subsequent skin grafts. The BTM showed good integration in most cases, allowing for split-skin grafting on a vascularised bed. Of the total area treated with BTM across all subjects (122% TBSA), less than 7% of the TBSA treated with BTM had to be removed due to non-integration, and 9% required replacement of BTM with complete subsequent integration. At 12 months, scar assessments using the Patient and Observer Scar Assessment Scale (POSAS) and the Matching Assessment using Photographs with Scars (MAPS) showed promising outcomes in both subjective and objective measures.

STUDY LIMITATIONS

The study's limitations include the small sample size of only five subjects, which restricts the generalisability of the findings. The follow-up duration, while adequate to observe initial integration and healing, may not fully capture long-term outcomes or potential late complications. Furthermore, the study was conducted in a single centre, which may introduce bias due to variations in clinical practice and patient management.

RELEVANT STUDIES

Since this publication, there are four other papers of interest and relevant to this. They are summarised below:

1. Long-Term Scarring Outcomes and Safety of Patients Treated with NovoSorb BTM: An Observational Cohort Study[1]
   - This cohort study focused on the long-term safety and scarring outcomes in patients treated with BTM. The patients reported good scar quality over a follow-up period of 18 months, with minimal adverse events. Using the Patient and Observer Scar Assessment Scale (POSAS), both patients and clinicians rated the scarring as favourable, supporting BTM's long-term effectiveness in promoting high-quality dermal regeneration. The study demonstrated good scar quality with minimal adverse effects. This is especially notable, as scarring is a major concern in burn treatment, and BTM proved effective in promoting wound closure and long-term aesthetic outcomes.
2. The Application of a Synthetic Biodegradable Temporizing Matrix in Extensive Burn Injury: A Unicenter Experience of 175 Cases[2]
   - This study analyzed 175 cases of patients with burns covering more than 10% of TBSA (average wound size was $30.3 \pm 19.8\%$ TBSA) treated with BTM. The study emphasised the importance of timely application of BTM, correlating better outcomes with early application post-debridement. The research demonstrated that BTM helped to minimise wound contraction and supported split-thickness skin grafting (STSG) with high take rates, contributing to the successful management of extensive burns, making it a reliable dermal substitute for large-scale burn injuries.

3. Wound Healing and Dermal Regeneration in Severe Burn Patients Treated with NovoSorb BTM: A Prospective Clinical Study[3]
   - This is a multicentre prospective study on 30 patients with severe burns treated with BTM. The study reported a high mean graft take rate at 81.9% and BTM take on the day of skin grafting relative to area of BTM implanted was 88.6%, demonstrating BTM's effectiveness in dermal regeneration, even in challenging wound conditions. Infection was recorded for 38.5% of patients between BTM implantation and SSG application. After SSG application, this infection reduced to 3.9% and no infection was recorded at 7–10 days after SSG. This supported BTM's utility in situations where infection risk is present, further validating its use in the management of severe burns compared to previously used dermal matrix.
4. Clinical Outcomes and Resource Utilization in Patients with Major Burns Treated with NovoSorb BTM[4]
   - This study retrospectively evaluated the clinical outcomes and resource use in 55 patients with major burns (≥40% TBSA) treated with BTM admitted to the Royal Brisbane and Women's Hospital Adult Burn Unit who survived their acute admission. The results showed a significant reduction in operative time for BTM-treated patients (median 1361.5 minutes compared to 1768 minutes for those treated with cadaveric allografts). Moreover, the study highlighted that the use of BTM led to cost savings due to the reduced need for cadaveric allografts, shorter operating times, and intensive care unit admissions. The cost estimate of treating a patient in the BTM group was 275,290 AUD, compared with 317,233 AUD in the non-BTM group (41,943 AUD reduction in the BTM group). This aspect of cost reduction is critical in managing extensive burn injuries, as it alleviates the financial burden associated with burn care, supporting the economic viability of BTM in clinical practice.

To summarise, these four studies reinforce the findings from the original paper, highlighting the clinical and economic benefits of BTM. The last study, in particular, underscores the cost-saving potential of BTM through reduced operative times and decreased reliance on cadaveric allografts, making it a valuable tool in modern burn care.

STUDY IMPACT

The development and use of BTM in burn care represents a significant advance in reconstructive surgery. BTM was the result of a collaboration between the Commonwealth Scientific and Industrial Research Organisation (CSIRO) and PolyNovo, with Professor John Greenwood from Adelaide, Australia, leading the clinical application efforts. Before its first human application in 2013, where it was used for reconstructing a free flap donor site,[5] numerous preclinical studies were conducted to evaluate its safety and efficacy in tissue regeneration.[6–11]

This pioneering study on the use of BTM in significant burn injuries marked a crucial turning point in burn management. Previously, other biological dermal matrices had been used for dermal regeneration, but they were associated with high costs and an increased risk of infection. BTM demonstrated superior resistance to wound contraction and infection, two critical factors that significantly influence healing outcomes in burn patients.

At the time of publication (2017), this was the first study to extensively evaluate BTM in the context of significant burn injury. The authors, who had spent over a decade developing and refining BTM, validated its ability to serve as a temporary scaffold. This scaffold stabilises the wound bed, offering a much-needed window for patient recovery before performing definitive skin grafting.

Since then, BTM has gained further recognition in burn treatment and other complex wound reconstructions. Additional studies have confirmed that BTM not only serves as an adjunct in complex wound care but also should be considered a critical part of the reconstructive surgeons' armamentarium.[12–14] The findings from these studies support the original research, showing that BTM facilitates subsequent skin grafting and improves overall burn management practices. BTM's role in burn care continues to be validated, with studies confirming its efficacy in enhancing patient outcomes. As a result, BTM is now considered a crucial component in modern reconstructive surgery, extending beyond burns to treat other complex wounds and defects.

As a reconstructive plastic surgeon, I have used BTM for 4 years now, treating over 60 patients in my series. My experience with BTM has significantly influenced my approach to complex wound and burn management. Here are the key observations from my practice:

- Grafts over BTM tend to be more robust within a shorter period compared to non-BTM cases.
- Once matured, the grafts are softer and more supple, which leads to better functional and aesthetic outcomes.
- In challenging anatomical areas like the bare skull, tendons, and irradiated tissues, BTM provides more consistent graft take, resulting in more stable scars. Interestingly, BTM has performed well over irradiated bone in my practice, but for reasons that are still unclear, it does not work effectively on irradiated skulls.
- BTM has become a reliable alternative to free flap reconstruction in many cases. In fact, several of my patients who might have required free flaps were able to avoid them, resulting in less donor site morbidity and fewer revision surgeries.
- In suitable cases, BTM has allowed me to preserve digital length during fingertip reconstructions, which has greatly improved functional and aesthetic outcomes for my patients.
- Like many studies have reported, I have found BTM to be more resistant to infection, making it a reliable option for complex wound care.
- The risks and financial costs associated with BTM are relatively low, especially when compared to the extensive procedures involved in free flap reconstruction, making it an excellent choice in appropriate cases.

BTM has undoubtedly changed the way I approach wounds and defects, offering versatility and flexibility in managing both burn injuries and other complex wound scenarios. Its effectiveness, combined with its lower cost and reduced risks, makes it an essential tool in my reconstructive surgery practice.

REFERENCES

1. Lo CH, Wagstaff MJD, Barker TM, *et al.* Long-term scarring outcomes and safety of patients treated with NovoSorb® Biodegradable Temporizing Matrix (BTM). *JPRAS Open.* 2023;37:42–51.
2. Tapking C, Panayi AC, Hundeshagen G, *et al.* The application of a synthetic biodegradable temporizing matrix in extensive burn injury: a unicenter experience of 175 cases. *J Clin Med.* 2024;13:2661–2673.
3. Lo CH, Brown JN, Dantzer EJG, Maitz PKM, Vandervord JG, Wagstaff MJD, Barker TM, Cleland H. Wound healing and dermal regeneration in severe burn patients treated with NovoSorb® Biodegradable Temporising Matrix: a prospective clinical study. *Burns.* 2022 May;48(3):529–538.
4. Betar N, Maher D, Wheatley L, Barker T, Brown J. Clinical outcomes and resource utilisation in patients with major burns treated with NovoSorb® BTM. *Burns.* 2023 Nov;49(7):1663–1669.
5. Wagstaff MJD, Schmitt BJ, Coghlan P, Finkemeyer JP, Caplash Y, Greenwood JE. A biodegradable polyurethane dermal matrix in reconstruction of free flap donor sites: a pilot study. *ePlasty.* 2015;15:102–118.
6. Greenwood JE Dearman BL. Comparison of a sealed, polymer foam biodegradable temporizing matrix against integra dermal regeneration template in a porcine wound model. *J Burn Care Res.* 2012;33(1):163–173.
7. Li A, Dearman BL, Crompton KE, Moore TG Greenwood JE.Evaluation of a novel biodegradable polymer for the generation of a dermal matrix. *J Burn Care Res.* 2009;30(4):717–728.
8. Greenwood JE, Li A, Dearman B, Moore TG. Evaluation of NovoSorbTM novel biodegradable polymer for the generation of a dermal matrix. Part 1: in-vitro studies. *Wound Pract Res.* 2010;18(1):14–22.
9. Greenwood JE, Li A, Dearman B, Moore TG. Evaluation of NovoSorbTM novel biodegradable polymer for the generation of a dermal matrix. Part 2: in-vivo studies. *Wound Pract Res.* 2010;18(1):24–34.
10. Greenwood JE, Dearman BL. Split-skin graft application over an integrating, biodegradable temporising polymer matrix: immediate and delayed. *J Burn Care Res.* 2012;33(1):7–19.
11. Dearman BL, Stefani K, Li A, Greenwood JE. 'Take' of a polymer-based autologous cultured composite 'skin' on an integrated temporising dermal matrix: proof of concept. *J Burn Care Res.* 2013;34(1):151–160.
12. Li H, Lim P, Stanley E, Lee G, Lin S, Neoh D, Liew J, Ng SK. Experience with NovoSorb® Biodegradable Temporising Matrix in reconstruction of complex wounds. *ANZ J Surg.* 2021 Sep;91(9):1744–1750.
13. Solanki NS, York B, Gao Y, Baker P, Wong She RB. A consecutive case series of defects reconstructed using NovoSorb® Biodegradable Temporising Matrix: Initial experience and early results. *J Plast Reconstr Aesthet Surg.* 2020 Oct;73(10):1845–1853.
14. Tapking C, Thomas BF, Hundeshagen G, Haug VFM, Gazyakan E, Bliesener B, Bigdeli AK, Kneser U, Vollbach FH. NovoSorb® Biodegradable Temporising Matrix (BTM): what we learned from the first 300 consecutive cases. *J Plast Reconstr Aesthet Surg.* 2024 May;92:190–197.

EDITOR COMMENTARY

We were the first in Asia to use Integra in 1995. Despite its efficacy in selected cases, its wider adoption was limited by its cost, availability, and susceptibility to infection. In 2015, we started using Nevelia (Symatese), which was cheaper, easier to handle particularly being able to hold sutures/ staples without tearing, but had similar susceptibility to infection. Unlike Nevelia, which was more of an evolutionary step over Integra, BTM represents a total paradigm shift (a term that I hate). I was dubious how a "simple" polyurethane foam devoid of collagen, etc. could function as a dermal substitute and be "resistant" to infection at the same time. However, clinical experience has confirmed these qualities and BTM has taken the place of Nevelia (and Integra) in our practice.

To add to N. Low's anecdotal points, we find that BTM:

- Significantly increases the success of Meek micrografting.

- Can substitute for cadaveric skin in coverage of debrided wounds when graft donor sites are insufficient and recovering for reharvest. The adhesion of BTM to the wound bed is much slower than cadaveric skin with a higher risk of interim infection but has the major advantage of providing a "dermal" layer when it is vascularised. This will support thin widely meshed/Meek grafts much better.

- Rather inexplicably, when a piece of BTM has to be removed because it looks infected/loose, etc., a second piece BTM (after wound preparation) vascularises much more quickly.

CHAPTER 13

Risk of Breast Implant Associated Anaplastic Large Cell Lymphoma (BIA-ALCL) in a Cohort of 3,546 Women Prospectively Followed Long Term after Reconstruction with Textured Breast Implants

Cordeiro PG, Ghione P, Ni A, Hu Q, Ganesan N, Galasso N, Dogan A, Horwitz SM. *J Plast Reconstr Aesthet Surg.* 2020 May;73(5):841–846

METHODS

A prospective cohort study was conducted in patients who underwent breast reconstruction by a single surgeon at Memorial Sloan Kettering Cancer Center (MSKCC) from December 1992 to December 2017. Major events related to implants were prospectively recorded. We identified cases of BIA-ALCL by cross-checking clinical, pathology, and external records data. Patients were followed until lymphoma occurrence or last follow-up. The primary outcomes were incidence rate per person-years and cumulative incidence.

RESULTS

From 1992 to 2017, 3,546 patients underwent 6,023 breast reconstructions, mainly after breast cancer removal or contralateral prophylactic mastectomy, using macro-textured surface expanders and implants. All reconstructions were performed by a single surgeon (PGC). Median follow-up was 8.1 years (range, 3 months–30.9 years). Ten women, 1/354, developed ALCL after a median exposure of 11.5 years (range, 7.4–15.8 years). Overall risk of BIA-ALCL in our cohort was 0.311 cases per 1,000 person-years (95% CI 0.118 to 0.503).

DISCUSSION

This study, the first to evaluate the risk of macro-textured breast implants from a prospective database with long term follow-up, demonstrates that the incidence rate

DOI: 10.1201/9781003413738-13

of BIA-ALCL may be higher than previously reported. These results can help inform implant choice for women undergoing breast reconstruction.

AUTHOR COMMENTARY

Paola Ghione and Peter G. Cordeiro

Introduction

Breast implant-associated anaplastic large cell lymphoma (BIA-ALCL) is a rare subtype of T-cell lymphoma, growing in the space between the breast implant and the fibrous capsule forming around it, and it is related to exposure to textured breast implants. Our paper[1] published in the *Journal of Plastic Reconstructive and Aesthetic Surgery* (JPRAS) in 2020 offers a critical evaluation of the incidence of BIA-ALCL within a large cohort of women who underwent breast reconstruction by surgeon Peter Cordeiro using macro-textured breast implants and followed long term at Memorial Sloan Kettering Cancer Center (MSKCC). This study provides essential insights into the long-term risks associated with these implants and has significant implications for clinical practice and patient safety.

SUMMARY OF THE STUDY

The research by Cordeiro and colleagues presents a prospectively enrolled cohort of patients who underwent breast implant reconstructive surgery and received macro-textured breast implants, followed for several decades to evaluate complications related to breast implants. The study investigates the risk of BIA-ALCL in these 3,546 patients who underwent 6,023 breast reconstructions between December 1992 and December 2017, with all procedures performed by a single surgeon at MSKCC. The study meticulously tracked patient outcomes, including any occurrence of BIA-ALCL, using a combination of clinical, pathological, and external records.

The cohort included patients who received macro-textured expanders and permanent implants for breast reconstruction following mastectomy for breast cancer or prophylactic mastectomy. The study excluded patients with smooth-surface implants, as BIA-ALCL has been primarily associated with textured implant exposure. Data collection was rigorous, involving regular follow-ups and detailed recording of complications and pathology reviews all performed at MSKCC. The incidence rate of BIA-ALCL was calculated based on the number of cases per 1,000 person-years, with cumulative incidence assessed through reverse Kaplan–Meier analysis.

The study identified 10 cases of BIA-ALCL arising within the cohort, yielding an incidence rate of 0.311 cases per 1,000 person-years (95% CI 0.118–0.503). The median time from implant placement to diagnosis was 11.7 years. The paper highlights that the observed incidence is higher than previous estimates, which had ranged from 1 in 2,832 to 1 in 30,000 women.

DISCUSSION

This study is pioneering for several reasons. First, it is the first study to provide a long-term, prospective evaluation of the risk associated with macro-textured implants, using a large, well-documented cohort. The higher-than-expected incidence of BIA-ALCL reported in this study highlights the importance of accurate risk assessment and comprehensive follow-up for patients with textured implants.

The study challenges earlier estimates of BIA-ALCL risk, which were based on approximations of the population at risk (based on sales records or other estimates) or shorter follow-up periods, mainly 2–3 years, which would have not been long enough to capture the cases that usually arise 7–10 years after exposure. For instance, the earlier risk estimates by the FDA were significantly lower, partly due to underreporting and shorter observation times. Cordeiro, Ghione et al. offer a more precise estimation of risk, which is critical for informing patient decisions and guiding implant choice.

The study also emphasizes the importance of continued vigilance and long-term monitoring in patients with textured implants. The relatively high incidence reported suggests that the risk of BIA-ALCL may be more significant than previously understood, potentially due to factors such as the specific texture of the implants, silicone particles, genetics, or the development of biofilm.

The findings of this study have implications for clinical practice. Given the higher-than-expected incidence of BIA-ALCL, surgeons must carefully weigh the risks and benefits of using textured implants for breast reconstruction after mastectomy for breast cancer. Patients should be informed of the potential risks and be followed for years to ensure early detection and correct management of BIA-ALCL.

CONCLUSION

The paper by Cordeiro et al. is a landmark in the field of plastic surgery and breast and lymphoma oncology, providing critical data on the risk of BIA-ALCL associated with macro-textured breast implants. Its comprehensive, long-term approach offers a more accurate assessment of risk, significantly impacting decision-making for breast reconstruction. By meticulously documenting the incidence of BIA-ALCL and challenging earlier risk estimates, this study has paved the way for more informed discussions about breast implant safety.

EDITOR COMMENTARY

This study is noteworthy given the large amount of prospective data from a single surgeon with median follow-up of 8.1 years and median "exposure" time of 11.7 years. All patients in the analysis had macrotextured implants (6020) and 10 developed BIA-ALCL, i.e., incidence of 1 in 602, which is somewhat higher than the Dutch (1/6,920) and Australian (1/3,817) studies. A total of 7 presented with a seroma. The calculated rate was 0.311 cases per 1,000 person-years. No cases developed after implant removal. This was the largest single surgeon series with meticulous record keeping (which tends to be better for reconstruction patients than for cosmetic patients), so it is probably a better measure than other papers.

Dr. Cordeiro was co-author in a follow-up study of sorts (Nelson JA et al., 2023) that looked at patients who had a temporary textured implant (n = 3,310) for a mean of 6.7 months before it was changed for a definitive smooth expander. There were no cases of BIA-ALCL in this cohort.

It is revealing that no cases of either BIA-ALCL or the even rarer breast implant-associated squamous cell carcinoma (BIA-SCC) were detected in Mentor and Allergan's 3-year outcomes studies, likely because of inherent weaknesses in the design of studies ironically intended to look at implant safety – the follow-up was too short (mean time to diagnosis is over 10 years) and the studies were underpowered to reveal what would have been rare diagnoses at the time. Data from the Patient Registry and Outcomes for Breast Implants and Anaplastic Large Cell Lymphoma Etiology and Epidemiology (PROFILE) registry (2018) found 186 cases in the United States starting from 2012 (the first case was reported in 1997), an average of 11 years from implant placement to diagnosis, and an association with textured devices. Soon after (2019), Allergan recalled Natrelle BIOCELL "macrotextured" breast implants at the request of the FDA. This would be the "1-point plan" alternative to the "14-point plan" (Adams et al., 2017). So far no cases have been reported in patients who have had smooth implants only – prior reports had included patients where smooth implants had replaced textured implants.

Adams et al.'s survey of 8 surgeons reported no cases of BIA-ALCL (presuming that failure to return equated to nothing being wrong), placing blame on technique rather than device. One of the co-authors, Mark Jewell (2020), speculated that Cordeiro's cases may be due to "surgical technique" or "poor institutional hygiene at MSKCC" or "ineffectual breast pocket irrigation with bacitracin." A more convincing explanation seems to be far better data for analysis due to meticulous records and follow-up (van Natta B, 2020).

Clemens et al. (2016) provided data on treatment, outcomes, and prognosis of BIA-ALCL. Limited somewhat by its retrospective design, small sample size, and short follow-up, there was support for complete surgical ablation at an early stage, which included removal of the breast implant, the scar capsule, and associated masses and which involved lymph nodes with negative margins. Late diagnosis and or incomplete surgical excision increases the risk of distant spread. Subsequent papers provided specific indications for adjunct treatments, such as chemotherapy. More patients are being detected at stage 1a (effusion limited) disease; how it is related to the capsular mass type of disease is unclear and some speculate that these may be different subtypes.

One particular topic that is hotly discussed is the recommendation (or not) for explantation; the FDA does not recommend explantation in asymptomatic women, arguing that the risks of surgery are higher than BIA-ALCL. However, this is based on lower estimates of risk and Santanelli di Pompeo et al. (2023b) found that there were no mortalities in 100,000 explantations over 8 years in Europe. Note that the FDA does not recommend against explantation either. A systematic review of 248 cases by Santanelli di Pompeo et al. (2023a) found that the incidence of BIA-ALCL decreased with implant removal/replacement.

REFERENCES

Adams WP Jr, Culbertson EJ, Deva AK, R Magnusson M, Layt C, Jewell ML, Mallucci P, Hedén P. Macrotextured breast implants with defined steps to minimize bacterial contamination around the device: experience in 42,000 implants. *Plast Reconstr Surg.* 2017 Sep;140(3):427–431. doi: 10.1097/PRS.0000000000003575.

Clemens MW, Medeiros LJ, Butler CE, *et al.* Complete surgical excision is essential for the management of patients with breast implant-associated anaplastic large-cell lymphoma. *J Clin Oncol.* 2016;34(2):160–168.

Jewell ML. Letter to the editor regarding; risk of breast implant associated anaplastic large cell lymphoma in a cohort of 3546 women prospectively followed long term after reconstruction with macro-textured breast implants [published online September 16, 2020]. *J Plast Reconstr Aesthet Surg.* doi:10.1016/j.bjps.2020.08.084.

Nelson JA, McKernan CD, Rubenstein RN, Shamsunder MG, Poulton R, Dabic S, Mehrara BJ, Disa JJ, Cordeiro PG, McCarthy CM. Risk of breast implant-associated anaplastic large cell lymphoma in patients with textured tissue expanders. *Plast Reconstr Surg.* 2023 Jul 1;152(1):32–37. doi: 10.1097/PRS.0000000000010195.

Santanelli di Pompeo F, Panagiotakos D, Firmani G, *et al.* BIA-ALCL epidemiological findings from a retrospective study of 248 cases extracted from relevant case reports and series: a systematic review. *Aesthet Surg J.* 2023a;43:545–555.

Santanelli di Pompeo F, Sorotos M, Clemens MW. Mortality rate in breast implant surgery: is an additional procedure worthwhile to mitigate BIA-ALCL risk? *Aesthetic Plast Surg.* 2023b;47:914–926.

Van Natta B. Letter to the editor regarding Jewell letter to the editor regarding: risk of breast implant associated anaplastic large cell lymphoma in a cohort of 3546 women prospectively followed long term after reconstruction with macro-textured breast implants [published online November 26, 2020]. *J Plast Reconstr Aesthet Surg.* doi:10.1016/j.bjps.2020.11.006.

CHAPTER 14

Latissimus Dorsi Musculocutaneous Flap without Muscle

Angrigiani C, Grilli D, Siebert J. *Plast Reconstr Surg.* 1995;96:1608–1614

AUTHOR COMMENTARY

Claudio Angrigiani

In the mid-1970s while in training I had the opportunity to actively undertake research in the Department of Anatomy at the University of Buenos Aires School of Medicine under the direction of Professor Elbio Cozzi. At the time, he had developed quite an original method for cadaveric intravascular injection with a coloured latex material that was flexible. Up to that point, we had only acrylic, which was brittle and did not allow precise dissection.

I was interested in flaps for limb reconstruction and this period was "dominated" by flaps of the axial random and musculocutaneous flap philosophy. I observed in my dissections that there were distinct "strong" branches to the skin that travelled through the muscles or around them, and, more interestingly, that the skin and subcutaneous tissue were "attached intimately to the underlying muscles." In 1980, I was awarded a Microvascular Fellowship in Japan by the Japanese government and I learned microvascular technique under Professors Kitaro Ohmori and Kyonori Harii. The surgical skills obtained in Japan provided me with more confidence to make use of my previous observations in the latex injected specimens in the clinical field. I started to perform flaps in the trunk and limbs without inclusion of the underlying muscles or fascia. When doing latissimus dorsi musculocutaneous flap for limb reconstruction, we tried several methods to diminish muscle bulkiness, most often using Marko Godina's muscle-tailoring technique. In 1985, I did the first thoracodorsal artery perforator (TDAP) free flap to reconstruct a traumatic forearm defect in a young patient, without prior Doppler or vascular study. Soon after, several cases were done as free or local flaps for burn sequelae.

From 1982 onwards, I presented these cases at local meetings, including the Argentinian Society of Plastic Surgery Meetings. Examples included "fasciocutaneous flaps of the anterior thigh" (1982); "reverse posterior interosseous forearm flap," together with Professor E. Zancolli (1985); "reverse flaps of the dorsum of the hand," together with C. Zaidemberg (1986); "latissimus dorsi musculocutaneous flap without muscle" (1987); and "adductor perforator flap" (1989). Several papers were submitted to English-language journals but were rejected.

DOI: 10.1201/9781003413738-14

In 1988, whilst I was a Visiting Fellow at the New York University Hospital Plastic and Reconstructive Unit under Professor Joseph McCarthy, I had the opportunity to present some of my anatomical and clinical research and received great support and assistance for publication in English-language journals. I will always be deeply grateful to Professor McCarthy, as well as Professors Charles Thorne, John Siebert, and Michael Longaker. "Anatomy of the LeFort I Osteotomized Segment" and "Vascularized Distal Radius Osseous Flap for Scaphoid Non-Union" were selected for presentation in meetings in the United States and for publication. Curiously, the possibility of harvesting the skin island of the latissimus dorsi flap was not considered of practical use at the time. Eventually, a 3-minute presentation was given at the 1993 ASPRS meeting in New Orleans and the paper was published in 1995.

Several years after the original description in Argentina, we presented the "Adductor Flap: A New Method for Transferring Medial and Posterior Thigh Skin" with my friends and colleagues Daniel Grilli and Charles Thorne at the 77th Annual Meeting of the American Association of Plastic Surgeons in Montreal, Canada (1988). The paper was eventually published in 2001. We used this flap for several cases of ipsilateral limb reconstruction where it can be done under localized unilateral limb block anaesthesia. In 1992 whilst I was Visiting Professor of the Plastic Surgery Educational Foundation – one of my greatest honours as a plastic surgeon – I presented this flap at the University of Miami Jackson Memorial Hospital by invitation of Professor R. Millard. Dr. Anthony Wolfe – a great and dear mentor and friend – was there and suggested using the adductor flap for breast reconstruction. I tried several times when I returned home, but the donor area was unacceptable for the patients in our area. The adductor flap was also presented at the 8th International Course in Perforator Flaps in São Paulo, Brazil, in 2004, and it was included in the first edition of the book *Perforator Flaps* (QMP, 2005). During the cadaver session of that course, I demonstrated the anatomical dissection of the flap. Bob Allen, who was co-faculty during that course, rediscovered the flap for use in breast reconstruction and it was named the PAP flap.

REFERENCES

Allen RJ Jr, Lee ZH, Mayo JL, Levine J, Ahn C, Allen RJ Sr. The profunda artery perforator flap experience for breast reconstruction. *Plast Reconstr Surg.* 2016 Nov;138(5):968–975. doi: 10.1097/PRS.0000000000002619.

Angrigiani C, Grilli D, Thorne CH. The adductor flap: a new method for transferring posterior and medial thigh skin. *Plast Reconstr Surg.* 2001 Jun;107(7):1725–1731. doi: 10.1097/00006534-200106000-00013.

EDITOR COMMENTARY

Claudio Angrigiani et al. combined anatomical study of fresh cadavers, demonstrating the musculocutaneous perforators with a small (five) retrospective clinical case series that showed that these perforators could be used for the safe harvest of large cutaneous flaps without including the LD muscle – what is known today as the thoracodorsal artery perforator (TDAP) flap. There was limited clinical data, including follow-up, complications, etc. In a separate article, Angrigiani had also described the dorsal scapular artery perforator flap based on a musculocutaneous perforator of the trapezius muscle, which was more versatile than the muscle flap.

It is interesting to note that the pioneers in perforator flap surgery at the time converged at the 2004 ICPF – Allen, Koshima, Angrigiani, and Blondeel. F.C. Wei was also at the 2004 ICPF talking about "free style flaps."

REFERENCE

Angrigiani C, Grilli D, Karanas YL, Longaker MT, Sharma S. The dorsal scapular island flap: an alternative for head, neck, and chest reconstruction. *Plast Reconstr Surg.* 2003 Jan;111(1):67–78. doi: 10.1097/01. PRS.0000037682.59058.6B.

CHAPTER 15

A Classification System and Algorithm for Reconstruction of Maxillectomy and Midfacial Defects

Cordeiro, Peter G., Santamaria, Eric. *Plast Reconstr Surg.* 2000;105:2331

AUTHOR COMMENTARY

Eric Santamaria and Peter G. Cordeiro

Given the complex interaction between form and function that maxillectomy defects present to the reconstructive surgeon, finding a universally accepted classification system that can be used to group maxillectomy defects according to tissue loss and potential reconstructive options has been difficult.

Unlike previous articles about the classification and management algorithm of post-maxillectomy defects, we described a reconstructive approach taking the maxillary bone and the 6 walls that compose it as the primary structure. Overlying this hexahedron bone there are different midfacial anatomical structures such as the cheek with the facial muscles, the oral sphincter, the nose, and the eyelids. Depending on whether they are resected and the extent of the defect, an algorithmic approach using free flaps was proposed to address both the bone and the soft tissues in the midface. Contiguous structures such as the lips, eyelids, or nose would be reconstructed separately, usually with local flaps, incorporating or not part of the free tissue transfer.

This article has been cited in most papers that have described maxillary and midfacial reconstruction in the intervening 24 years, and it has been considered a landmark in microsurgical reconstruction of the head and neck. This classification has also been proposed as a guide for defects that must be reconstructed with facial transplantation.[1]

The senior author (PGC) subsequently published a larger series (2012) describing his experience with 100 free flaps performed in 96 patients with maxillectomy defects. He also added a subclassification of Type II (subtotal maxillectomy) defects, into IIA and IIB defects. The former includes defects with less than 50% loss of the transverse palate, and Type IIB defects include greater than 50% of the transverse palate and/or the anterior arch of the maxilla. Both Type IIA and Type IIB maxillectomy defects are moderate-volume deficiencies with large surface area requirements, which usually need two skin islands.

DOI: 10.1201/9781003413738-15

For Type IIA defects, reconstruction may involve either a free flap or a skin graft and an obturator, depending on patient and surgeon preference. If a free flap is selected to avoid the inconvenience and maintenance of a palatal obturator, the authors' flap of choice is the radial forearm fasciocutaneous free flap. They advocate that the skin inset is critical, and the skin paddle must be equal to or smaller than the original defect to keep the soft palate taut, re-create the buccal sulcus, and avoid prolapse into the oral cavity. If adequate teeth or bone stock remains, dentures or osseointegrated dental implants may be used.

For Type IIB defects, an osteocutaneous free flap is needed as these defects require bone for structural support as well as the skin lining of the (neo)palate and nasal floor. A prosthesis is inadequate because support to the upper lip is better with bone. The authors' flap of choice is the radial forearm osteocutaneous sandwich flap. The bone segment can be shaped to re-create the maxillary alveolar arch and support the upper lip, and the thin pliable skin can be wrapped around the bone to replace the lining of the palate and nose.[2]

In a further paper, Cordeiro et al. (2012) described technical improvements in these same 100 free flaps used for oncologic midface/maxillectomy reconstructions over 15 years. They focused mostly on the following areas: palate, dental implants and prosthesis, orbital floor, eyelid, nasal sidewall, lips, cranial base and dura, and pedicle anastomosis. In addition, the authors compared the functional and aesthetic outcomes of the first 50 flaps and the second 50 flaps.

They demonstrated that with improvements in palatal reconstruction, the proportion of patients who achieved normal speech increased from 38.9% in the first half of the series (1992 to 2000) to 50% in the second half of the series (2001 to 2006). Patients who tolerated an unrestricted diet, increased from 44.4% to 52%. The use of a modified access incision, new methods to reconstruct the orbital floor, and medial canthal tendon reconstruction also lowered the ectropion rate from 71.4% in the first half of the series to 47.6% in the second half of the series. Finally, the percentage of patients whose aesthetic results were judged as "excellent" increased from 12% to 58.6%.[3]

With the increasing refinement of reconstructive microsurgical procedures, several authors have described other free flaps to reconstruct the same maxillectomy defects, such as the ALT, the fibula, and the scapular or iliac crest osteocutaneous free flap.[4–7] Many of these variants arise because different authors have included patients with other types of defects, which are not caused by malignant tumors but rather by trauma, benign pathologies, or even congenital craniofacial defects.[7–9] Nevertheless, the ALT and the fibula free flap have largely replaced the radial forearm fasciocutaneous and osteocutaneous free flap due to the latter's higher morbidity and potentially poor aesthetic outcome at the donor site.

Likewise, some articles have included the reconstruction of delayed defects, in contrast to our original article, which discussed only immediate reconstruction in cancer patients. Santamaria and De la Concha (2016) compared a group of 13 patients who underwent immediate reconstruction of maxillectomy defects with a group of 24 patients who had delayed reconstruction of defects due to malignant and benign tumors or trauma sequelae. They used more fibula osteocutaneous and ALT free flaps, instead of rectus abdominis or radial forearm flaps for Types II and IIIa maxillectomy defects. They found that delayed reconstruction was associated with a higher incidence of complications and free flap failures, especially when the tumor resection was followed by postoperative radiotherapy. Therefore, multiple free and local flaps were required in delayed reconstruction patients to address wound dehiscence with hardware exposure, oronasal fistula, and upper lip or partial nasal retraction and to provide stable skeletal and soft tissue reconstruction.[7]

Recently, the introduction of computer-assisted design and computer-assisted modeling (CAD/CAM) has been a major step forward in bony free flap reconstruction of maxillectomy defects. Pre-preoperative planning of the osteotomies improves accuracy and the outcome is more predictable, often allowing immediate insertion of osseointegrated dental implants in selected patients.[10,11]

In conclusion, reconstruction of maxillectomy and midfacial defects is one of the most challenging operations performed by reconstructive microsurgeons. While several classification systems have been described, many midface defects are unique and sometimes may not fall into a specific type of category. This article has been accepted as one of the simplest and most useful classifications for post-maxillectomy defects reconstruction as it describes the fundamental principles and management algorithm to restore form and function, which are essential to achieve optimal results.

REFERENCES

1. Gastman B, Djohan R, Siemionow M. Extending the cordeiro maxillofacial defect classification system for use in the era of vascularized composite transplantation. *Plast Reconstr Surg.* 2012;130:419.
2. Cordeiro PG, Chen CM: A 15-year review of midface reconstruction after total and subtotal maxillectomy: Part I. Algorithm and outcomes. *Plast Reconstr Surg.* 2012;129:124–136.
3. Cordeiro PG, Chen CM. A 15-year review of midface reconstruction after total and subtotal maxillectomy: Part II. Technical modifications to maximize aesthetic and functional outcomes. *Plast Reconstr Surg.* 2012;129:139–147.
4. Bianchi B, Ferri A, Ferrari S, *et al.* Maxillary reconstruction using anterolateral thigh flap and bone grafts. *Microsurgery.* 2009;29(6):430–436.
5. Cho M-J, Padilla PL, Skoracki RJ, Hanasono MM. Maxillary reconstruction with free vascularized fibula: 15-year experience. *Plast Reconstr Surg.* 2025 Mar 1;155(3):597e–609e.
6. Haring CT, Marchiano EJ, Stevens JR, *et al.* Osteotomized folded scapular tip free flap for complex midfacial reconstruction. *Plast Aesthet Res.* 2021;8:21–44.
7. Santamaria E, De la Concha E. Lessons learned from delayed versus immediate microsurgical reconstruction of complex maxillectomy and midfacial defects: experience in a tertiary center in Mexico. *Clin Plast Surg.* 2016 Oct;43(4):719–727.
8. Rodriguez ED, Martin M, Bluebond-Langner R, Khalifeh M, Singh N, Manson PN. Microsurgical reconstruction of posttraumatic high-energy maxillary defects: establishing the effectiveness of early reconstruction. *Plast Reconstr Surg.* 2007;120(7 Suppl 2):103S–117S.
9. Santamaria E, Correa S, Bluebond-Langner R, Orozco H, Ortiz-Monasterio F. A shift from the *Osteocutaneous fibula* flap to the prelaminated osteomucosal fibula flap for maxillary reconstruction. *Plast Reconstr Surg.* 2012 Nov;130(5):1023–1030.
10. Chang EI, Hanasono MM. State-of-the-art reconstruction of midface and facial deformities. *J Surg Oncol.* 2016 Jun;113(8):962–970.

11. Chiapasco M, Biglioli F, Autelitano L, *et al.* Clinical outcome of dental implants placed in fibula-free flaps used for the reconstruction of maxillomandibular defects following ablation for tumors or osteoradionecrosis. *Clin Oral Implants Res.* 2006;17:220–228.

EXPERT COMMENTARY

Terence Poon

The research objective was to devise a simple classification system for maxillectomy/midfacial defects and describe a systematic algorithm for reconstruction of these complex defects.

STUDY DESIGN

- Retrospective Review

SAMPLE SIZE

- 60 patients

FOLLOW-UP

- 50 patients evaluated a minimum of 6 months after reconstruction. Mean follow-up 27.7 months (range 6–62 months).

RESULTS

- 60 flaps in 5 years

In summary, defects were classified into:

- Type I, limited maxillectomy ($n = 7$)
- Type II, subtotal maxillectomy ($n = 12$)
- Type IIIA, total maxillectomy with preservation of the orbital contents ($n = 13$)
- Type IIIB, total maxillectomy with orbital exenteration ($n = 18$)
- Type IV, orbitomaxillectomy ($n = 10$)

Reconstructions

- Free flaps in 55 patients (91.7%)
  - 45 rectus abdominis
  - 10 radial forearm
- Temporalis muscle in 5 patients deemed not candidates for free flaps
- Bony reconstruction
  - Vascularized (radial forearm osteocutaneous) bone flaps in 4/60 patients (6.7%)
  - Non-vascularized bone grafts in 17 (28.3 %)
  - Estlandler flap in 10 patients with maxillectomy and through-and-through soft tissue defects

Surgical Outcomes

- Free flap survival: 100%
  - Re-exploration rate: 9.1%
  - 1 partial-flap necrosis
  - Systemic complications: 7/60 patients (11.7%)
- Mortality within 30 days: 4
- Postoperative radiotherapy: 64%

Functional Assessment

- Chewing and speech functions assessed in 36 patients with Types II, IIIA, and IIIB defects
  - Prosthetic denture: 41.7%
- Chewing
  - Return to an unrestricted diet: 44.4%
  - Soft diet: 47.2%
  - Liquid diet: 8.3%
- Oral competence
  - Good in all 10 patients with excision/reconstruction of the oral commissure
  - Two patients (20%) developed microstomia after receiving radiotherapy
- Speech
  - Normal: 38.9%
  - Near normal: 41.7%
  - Intelligible: 16.7%
  - Unintelligible: 2.8%
- Globe and periorbital soft tissue position assessed in 14 patients with Type I and Type IIIA defects
  - Enophthalmos = 0
  - Vertical dystopia = 1
  - Ectropion: 71.4%
- Aesthetic results (evaluated at least 6 months after reconstruction in 50 patients)
  - Good to excellent: 58% (cheek skin and lip were not resected)
  - Poor to fair: 42% (external skin or orbital contents were excised)
  - Secondary procedures were required in 16 of 50 patients: 32%

STUDY IMPACT

For plastic surgeons involved in head and neck reconstructions, maxillectomy and midface defects are encountered from time to time. This article by Peter Cordeiro and Eric Santamaria along with Brown's classification have been the most cited articles[1] for the classification for maxillary and midface reconstructions, and thus familiarity with them is essential.

The paired maxillae, as described in this article, are indeed complex and unique structures with their hexahedrium form, which interact closely with adjacent cavities of the facial skeleton, namely, the orbit, nasal, and oral cavities. In addition, they are integral components of important functions, such as dental occlusion for chewing, as well as velopharyngeal competency for speech and swallowing functions.

With such anatomical complexity, as well as with different indications and thus different extent of resection in each individual case, it would be easy to become confused without an appropriate classification system to assist decision-making on the most appropriate method of reconstruction for patients.

To be able to guide management decisions, an ideal classification system should be systematic, user-friendly, and without being overly complicated, as well as being in common use to facilitate communication between surgeons. The classification described in this article serves these purposes well and excels among the numerous alternative classifications.

DISCUSSION

The two main free flap options preferred by the authors are the free radial forearm flap (either as a fasciocutaneous flap or as an osteocutaneous flap when bone is also harvested and inset in a "sandwich" manner) and the free rectus abdominis musculocutaneous flap, which is often used for higher class maxillectomy defects when bulk is needed.

The radial forearm flap provides a thin and reliable skin island, together with a long and robust pedicle that can be tunneled to the neck for microvascular anastomosis, but use of the osteocutaneous variant, in particular, has decreased significantly. The free fibular flap provides excellent bone quality that is particularly suitable for multiple osteotomies needed to match the shape of the dental arch, which not only serves as optimal support for the facial profile but also provides an ideal foundation for dental rehabilitation[2]. The need for a free bone graft can be eliminated with vascularized fibula flaps, reducing concerns over potential bone necrosis after postoperative radiotherapy that is often needed. The donor site in the leg is also usually considered to be superior when compared to the forearm.

For reconstruction with soft tissue only flaps, the anterolateral thigh (ALT) flap offers a good alternative to the free rectus abdominis musculocutaneous flap. The ALT flap can provide a sufficient volume of tissue as well as a large skin island. If more bulk is needed in thin patients, areas of the skin flap can be de-epithelialized and turned over at its deep surface to be inset, or, if there is more than one perforator to the flap, multiple skin islands based on the same pedicle can be used to create a robust "sandwich" (like "stacked flaps" in breast reconstruction). The pedicle of the ALT is usually longer than that of the rectus abdominis flap. An inner lining for the nasal cavity may not be strictly necessary in most cases since surface usually mucosalizes well even in the absence of an epithelial flap surface. However, where needed/desired, an inner epithelial lining can be provided with multiple skin islands/perforators or by folding the flap and de-epithelialization of the central bridging segment. The ALT flap can be raised in a suprafascial plane if a thin flap is needed, but this increases the risk of partial loss by making the skin more reliant on the subdermal supply. Some choose to postpone flap thinning to a second-stage revision procedure after completion of any oncological treatments. This approach would minimize flap complications and facilitate timely adjuvant treatment, which is also an important target of reconstruction from an oncological safety point of view.

The authors prefer non-vascularized bone graft for orbital floor reconstruction. We often use titanium mesh or a PTFE sheet implant (Medpor), which are often amenable to shaping to fit the orbital floor contour in a more refined manner when compared to bone grafting and which also obviates the need for a bone graft donor site.

In conclusion, this is a fundamental classification system that reconstructive surgeons should be familiar with. It has stood the test of time; continuous advances in reconstructive microsurgery and emerging novel reconstructive options, such as the recent developments of 3D planning and printing, will add to the armamentarium of reconstructive surgeons.

REFERENCES

1. Alqarni H, Alfaifi M, Ahmed WM, Almutairi R, Kattadiyil MT. Classification of maxillectomy in edentulous arch defects, algorithm, concept, and proposal classifications: a review. *Clin Exp Dent Res.* 2023 Feb;9(1):45–54. doi: 10.1002/cre2.708.
2. Joshi S, Salema HJ, Pawar S, Nair VS, Koranne V, Sane VD. Patient-specific implants in maxillofacial reconstruction: a case report. *Ann Maxillofac Surg.* 2023 Jul–Dec;13(2):258–261. doi: 10.4103/ams. ams_126_23.

EDITOR COMMENTARY

The authors introduced a classification system and an algorithm for the reconstruction of maxillectomy defects. The classification is relatively simple to follow, providing guidelines for flap reconstruction of various complex maxillectomy defects. However, it does not adequately address composite defects, particularly those requiring dental reconstruction. The paper can be regarded as the beginning of a series of papers elegantly showing the evolution of the senior author's technique, demonstrating how specific issues can be addressed by altering technique/strategy.

It has been widely adopted though not universally. It coexists with Brown (2000) and Okay (2001), which confirms that no single (but relatively simple) system can be comprehensive enough to address the almost unlimited types of defects possible in such a key region. It has provided a solid foundation for more complex patient- and defect-centric algorithms, including Gastman, used for defects best addressed with facial transplants.

As discussed in the author commentary, though the classification scheme itself has held up very well in the 25 years since, reconstructive methods have continued to evolve – flaps such as the ALT and fibular have found more favour in the interim whilst some advocate for flaps from the subscapular system, which can provide a variety of chimeric configurations, but positioning needs can hinder a two-team approach. Other developments, such as CAD/CAM, virtual surgical planning, cutting guides, and patient-specific implants, are particularly well suited to reconstruction of these defects.

Finally, a hexahedron is any polyhedron with six faces and includes cubes but also many other shapes. The closest description that matches the maxilla might be an asymmetric inverted quadrilateral frustum (top-truncated square pyramid). The term "hexahedrium" seems to have been used in reference only to the maxilla, possibly first appearing in this paper.

CHAPTER 16

Clinical Treatment of Radiotherapy
Tissue Damage by Lipoaspirate
Transplant: A Healing Process Mediated
by Adipose-Derived Adult Stem Cells

Rigotti G, Marchi A, Galiè M, Baroni G, Benati D, Krampera M, Pasini A, Sbarbati A.
Plast Reconstr Surg. 2007 Apr 15;119(5):1409–1422
doi: 10.1097/01.prs.0000256047.47909.71. PMID: 17415234

EXPERT COMMENTARY

Marcela Sánchez-Vargas and Andrea Donoso-Samper

Autologous fat grafting has become one of the main tools in breast reconstruction and aesthetic surgery. This article is a perfect example of bench to bedside research in this area.

The authors demonstrated the presence of mesenchymal cells in the lipoaspirate-derived stromal-vascular fraction, their density, and their potential differentiation to chondrocytes, osteoblasts, and adipocytes. Then using a computer-guided software, the lipoaspirate was injected uniformly into severely irradiated areas in patients with a history of breast cancer with two outstanding outcomes. Clinically, measured with the LENT-SOMA scale, patients experienced significant reduction of the symptoms. Histologically, there was detailed documentation of tissue regeneration, neovascularization, and progressive maturation of new adipocytes.

Even though differentiation of lipoaspirate cells had been previously described (Mizuno H et al. 2002; Zuk PA et al. 2002), the clinical and ultrastructural results of this study drew the attention of plastic surgeons. This article has had a noticeable impact in this area, having been cited 288 times since its publication, not only in our field but also in neurosurgery, gastrointestinal surgery, and urology.

Currently, the indications for autologous fat grafting (AFG) in reconstructive breast surgery include small-to-moderate volume augmentation, correction of localized deformities following either implant-based reconstruction or breast-conserving therapy, and complete reconstruction of the small breast with autologous fat (Vindigni V et al. 2024). AFG in breast reconstruction has been proven to be an oncologically safe and

DOI: 10.1201/9781003413738-16

effective procedure with a 93.3% satisfaction and a 7% complication rate in irradiated breasts and 15.5% in non-irradiated breasts (Chen Y and Li G 2021; Lo Torto F et al. 2024). Recent research has centered on optimization of graft survival, maximizing cell differentiation and neovascularization (Hivernaud V et al. 2015; Debuc B et al. 2023). Nevertheless, a translational medicine approach, like the one proposed by Rigotti et al., might give a more complete perspective of the molecular and clinical applications, promoting the wider use of adjuvants in autologous fat grafting.

REFERENCES

Chen Y, Li G. Safety and effectiveness of autologous fat grafting after breast radiotherapy: a systematic review and meta-analysis. *Plast Reconstr Surg.* 2021 Jan 1;147(1):1–10. doi: 10.1097/PRS.0000000000007416.

Debuc B, Gendron N, Cras A, Rancic J, Philippe A, Cetrulo CL Jr, Lellouch AG, Smadja DM. Improving autologous fat grafting in regenerative surgery through stem cell-assisted lipotransfer. *Stem Cell Rev Rep.* 2023 Aug;19(6):1726–1754.

Hivernaud V, Lefourn B, Guicheux J, Weiss P, Festy F, Girard AC, Roche R. Autologous fat grafting in the breast: critical points and technique improvements. *Aesthetic Plast Surg.* 2015 Aug;39(4):547–561. doi: 10.1007/s00266-015-0503-y.

Lo Torto F, Patanè L, Abbaticchio D, Pagnotta A, Ribuffo D. Autologous Fat Grafting (AFG): a systematic review to evaluate oncological safety in breast cancer patients. *J Clin Med.* 2024 Jul 26;13(15):4369. doi: 10.3390/jcm13154369.

Mizuno H, Zuk PA, Zhu M, Lorenz HP, Benhaim P, Hedrick MH. Myogenic differentiation by human processed lipoaspirate cells. *Plast Reconstr Surg.* 2002 Jan;109(1):199–209; discussion 210–211. doi: 10.1097/00006534-200201000-00030.

Vindigni V, Marena F, Zanettin C, Bassetto F. Breast reconstruction: the oncoplastic approach. *J Clin Med.* 2024 Aug 12;13(16):4718. doi: 10.3390/jcm13164718.

Zuk PA, Zhu M, Ashjian P, De Ugarte DA, Huang JI, Mizuno H, Alfonso ZC, Fraser JK, Benhaim P, Hedrick MH. Human adipose tissue is a source of multipotent stem cells. *Mol Biol Cell.* 2002 Dec;13(12):4279–4295. doi: 10.1091/mbc.e02-02-0105.

EDITOR COMMENTARY

The introduction of autologous fat grafting has been a paradigm shift (that phrase again) in the management of soft tissue deficits. The publication of Dr. Sydney Coleman in 1995 could be regarded as a landmark paper in its own right, as it meticulously detailed his thinking and his technique and contributed to wider acceptance of the technique. He emphasized gentle handling to maximize the viability of the fat cells by minimizing trauma throughout the steps of harvest, processing, and reinjection. Results were shown to be efficacious and consistent, but this did not stop the ASPS fat graft task force in 1987 from unaminously "deploring" the use of fat injection in the breast. Inevitably, there was an about turn in Gutowski (2009), after further clinical evidence from outside the United States as well as Coleman.

It was found that although fat is rich in mesenchymal stem cells, often called adipose-derived stem cells (ADSC), most of them are localized to the region around the stroma and blood vessels and are mostly "left behind" when fat is harvested by aspiration; thus, aspirated fat is actually *relatively* stem cell poor, volume for volume. Yoshimura et al. (2008) described how they would enrich the fat before injection – half of the aspirated fat would be processed in a dedicated laboratory to isolate the stem cells into a small volume that was then added to other half of the fat processed as per usual to be injected together into the patient – this was called cell-assisted lipotransfer (CAL). The rationale was that increasing the concentration of stem cells with the stem cell–rich stromal vascular fraction (SVF) would improve results, generally the percentage survival. In this study the SVF is obtained by a different strategy – aspirated fat was spun at 2,700 RPM for 15 minutes ostensibly to deliberately cause "lesions" in the mature adipocytes to accelerate their clearance after injection while sparing stem cells, which was confirmed by in vitro studies with the fraction. There are automated SVF machines that are becoming smaller, quicker, and easier to use; our first unit (Cha Station) was the size of a refrigerator.

Radiation injury is a difficult clinical problem with progressive tissue ischaemia due to fibrotic changes in the vessels; radionecrosis is a particularly challenge. Rigotti et al. used their stem cell–rich lipoaspirate in a variety of recalitrant wounds related to radiation injury. After debridement and repeated injections, there was gradual, albeit slow, healing that was persistent at 2-year follow-up. The author postulated that the stem cells promoted neovascularization; Rudolph (2008) suggested that replacement of stem cells may be a better explanation than reversal of ischaemia. The ability of fat grafting to reverse chronic radiation damage has since been confirmed in multiple clinical studies. A review in 2020 by Krastev et al. found 45 studies suitable for the meta-analysis. They found that fat transfer increased patient satisfaction scores with measurable improvement in scar assessment scores, particularly for stiffness, pliability, and pain.

Fat has been used to "soften" irradiated tissues in the neck (Masia-Gridilla J et al., 2023). Breast implants have been "successfully" placed in irradiated tissues along with fat grafting; Sarfati et al. (2011) injected fat (average 2 times) 6 months after radiotherapy – one implant required explantation out of 28 with an average follow-up of 17 months. A follow-up study 2 years later had seen numbers increase to 68 and follow-up to 23 months, and the same single explantation; no cancer recurrence was found. Barone Adesi et al. (2024) randomized breast cancer patients to have fat injections (n = 22) or not (n = 27) before implant insertion after NSM/SSM and RT. They found a lower rate of capsular contracture and higher patient satisfaction with the aesthetic results, but mean LENT-SOMA scores showed no significant difference.

BIBLIOGRAPHY

Barone Adesi L, Taraschi F, Macrì G, Scardina L, Di Leone A, Franceschini G, Salgarello M. Fat grafting and prepectoral prosthetic reconstruction with polyurethane-covered implants: protective role against adjuvant radiotherapy. *J Clin Med.* 2024 Aug 23;13(17):4982.

Coleman SR. Long-term survival of fat transplants: controlled demonstrations. *Aesthetic Plast Surg.* 1995;19:421–425.

Gutowski KA, ASPS Fat Graft Task Force. Current applications and safety of autologous fat grafts: a report of the ASPS fat graft task force. *Plast Reconstr Surg.* 2009;124:272–280.

Krastev TK, Schop SJ, Hommes J, Piatkowski A, van der Hulst RRWJ. Autologous fat transfer to treat fibrosis and scar-related conditions: a systematic review and meta-analysis. *J Plast Reconstr Aesthet Surg.* 2020 Nov;73(11):2033–2048. doi: 10.1016/j.bjps.2020.08.023.

Masià-Gridilla J, Gutiérrez-Santamaría J, Álvarez-Sáez I, Pamias-Romero J, Saez-Barba M, Bescós-Atin C. Outcomes following autologous fat grafting in patients with sequelae of head and neck cancer treatment. *Cancers (Basel)*. 2023 Jan 28;15(3):800. doi: 10.3390/cancers15030800.

Rudolph R. Lipoaspirated stem cells may not have been placed in ischemic tissue. *Plast Reconstr Surg*. 2008 Aug;122(2):680. doi: 10.1097/PRS.0b013e31817d637d.

Sarfati I, Ihrai T, Kaufman G, Nos C, Clough KB. Adipose-tissue grafting to the post-mastectomy irradiated chest wall: preparing the ground for implant reconstruction. *J Plast Reconstr Aesthet Surg*. 2011 Sep;64(9):1161–1166. doi: 10.1016/j.bjps.2011.03.031.

Sarfati I, Ihrai T, Duvernay A, Nos C, Clough K. Transfert de tissu adipeux autologue préalable à la reconstruction mammaire par implant après mastectomie et irradiation: à propos d'une série de 68 cas [Autologous fat grafting to the postmastectomy irradiated chest wall prior to breast implant reconstruction: a series of 68 patients]. *Ann Chir Plast Esthet*. 2013 Feb;58(1):35–40. French. doi: 10.1016/j.anplas.2012.10.007.

Yoshimura K, Sato K, Aoi N, Kurita M, Hirohi T, Harii K. Cell-assisted lipotransfer for cosmetic breast augmentation: supportive use of adipose-derived stem/stromal cells. *Aesthetic Plast Surg*. 2008 Jan;32(1):48–55; discussion 56–57. doi: 10.1007/s00266-007-9019-4.

Laser Resurfacing and Remodeling of Hypertrophic Burn Scars: The Results of a Large, Prospective, Before-After Cohort, with Long-Term Follow-Up

Hultman CS, Friedstat JS, Edkins RE, Cairns BA, Meyer AA.
Ann Surg. 2014;260(3):519–532

EXPERT COMMENTARY

Wenjing Xi

Research Objective

Study the long-term impact of laser therapy on hypertrophic burn scars.

Study Design

Prospective, before-after, single-cohort study of the hypertrophic burn scar patients treated by the author in 2011.

Sample Size

147 patients (short-term follow-up), 35 patients (long-term follow-up).

Follow-Up

Short term: 4.65 months (standard deviation (SD) 3.14, median 4.45), long term: 30.7 months (SD 4.7,median 29).

Inclusion/Exclusion Criteria

Burn patients who received laser treatment of hypertrophic burn scars in the author's clinic in 2011.

Intervention or Treatment Received

- *Endpoint of the treatments and number of treatments*: Symptomatic scars were treated until both the patient and the provider agreed that scar improvement had plateaued. All patients (n = 147) received 3.82 treatments on average
- *Treatment interval*: 4–6 weeks

DOI: 10.1201/9781003413738-17

Treatment Protocol

1. Vascular-specific, 595 nm wavelength, pulsed dye laser (PDL) (Candela V-beam, Wayland, MA) to reduce hyperaemia and oedema of the immature burn scar.
2. Fractional, 10,600 nm wavelength CO2 laser (Lumenis UltraPulse, ActiveFX and DeepFX hand pieces, Santa Clara, CA) to correct abnormal texture, thickness, and stiffness of the more mature scar through ablative destruction and resurfacing followed by remodeling.
3. Noncoherent intense pulsed light (Lume 1 Workstation with IPL/Nd:YAG/ light sheer diode, Santa Clara, CA) to improve burn scar dyschromia and mild persistent inflammation.
4. 755 nm wavelength Alexandrite laser (Cynosure, Westford, MA) to destroy ingrown hair follicles and obstructed sweat glands.

Results

The Vancouver Scar Scale (VSS) decreased from 10.43 (SD 2.37) to 6.67 (SD 2.11) after the first session, to 5.16 (SD 1.92) by the end of treatments and subsequently decreased to 3.29 (SD 1.24) at a follow-up of 25 months.

The University of North Carolina "4P" Scar Scale (UNC4P) fell from 5.40 (SD 2.54) to 2.89 (SD 1.91) after the first session, to 2.05 (SD 1.67) at the end of treatments, and further decreased to 1.74 (SD 1.72) after 2 years.

Study Limitations

The main limitation of this study was the lack of a control group. Most hypertrophic burn scars tend to gradually mature on their own over the course of several years, as such a single cohort study cannot provide direct evidence that the improvements in VSS and UNC4P were the results of laser intervention alone.

Relevant Studies

1. Alster et al. (1995). Split-scar study of 16 hypertrophic median sternotomy scars (scar duration more than 6 months) 6 months after 2 PDL treatments (treatment interval 6–8 weeks), the treated half saw improvement in pain and pruritis, erythema, thickness, and stiffness. This study offered solid evidence of the effect of PDL on hypertrophic linear scars and the laser parameters used in this study served as a useful reference for the treatment of hypertrophic burn scars.
2. Miletta et al. (2019). A prospective study of hypertrophic burn scars in 22 subjects (scar duration > 1 year). The stability of the scars was established by a 3-month period of pretreatment observation. The subjects were excluded if they had a >10% change in objective measurements of their scars during this observation period. Included subjects underwent 3-monthly fractional CO_2 laser treatments and followed up 6 months after the last intervention. The elasticity of the scar, objectively measured by a dermal torque meter,

demonstrated 16%–46% improvement (P < 0.01). The thickness of the scar, measured by ultrasound saw 21%–22% improvement (P < 0.01). Changes in erythema and pigmentation, measured by DSM II ColoriMeter were not significant. Patient- and physician-reported pain/pruritus were significantly improved (P < 0.01). This carefully designed study provided more support that fractional CO_2 can be beneficial for mature hypertrophic scars.

Study Impact

This paper was the earliest report on burn scar laser treatment with a reasonably large sample size and long-term follow-up. Compared to conventional modalities, such as silicone sheet and presssure therapy, the history of the application of lasers in burn scar management has been rather brief. This study[1] supported the application of this modality by demonstrating a successful practice and a working protocol. Currently, approximately 10 years after the publication of the study, laser treatment has been incorporated into protocols for burn scar management in many burn units, scar clinics, and plastic surgery departments.

There have been doubts that the improvement observed in single-arm cohort studies was due to a treatment effect instead of the result of natural evolution of the scar. As research on the topic has accumulated over time, some of the best evidence that has emerged so far came from Miletta et al.,[2] who confirmed the beneficial effect of fractional CO_2 laser on *mature* hypertrophic scars. The authors having meticulously established the mature status of scar before fractional CO_2 laser intervention (scar duration > 1 year, scar objective measurements did not change in 3-month observation period), then evaluated the outcome with objective measures and confirmed that CO_2 laser intervention enhanced elasticity and reduced the thickness of the hypertrophic scar.

The exact mechanisms underlying the effects of scar laser treatment are not yet totally clear. Theoretically PDL selectively damages the vasculature in hypertrophic scars. Molecular and histological studies[3,4] showed that fractional CO_2 intervention affects collagen production and initiates collagen remodeling.

Though the acceptance of laser treatment in hypertrophic burn scars is increasing, many unresolved problems on this topic remain to be investigated. First, it is much more challenging to treat *immature* hypertrophic burn scar with lasers – more sessions are needed and less progress is observed during the process. This situation would be more complex than described in the papers of Hultman and Miletta, both of which included more mature scars (median scar duration in Hultman's study was 18 months). Second, it is unclear if fractional CO_2 has the same beneficial effects in immature scars as mature scars and how variations in laser parameter settings affect treatment results in immature scars, etc. On the other hand, although Alster[5] confirmed the efficacy of PDL in hypertrophic linear scars, there has been contrary reports on PDL effect on hypertrophic burn scars.[6] Though parameter settings may contribute to some of the negative results as discussed in literature, there may be difficult situations where progressing immature hypertrophic scars appear to be more resistant to laser treatment. Third, there are different opinions on the best practice in terms of treatment details, such as treatment interval, parameter setting, intervention timing, end point, etc. Hence, more studies are required to seek the best practice and understand the limitations of scar laser treatment.

REFERENCES

1. Hultman, C. S., Friedstat, J. S., Edkins, R. E., Cairns, B. A., & Meyer, A. A. (2014). Laser resurfacing and remodeling of hypertrophic burn scars: the results of a large, prospective, before-after cohort study, with long-term follow-up. *Annals of Surgery*, *260*(3), 519–532.
2. Miletta, N., Siwy, K., Hivnor, C., Clark, J., Shofner, J., Zurakowski, D., ... & Donelan, M. (2021). Fractional ablative laser therapy is an effective treatment for hypertrophic burn scars: a prospective study of objective and subjective outcomes. *Annals of Surgery*, *274*(6), e574–e580.
3. Ozog, D. M., Liu, A., Chaffins, M. L., Ormsby, A. H., Fincher, E. F., Chipps, L. K., ... & Moy, R. L. (2013). Evaluation of clinical results, histological architecture, and collagen expression following treatment of mature burn scars with a fractional carbon dioxide laser. *JAMA Dermatology*, *149*(1), 50–57.
4. Qu, L., Liu, A., Zhou, L., He, C., Grossman, P. H., Moy, R. L., ... & Ozog, D. (2012). Clinical and molecular effects on mature burn scars after treatment with a fractional CO2 laser. *Lasers in Surgery and Medicine*, *44*(7), 517–524.
5. Alster, T. S., & Williams, C. M. (1995). Treatment of keloid sternotomy scars with 585 nm flashlamp-pumped pulsed-dye laser. *The Lancet*, *345*(8959), 1198–1200.
6. Chan, H. H., Wong, D. S., Ho, W. S., Lam, L. K., & Wei, W. (2004). The use of pulsed dye laser for the prevention and treatment of hypertrophic scars in Chinese persons. *Dermatologic Surgery*, *30*(7), 987–994.

EDITOR COMMENTARY

Burn scars contribute a great deal to the morbidity of burn survivors and are notoriously difficult to treat. As Dr. Xi alludes to, there is some contradictory evidence for the role of PDL in hypertrophic scars. Allison et al. (2003) and Chan (2004) found that PDL effectively reduced pruritis but that changes in redness, height, and texture of the scar were not significant, in contrast to Alster et al. (1995). Allison suggested that this may be related to the smaller size of vessels seen in HTS compared to the PWS they were originally intended to treat; furthermore, PDL is less likely to be effective in thick burn scars (>1 cm) as the depth of PDL penetration is ~1.2 mm. A review by Parrett et al., (2010) provided some generic guidelines and did not address the lack of significant results in these studies. Recent systematic reviews (Vrijman C et al., 2011; Kafka M et al., 2017) seem to confirm the usefulness of PDL, but, overall, there is a lack of newer robust properly controlled trials to shore up the evidence levels.

Li N. (2018) compared PDL with fractional CO_2 laser for the treatment of burn HTS; both were efficacious, but PDL was preferred by patients due to less treatment pain and faster recovery, being particularly suited for children. There has been a recent trend of combining PDL and fractional CO_2 lasers, particularly in China, but the results are difficult to interpret (Lei Y, 2020).

The use of deeper mode fractional CO_2 laser, e.g., SCAAR FX Ultrapulse, seemed to have an exciting moment with reported functional improvements in the form of contracture relaxation (Uebelhoer NS et al., 2012) and healing of scar associated wounds (Shumaker PR et al., 2012), presumably due to the remodeling. However, despite formulation of consensus statements in 2014 and 2020, little progress with controlled trials defining the effect of these lasers seems to have been made. Issler-Fisher et al. (2020) reported that incorporation of ablative fractional lasers reduced the use of elective burn reconstruction surgery for burn scars by 23.9% (2020). Liu H et al. (2022) reported an improvement in the quality of life in those with extensive burn scars.

REFERENCES

Allison KP, Kiernan MN, Waters RA, Clement RM. Pulsed dye laser treatment of burn scars. Alleviation or irritation? *Burns.* 2003;29:207–213.

Chan HH, Wong DS, Ho WS, Lam LK, Wei W. The use of pulsed dye laser for the prevention and treatment of hypertrophic scars in Chinese persons. *Dermatol Surg.* 2004;30:987–994.

Issler-Fisher AC, Fisher OM, Clayton NA, Aggarwala S, Haertsch PA, Li Z, Maitz PKM. Ablative fractional resurfacing for burn scar management affects the number and type of elective surgical reconstructive procedures, hospital admission patterns as well as length of stay. *Burns.* 2020 Feb;46(1):65–74. doi: 10.1016/j.burns.2019.01.004.

Kafka M, Collins V, Kamolz LP, Rappl T, Branski LK, Wurzer P. Evidence of invasive and noninvasive treatment modalities for hypertrophic scars: a systematic review. *Wound Repair Regen.* 2017 Jan;25(1):139–144. doi: 10.1111/wrr.12507.

Lei Y, Ouyang HW, Tan J. [Effect of pulsed dye laser in combination with ultra-pulsed fractional carbon dioxide laser in treating pediatric burn scars at early stage]. *Zhonghua Shao Shang Za Zhi.* 2020;36:357–362.

Li N, Yang L, Cheng J, Han JT, Hu DH. [Clinical comparative study of pulsed dye laser and ultra–pulsed fractional carbon dioxide laser in the treatment of hypertrophic scars after burns]. *Zhonghua Shao Shang Za Zhi.* 2018;34:603–607.

Liu H, Shu F, Xu H, Ji C, Wang Y, Lou X, Luo P, Xiao S, Xia Z, Lv K. Ablative fractional carbon dioxide laser improves quality of life in patients with extensive burn scars: a nested case-control study. *Lasers Surg Med.* 2022 Nov;54(9):1207–1216. doi: 10.1002/lsm.23603.

Parrett BM, Donelan MB. Pulsed dye laser in burn scars: current concepts and future directions. *Burns.* 2010 Jun;36(4):443–449. doi: 10.1016/j.burns.2009.08.015.

Shumaker PR, Kwan JM, Badiavas EV, Waibel J, Davis S, Uebelhoer NS. Rapid healing of scar-associated chronic wounds after ablative fractional resurfacing. *Arch Dermatol.* 2012 Nov;148(11):1289–1293. doi: 10.1001/2013.jamadermatol.256.

Vrijman C, van Drooge AM, Limpens J, Bos JD, van der Veen JP, Spuls PI, Wolkerstorfer A. Laser and intense pulsed light therapy for the treatment of hypertrophic scars: a systematic review. *Br J Dermatol.* 2011 Nov;165(5):934–942. doi: 10.1111/j.1365-2133.2011.10492.x.

Uebelhoer NS, Ross EV, Shumaker PR. Ablative fractional resurfacing for the treatment of traumatic scars and contractures. *Semin Cutan Med Surg.* 2012 Jun;31(2):110–120. doi: 10.1016/j.sder.2012.03.005.

CHAPTER 18

Digital Artery Perforator Flaps for Fingertip Reconstructions

Koshima I, Urushibara K, Fukuda N, Ohkochi M, Nagase T, Gonda K, Asato H, Yoshimura K. *Plast Reconstr Surg.* 2006 Dec;118(7):1579–1584 doi: 10.1097/01.prs.0000232987.54881.a7. PMID: 17102731

EXPERT COMMENTARY

Josephine Yip

Introduction

The use of perforator flaps in the fingers is gaining popularity as a method of reconstruction as the main digital vessels can be preserved. The design of perforator flaps can be very versatile in general and can be considered almost as free style flaps. This paper discusses the new landmark technique of perforator flaps in the management of fingertip injuries.

DESIGN: ANATOMICAL STUDY AND RETROSPECTIVE CASE SERIES

In this paper, the surgical anatomy of digital perforator flaps was studied through cadaveric dissection. It was found that there are many branches from the digital arteries in the lateral aspect of the fingers. These branches perforate the thin fascia and adipose tissue and terminate as multiple arterioles in the subdermal layer. Rich perforating arterioles and venules between these perforators exist in the subcutaneous tissue across the midline of the fingers.

A clinical series of 5 cases using digital artery perforator flaps for fingertip injuries were described. The author tried to design the flaps in a manner to avoid the need for skin grafting; conversely, the need for skin grafting, e.g., for a large flap, was considered a contraindication to this treatment option.

DISCUSSION

Fingertip injuries are common hand injuries as the fingertips are the most distal part of the upper limb and are prone to injuries during activities of daily life and work. The anatomy of the fingertip is specialized for the manipulation of objects and for

DOI: 10.1201/9781003413738-18

sophisticated sensation. The volar pulp tissue consists of multiple compartments formed by fascial layers connecting skin to distal phalanx while the dorsal aspect consists of nail and nail bed.

Fingertip injuries can be difficult to manage, which is reflected in the numerous options described in the literature. Optimal treatment should preserve length, cosmesis, function, and sensation of the digit, with minimization of pain and hypersensitivity. The use of digital perforator flaps has definite advantages in certain situations.

A local flap is a technique that mobilizes skin and soft tissue from the injured digit (or sometimes an adjacent digit) to cover up the fingertip defect. It is a common option when the defect size is big and the bone end is significantly exposed. Local flaps can cover the defect with skin and subcutaneous tissue, which is more durable than skin graft alone with preservation of bone length. If the nerve supply of the flap is preserved, the flap can be (potentially) sensate. The choice of flap in individual cases depends on the defect size and complexity, the availability of tissue in the same digit, functional demand of the injured digit, patient's choice, and surgeon's preference. In general, flaps from the same digit have the least impact to the patient.

Perforator flaps are a subtype of local flap that use skin and soft tissue supplied by a perforator from the digital vessel. There is no disturbance of the digital arteries and the donor site can be closed primarily without tension if it is small or can be grafted. Based on this index paper, there was good sensory recovery of the flaps. Skin grafting was considered a contraindication of this flap and primary closure of the donor site was preferred.

For well-designed flaps, the healing is usually uneventful. The vascularity of the finger/hands is good, in general, unless the patient is a smoker or has underlying peripheral vascular disease. Most patients require a course of rehabilitation in terms of desensitization, oedema control, shaping of fingertip with pressure garments, scar management, range of motion exercise, and strengthening programs. Even insensate flaps achieve some transmitted sensation. The prognosis is usually favorable.

EDITOR COMMENTARY

Conventional homodigital flaps are useful for fingertip reconstruction, but, in general, they are quite limited in their reach and size, relying largely on VY closure. Other options, such as cross finger flaps and hypo/thenar flaps, are two-staged and may result in some stiffness. The author describes techniques for closure of fingertip injuries that rely on the small "perforator" vessels that come off the main axial vessel of the digits. The flaps do not rely on reverse flow, such as those based on the transverse arches, and require division of the ipsilateral digital artery proximally (Kim KS et al., 2001).

A series of cadaveric dissections and injection studies were made to define these digital artery perforators and how they supplied the subdermal plexus. They found a rich network of arterioles, venules, and nerves that allowed flaps to be raised without sacrifice of the digital arteries; flaps were usually based on the sides of the finger (non-dominant/ non pressure side preferred). These perforator branches have been found at fairly predictable intervals from landmarks such as the PIPJ (Strauch B et al., 1990; Braga-Silva J et al., 2002) or eponychial fold (Delia G et al., 2018). Koshima I et al. used the handheld Doppler for pre/intraoperative perforator localization in some cases, while later they (Mitsunaga N et al., 2010) used CT imaging in severe injuries. Shintani K et al. (2016) used color Doppler ultrasound, while many do not use any imaging, "relying" on the predictable patterns as noted above.

Flap elevation proceeds using digital block and a tourniquet while preserving the digital neurovascular bundle, and a dominant perforator is used as the pedicle base. The dissection is best performed under magnification. Choosing a perforator close to the defect edge will allow 180-degree rotation like a propellor flap, and skeletonization of the perforators should be avoided, with a cuff of tissue left to preserve venous return. Venous congestion seen in about 8% is usually transient but may take a week or more to resolve. Defects <1 cm wide (and <2 cm long) can often be closed directly; a main perforator from the digital artery can sustain a flap as large as 4×2 cm. In their follow-up study (Mitsunaga N et al., 2010), Mitsunaga et al. used dermal substitutes for the donor site, without the need for further skin grafting. Even if a perforator is not seen, leaving a substantial soft tissue pedicle at the base may preserve sufficient vascularity.

The authors present a series of 5 cases where all the flaps survived and the patients had good sensation, with no hypersensitivity or cold intolerance. The harvest is somewhat "freestyle" and the vessels are small, but the principles are similar to the usual larger propellor flaps. The technique is versatile and a useful option for fingertip amputations with exposed bone. It is simple/quick, replaces "like for like," and preserves the main digital NVB, but it requires magnification and a familiarity with the smaller vessels of the fingers.

The follow-up paper by Mitsunaga N et al (2010) provided an update following 10 years of experience. A new variant was the harvest of adiposal-only DAP flap, using skin graft from a crushed fingertip for cover, for example. A total of 2 flaps were "supercharged" by perforator-to-perforator anastomoses (0.2–0.3 mm). Pin-cushioning was one of the more common problems reported by the authors, but curiously it is not mentioned by others using DAP flaps.

Koshima described the propeller type DAP, and, since then, variants such as bilobed DAP, rotational DAP, VY DAP, etc. have appeared in the literature. The majority of reports describe the use of pedicled DAP flaps for tip defects of the digits and sometimes the thumb. The DAP flap is an elegant effective option for a very specific defect – the trick is knowing when best to use them.

REFERENCES

Braga-Silva J, Kuyven CR, Fallopa F, Albertoni W. An anatomical study of the dorsal cutaneous branches of the digital arteries. *J Hand Surg. [Br]* 2002;27:577–579. doi: 10.1054/jhsb.2002.0830.

Delia G, Battaglia F, Colonna MR, Barresi V, d'Alcontres FS. Is the adipofascial flap the key to regenerative surgery? *JPRAS Open*. 2018 Jul 31;18:49–58. doi: 10.1016/j.jpra.2018.07.004. Erratum in: JPRAS Open. 2021 Sep 24;30:174–175. doi: 10.1016/j.jpra.2021.09.007.

Kim KS, Yoo SI, Kim DY, Lee SY, Cho BH. Fingertip reconstruction using a volar flap based on the transverse palmar branch of the digital artery. *Ann Plast Surg*. 2001 Sep;47(3):263–268. doi: 10.1097/00000637-200109000-00008.

Mitsunaga N, Mihara M, Koshima I, Gonda K, Takuya I, Kato H, Araki J, Yamamoto Y, Yuhei O, Todokoro T, Ishikawa S, Eri U, Mundinger GS. Digital artery perforator (DAP) flaps: modifications for fingertip and finger stump reconstruction. *J Plast Reconstr Aesthet Surg*. 2010 Aug;63(8):1312–1317. doi: 10.1016/j.bjps.2009.07.023.

Shintani K, Takamatsu K, Uemura T, et al. Planning digital artery perforators using color Doppler ultrasonography: a preliminary report. *J Plast Reconstr Aesthet Surg*. 2016 May;69(5):634–639. doi: 10.1016/j.bjps.2016.01.003.

Strauch B, de Moura W. Arterial system of the fingers. *J Hand Surg Am*. 1990 Jan;15(1):148–154. doi: 10.1016/s0363-5023(09)91123-6.

CHAPTER 19

Simultaneous Transposition of Anterior Thigh Muscle and Fascia Flaps: An Introduction of the Chimera Flap Principle

Hallock GG. *Ann Plast Surg.* 1991;27:126–131

AUTHOR COMMENTARY

Geoffrey G. Hallock

> **Chimera** was a fire-breathing monster with a lion's head, a goat's body, and the tail of a serpent … dissimilar tissues … but joined together for survival.[1,2]

Extremely complex multidimensional defects challenge the ingenuity of all reconstructive surgeons. Not just coverage, but volume, contour, structural stability, and perhaps dynamic function may have to be restored; and all this while minimizing donor site morbidity using preferably autogenous tissues. Multiple discrete and altogether unrelated flaps could be a solution. Yet, instead, a compound flap, which, by definition, consists of diverse tissue components and parts that remain in some fashion all dependent often will satisfy the aforementioned prerequisites with the advantage that but a single donor region need be violated.[1] One subtype permits the transfer of multiple flaps, each with their own intrinsic vascular supply, that are independent of any physical interconnection except where ultimately their circulation arises from a common source pedicle.[1,3,4] Yesterday, and still today, combinations fulfilling such a profile have been termed chain flaps,[5] polyflaps,[6] double flap designs,[7] quadrifoliate flaps,[8] split-cutaneous flaps,[9] double skin paddle flaps,[10,11] dual-skin paddle flaps,[12] or chain-linked flaps.[13]

This potpourri of appellations used for what seems to be a single entity was and is by itself confusing and unclear. An improvement in the nomenclature that should be used seemed essential to better facilitate collegial communication, establish guidelines, and foster innovation for what appeared to be an appealing, efficient solution for, indeed, complicated but unusual circumstances. That alone was the basis for this manuscript here commentated – to introduce a *principle* and not a surgical technique. So a name had to be chosen that would easily be remembered, sought from the Greek mythology studied in this author's elementary school days as a logical place for this quest. As the introductory quotation stated, did not the **Chimera** have multiple independent parts each sustained ultimately by a single source of circulation, thereby apropos to name this compound flap subtype to be the same? And so it was.

DOI: 10.1201/9781003413738-19

The report of a single case from the anterior thigh was selected solely to demonstrate the application of the chimera principle as a potential solution. The perforator flap concept had not yet been realized, although Pontén's[14] longitudinally oriented peninsular fasciocutaneous flaps represented a recent evolution away from the use of a musculocutaneous flap where the "viability of the cutaneous portion relies on perforators from the underlying muscle,"[1] and so as quoted perhaps foresaw the future. Yet simultaneously a muscle flap was also needed to capture its greater malleability for wrapping about the femur in a deep recess – some things still remain the same today.[15]

The individual parts of a chimeric flap "may consist of only a single different tissue form,"[1] but "each may also be a composite flap,"[1] implied not as Agarwal, et al.,[16] but as many other critics have since stated that a "true" chimeric flap must have completely different tissue types. Instead, combinations of muscle flaps,[17] and especially now perforator flaps alone,[18,19] are acceptable choices. Although the given clinical example involved the transposition of local flaps using indigenous tissues, a suggestion was made that even more versatile variations, such as an "island chimera flap or free-flap transfer[1]" would be possible (Figure 19.1). After all, Koshima, et al.[20] just 2 years later (1993) also introduced the chimeric flap principle, but they used a microanastomosis in some form in all cases for fabricating the interconnections of their numerous flap components.

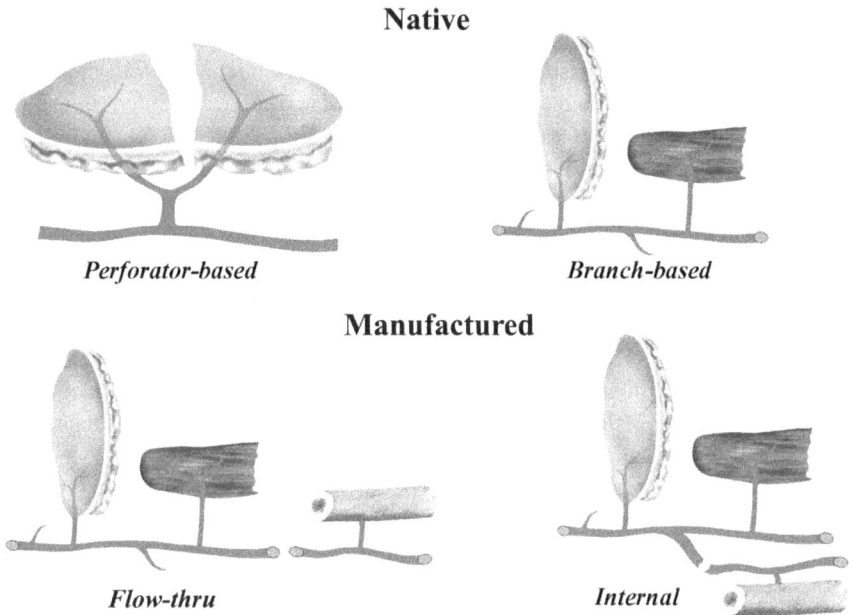

Native

Perforator-based   *Branch-based*

Manufactured

Flow-thru   *Internal*

Figure 19.1   Chimeric flaps can be indigenous [native] or naturally available, with each flap component then based on a discrete perforator [perforator-based] or branch [branch-based] of the main source vessel. They can also be fabricated [manufactured], connected via a microanastomosis to a branch of the source vessel [internal] or added sequentially as a flow-through. (Modified from Hallock, GG, The Chimera Flap: A Quarter Century Odyssey, *Ann Plast Surg*, 2017;78:223–229.)

Table 19.1   Top 10 attributes of the chimeric flap[1,4]

---
1. Synchronous or metachronous transfer of multiple combinations of independent flaps.
2. Composition may include identical or diverse tissue formats.
3. Independent insetting of each component.
4. Extraordinarily large surface area coverage is possible.
5. 3-dimensional restoration of volume and contour.
6. Permits recovery of function simultaneously with form.
7. Only a single recipient vascular site is required if transferred as a free flap.
8. Provides means for monitoring the primary flap used for the reconstruction.
9. Enables relief of tension at the recipient site, if free flap or otherwise.
10. Donor site morbidity will be restricted to a single body region.

This versatility of the "Chimera Flap Principle" a quarter century later reiterated what this initial presentation suggested would be the expected value (Table 19.1).[4] Proselytization of this concept has crept into all the major journals.[11,17,21–24] Indeed, it is understanding "the principle of designing multiple independent flaps of different tissue types within the same cutaneous territory that deserves emphasis,"[1] and how even this basic principle continues to evolve, e.g., the chimeric propeller flap[21] or perforator chimerism.[22] Albeit rarely required except for an unusual situation, remember that "the chimeric flap concept has some practical merit that deserves occasional consideration."[1] Indeed, the chimeric flap and the appellation so thrust upon it have withstood the test of time.

REFERENCES

1. Hallock GG. Simultaneous transposition of anterior thigh muscle and fascia flaps: an introduction to the chimera flap principle. *Ann Plast Surg.* 1991;27:126–131.
2. D'Aularie I, D'Aularie EP. *Book of Greek Myths.* Garden City, New York: Doubleday; 1962.
3. Hallock GG. Further clarification of the nomenclature for compound flaps. *Plast Reconstr Surg.* 2006;117:151e–160e.
4. Hallock GG. The chimera flap: a quarter century odyssey. *Ann Plast Surg.* 2017;78:223–229.
5. Chen HC, Tang, YB, Noordhoff MS. Reconstruction of the entire esophagus with "Chain Flaps" in a patient with severe corrosive injury. *Plast Reconstr Surg.* 1989;84:980–984.
6. Belousov AE, Kishemasov SD, Kochish AY, Pinchuk VD. A new classification of vascularized flaps in plastic and reconstructive surgery. *Ann Plast Surg.* 1993;31:47–52.
7. Sawaizumi M, Maruyama Y, Kawaguchi N. Vertical double flap design for repair of wide defects of the lower limb, using combined ascending scapular and latissimus dorsi flaps. *J Reconstr Microsurg.* 1995;11:407–414.
8. Bakhach J, Peres JM, Scalise A, *et al.* The quadrifoliate flap: a combination of scapular, parascapular, latissimus dorsi, and scapula bone flaps. *Br J Plast Surg.* 1996;49:477–481.
9. Tsai FC, Yang JY, Mardini S, Chuang SS, Wei FC. Free split-cutaneous perforator flaps procured using a three-dimensional harvest technique for the reconstruction of postburn contracture defects. *Plast Reconstr Surg.* 2004;113:185–193.
10. Marsh DJ, Chana JS. Reconstruction of very large defects: a novel application of the double skin paddle anterolateral thigh flap design provides for primary donor-site closure. *J Plast Reconstr Aesthet Surg.* 2010;63:120–125.
11. Loeffelbein DJ, Hölzle F, Wolff K-D. Double-skin paddle perforator flap from the lateral lower leg for reconstruction of through-and-through cheek defect – a report of two cases. *Int J Oral Maxillofac Surg.* 2006;35:1016–1020.

12. Qing L, Wu P, Yu F, Zhou Z, Tang J. Use of dual-skin paddle anterolateral thigh perforator flaps in the reconstruction of complex defect of the foot and ankle. *J Plast Reconstr Aesthet Surg.* 2018;71:1231–1238.
13. Qing L, Li X, Wu P, Zhou Z, Yu F, Tang C. Customized reconstruction of complex soft-tissue defect in the hand and forearm with individual design of chain-linked bilateral anterolateral thigh perforator flaps. *J Plast Reconstr Aesthet Surg.* 2019;72:1909–1916.
14. Pontén B. The fasciocutaneous flap: its use in soft tissue defect of the lower leg. *Br J Plast Surg.* 1981;34:215–220.
15. Lee KT, Wiraatmadja ES, Mun GH. Free latissimus dorsi muscle-chimeric thoracodorsal artery perforator flaps for reconstruction of complicated defects: does muscle still have a place in the domain of perforator flaps? *Ann Plast Surg.* 2015;74:565–572.
16. Agarwal JP, Agarwal S, Adler N, et al. Refining the intrinsic chimera flap: a review. *Ann Plast Surg.* 2009;63:462–467.
17. Hallock GG. The extended latissimus dorsi–serratus anterior chimeric local free flap for salvage of the complicated posterolateral thoracotomy incision. *Injury.* 2019;50(Supplement 5):S8–S10.
18. Huang WC, Chen HC, Wei FC, *et al.* Chimeric flap in clinical use. *Clin Plast Surg.* 2003;30:457–467.
19. Hallock GG. The complete nomenclature for combined perforator flaps. *Plast Reconstr Surg.* 2011;127:1720–1729.
20. Koshima I, Yamamoto H, Hosoda M, *et al.* Free combined composite flaps using the lateral circumflex femoral system for repair of massive defects of the head and neck regions: an introduction to the chimeric flap principle. *Plast Reconstr Surg.* 1993;92:411–420.
21. Hallock GG. The chimeric propeller flap. *Sem Plast Surg.* 2020;34:207–209.
22. Kim JT, Kim YH, Ghanem AM. Perforator chimerism for the reconstruction of complex defects: a new chimeric free flap classification system. *J Plast Reconstr Aesthet Surg.* 2015;68:1556–1567.
23. Sano K, Hallock GG, Ozeki S, *et al.* Devastating massive knee defect reconstruction using the cornucopian chimera flap from the subscapular axis: two case reports. *J Reconstr Microsurg.* 2006;22:25–32.
24. Xie Z, Cao Z, Yang Y, Lu YL, Qing LM, Wu PF, Tang J. Clinical effect of free chimeric anterolateral thigh flap and chimeric thoracodorsal artery perforator flap in chronic osteomyelitis. *J Plast Reconstr Aesthet Surg.* 2024;98:272–280.

EDITOR COMMENTARY

The chimeric flap is a concept or principle more than a technique. The author describes the concept and expands upon it eloquently. Definitions are not set in stone, but, for the editor, the baseline characteristic of a chimeric flap is that the individual components are inset independently and have independent functions. A dual skin paddle anterolateral thigh flap would be a chimera but a standard TRAM flap would not.

The chimeric flap when well designed is elegant, and the surgeon can be seen to be pushing the boundaries a bit further, at least in their own mind. There are some advantages that can be espoused, such as saved time and minimization of donor site(s), though neither would constitute a "game changer." Microanastomoses are routine and a double free flap might not take that much longer, particularly if you can work effectively with multiple teams (something facilitated by using loupes instead of microscopes) (Mo et al., 2014). Certainly, needing only one set of anastomoses would be very welcome in cases of redo or (re-redo) necks, particularly after recurrences/radiotherapy where there is a severe lack of recipient vessels. Overall, the utilization of chimeric flaps requires some thought in the design, a bit more patience in the dissection, but they are otherwise unremarkable and should be regarded as a variant in our free flap armamentarium.

One particular point is to take extra care during inset to ensure that the pedicles are not twisted around each other.

A prerequisite of sorts to a chimeric flap is having an arterial system supplying different components and, as such, the subscapular, deep circumflex iliac, and lateral circumflex iliac artery flaps are the most common sources for chimeric flaps. In the editor's practice, the most common chimeric flaps are:

- *Two skin paddles* – they may or may not be regarded as a chimera but they are often serve different "functions" with one being skin cover, the other being mucosa, e.g., full thickness buccal defects, pharyngeal defects with loss of neck skin. The mythological monster as described in the Iliad had the front of a lion with an extra (goat's) head from its back and a snake's head at its tail.

- *Pharyngeal reconstruction* – when a second skin paddle is not available to facilitate monitoring of the buried flap, a little nubbin of muscle less than 1 × 1 × 1 cm is taken on a distal branch and exteriorized. This might be regarded as a "'mini" chimera.

- *Nasopharynx/ skull base/ orbit* – where the resecting surgeon often asks for a "bit of muscle" to plug up a hole in the dura.

- *Radical parotidectomy* – combining skin and vascularized innervated muscle for combined soft tissue cover and facial reanimation (Hasmat S, 2019).

REFERENCES

Mo KW, Vlantis A, Wong EW, Chiu TW. Double free flaps for reconstruction of complex/composite defects in head and neck surgery. *Hong Kong Med J.* 2014 Aug;20(4):279–284. doi: 10.12809/hkmj134113.

Hasmat S, Low TH, Krishnan A, Coulson S, Ch'ng S, Ashford BG, Croxson G, Clark JR. Chimeric vastus lateralis and anterolateral thigh flap for restoring facial defects and dynamic function following radical parotidectomy. *Plast Reconstr Surg.* 2019 Nov;144(5):853e–863e. doi: 10.1097/PRS.0000000000006183.

CHAPTER 20

An Updated Evaluation of the Management of Nerve Gaps: Autographs, Allografts, and Nerve Transfers

Johnson AR, Said A, Acevedo J, Taylor R, Wu K, Ray WZ, Patterson JM, Mackinnon SE. *Semin Neurol.* 2025 Feb;45(1):157–175 doi: 10.1055/s-0044-1791665. Epub 2024 Oct 11. PMID: 39393799

AUTHOR COMMENTARY

Anna Rose Johnson, Kitty Wu, and Susan E. Mackinnon

Study Design

This manuscript provides a critical analysis of advancements in the field of nerve surgery for management of nerve gaps – specifically autografts, allografts, and nerve transfers. It focuses on fundamental advancements since 2010 which have furthered the field.

Follow-Up

N/A

Inclusion/Exclusion Criteria

N/A

Study Limitations

This paper serves as a critical review which analyzes updates in nerve surgery. It was not designed to be a systematic review with strict inclusion/exclusion criteria. Therefore, there may be studies which were not captured since the publication of the Ray et al. (2010) study.[1]

Relevant Studies

This study was designed to critically update the 2010 publication by Ray et al.[1] and outline key advancements in the field. This initial publication included algorithms for classification of nerve injuries, management of injuries of varying degree, reviewed nerve transfers for various pathologies (with a focus on end to end and end to side), and it discussed the role and utility of allografts. It has been cited 590 times since publication. Since this time, there have been many changes which have transformed the field.

    DOI: 10.1201/9781003413738-20

Study Impacts

Within the past decade, numerous innovations in the field of nerve have revolutionized the field. This paper highlights critical advancements, including introduction of an expanded classification system for nerve injury, a refined understanding of electrodiagnostic (EDX) studies to guide patient selection, changes in the approach to the management of nerve gaps (including a defined utility and limitations for the role of acellular nerve allograft [ANA]), and review of the evolution and adaptation of nerve transfers. Furthermore, we have a more nuanced understanding of axonal regeneration and its relationship with functional recovery and have defined a critical plateau for functional recovery (CPFR), which can help inform decision-making for nerve surgery and provides a timeline for expected recovery.

The revised classification schema of nerve injury includes new degrees of injury and associated recovery/prognoses. A Sunderland 0 is an ischaemic nerve dysfunction with rapid and reversible recovery following decompression at the entrapment point.[2] A Sunderland 0 cannot be identified by electrodiagnostic (EDX) studies, but it can be elicited by physical exam maneuvers (positional or pressure provocative testing). Additionally, it is noted postoperatively by rapid (even immediate) sensory or motor recovery prior to the 2-month time point for remyelination. A Sunderland 6 is a mixed nerve injury which is comprised of different degrees of injury and can even include normal fascicles. Its recovery is not as predictable as it depends on the variable degree of fascicular injury. Figure 20.1 provides an overview of the six degrees of injury and their respective anticipated recovery, rate of recovery, prognosis, and corresponding EDX findings. This arms the provider with a concrete guide to help classify presence of nerve(s) injury and predict time for recovery. One critical finding to differentiate grade III and IV injuries is the presence of motor unit potentials (MUPs) at different time points. If an injury has no MUPs at 3 months, repeat testing should be performed at month 4. If there are MUPs present, the injury is a grade III injury with variable, slow partial recovery anticipated. In contrast, an absence of MUPs at month 4 would be consistent with a neurotmetic injury with unfavorable recovery. These findings have important surgical considerations. A grade III injury would be amenable to an end-to-side nerve transfer to facilitate the opportunity for axons to reach the target, whereas a grade IV injury would require a procedure to establish neural continuity (nerve repair with or without grafting, end-to-end transfer).

The critical plateau for functional recovery (CPFR) is introduced in this review and its importance cannot be overlooked. The most important factor that influences recovery is time to reinnervation of the distal motor endplate and sensory receptors.[3] The authors build upon this and define the CPFR, which supports that at least 30% of original motor neurons must meet their target endplate for ability to establish full sensorimotor recovery (Figure 20.1). This concept is critical to our understanding of nerve transfers. Specifically, the authors demonstrate how a supercharged end-to-side (SETS) nerve transfer can be performed to help redirect axons to reach the CPFR in patients with a Sunderland III grade injury.[4]

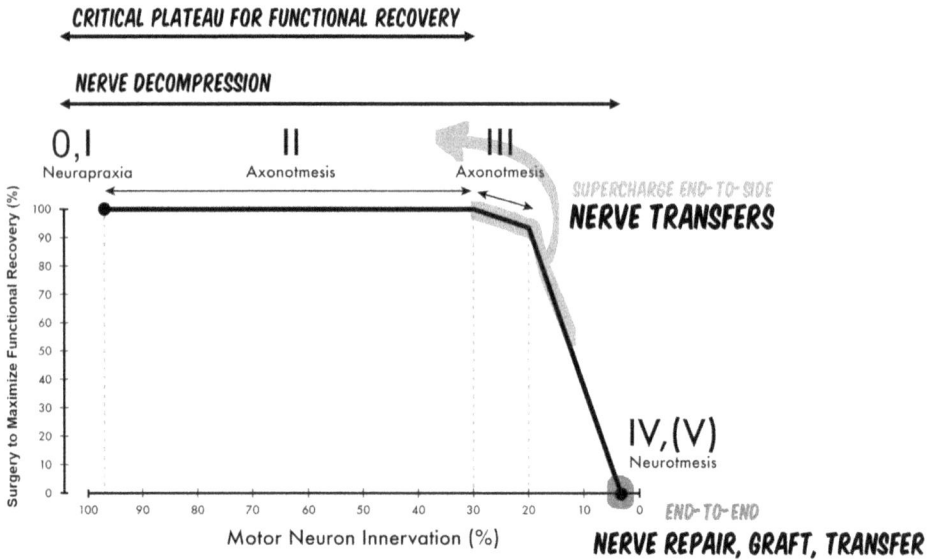

Figure 20.1   Potential for functional recovery based on motor neuron innervation. Relationship between functional recovery and percentage of intact motor neurons. Sunderland 0 injury is associated with ischemic block. A Sunderland I injury is associated with demyelination and has no axonal loss. A Sunderland II (axonotmesis) has adequate uninjured axons to ensure full function with collateral sprouting of uninjured axons (physiological nerve transfer) and regenerating injured axons, whereas a Sunderland III has substantial axonal loss and endoneurial scar such that recovery is variable. The Sunderland IV and V injuries (neurotmesis) have no function, as the axonal loss is severe to complete. The bracket denotes the "critical plateau for function recovery" which indicates the potential for recovery with or without surgery. In this figure, SETS transfers are shown to help redirect axons to assist in reaching the CPFR in patients with Sunderland III injuries. In patients with Sunderland IV and V injuries, nerve grafting and end-to-end nerve transfers can be considered. (Reprinted with permission, Copyright 2021, nervesurgery.wustl.edu.)

The authors have expanded on the evolution of nerve transfers and describe procedures to augment the number of the axons to meet the CPFR. One example is the super turbocharged end-to-side (STETS) transfer for ulnar reinnervation, which builds upon the SETS transfer. This includes an additional abductor digiti minimi transfer to the ulnar deep motor to optimize the number of axons reaching the CPFR. This fundamental concept illustrates how an uninjured nerve with relative expendability is rerouted to direct axons to a more critical distal function (ulnar intrinsic function). The authors introduce the turbocharged end-to-side (TETS) transfer, which utilizes expendable donor nerves (i.e., supinator in the forearm) and reroutes its axons to an adjacent motor nerve with a more critical function (posterior interosseus nerve). These transfers have been increasingly adopted since their initial descriptions.[5,6] Additionally, the use of side-to-side sensory cross-palmar grafting has been described to help restore ulnar sensation in the palm.[7]

The clinical utility of the nerve allograft has been narrowly defined by the authors in this study. This is timely, as its application has been a topic of intense interest and contention. The authors advocate for the use of acellular nerve allograft (ANAs) for short-gap (<3 cm) non-critical, small diameter sensory nerves. This is supported by research that compares autografts to acellular nerve allografts. Autografts have been shown to fail with increasing length (up to 6 cm). This is in stark contrast to the ANA, which fail at shorter distances (<3 cm and with larger diameters).[8,9] The authors implore readers to be scrupulous in evaluation of studies assessing ANAs as many are industry funded and often conclude equivalence in many applications of nerve surgery.[10,11] As more objective data emerges, we will be even better poised to evaluate their true efficacy in nerve surgery.

Electrodiagnostic studies are a critical tool in the nerve surgeon's armamentarium. An ability to interpret these studies constitutes a paradigm shift for management of patients with nerve injuries.[12] In this paper, the authors provide an overview of critical findings in the EDX and relate them to existing schema for nerve injury classification. There are algorithms provided, supplemented with real-world patient scenarios (i.e., clinical diagnosis of cubital tunnel syndrome) to further illustrate how findings are critical in evaluation, diagnosis, and management.[4,13]

This paper provides a timely review of critical advancements in the field of nerve surgery, a field which has seen tremendous innovation and change since the publication of the Ray et al. paper in 2010. The development of a refined nerve classification schema has broadened our understanding of nerve injuries and provided a means to classify degree of injury and prognosis, and to inform surgical planning. The CPFR marks a critical advancement in axonal quantification for meaningful functional recovery, which illustrates the utility of nerve transfers including STETS to help augment recovery.

REFERENCES

1. Ray WZ, Mackinnon SE. Management of Nerve Gaps: Autografts, Allografts, Nerve Transfers, and End-to-Side Neurorrhaphy. *Exp Neurol.* 2010;223(1):77–85. doi:10.1016/j.expneurol.2009.03.031
2. Peters BR, Pripotnev S, Chi D, Mackinnon SE. Complete Foot Drop with Normal Electrodiagnostic Studies: Sunderland "Zero" Ischemic Conduction Block of the Common Peroneal Nerve. *Ann Plast Surg.* 2022;88(4):425. doi:10.1097/SAP.0000000000003053
3. Kobayashi J, Mackinnon SE, Watanabe O, *et al.* The Effect of Duration of Muscle Denervation on Functional Recovery in the Rat Model. *Muscle Nerve.* 1997;20(7):858–866. doi:10.1002/(sici)1097-4598(199707)20:7<858::aid-mus10>3.0.co;2-o
4. Power HA, Kahn LC, Patterson MM, Yee A, Moore AM, Mackinnon SE. Refining Indications for the Supercharge End-to-Side Anterior Interosseous to Ulnar Motor Nerve Transfer in Cubital Tunnel Syndrome. *Plast Reconstr Surg.* 2020;145(1):106e–116e. doi:10.1097/PRS.0000000000006399
5. Peters BR, Jacobson L, Pripotnev S, Mackinnon SE. Abductor Digiti Minimi and Anterior Interosseous to Ulnar Motor Nerve Transfer: The Super Turbocharge End-to-Side Transfer. *Plast Reconstr Surg.* 2023;151(4):815–820. doi:10.1097/PRS.0000000000010003
6. Bazarek S, Sten M, Nin D, Brown JM. Supinator to Posterior Interosseous Nerve Transfer for Restoration of Finger Extension. *Oper Neurosurg Hagerstown Md.* 2021;21(5):E408–E413. doi:10.1093/ons/opab263
7. Felder JM, Hill EJR, Power HA, Hasak J, Mackinnon SE. Cross-Palm Nerve Grafts to Enhance Sensory Recovery in Severe Ulnar Neuropathy. *Hand N Y.* 2020;15(4):526–533. doi:10.1177/1558944718822851

8. Saheb-Al-Zamani M, Yan Y, Farber SJ, *et al.* Limited Regeneration in Long Acellular Nerve Allografts is Associated with Increased Schwann Cell Senescence. *Exp Neurol.* 2013;247:165–177. doi:10.1016/j.expneurol.2013.04.011

9. Peters BR, Wood MD, Hunter DA, Mackinnon SE. Acellular Nerve Allografts in Major Peripheral Nerve Repairs: An Analysis of Cases Presenting with Limited Recovery. *Hand N Y.* 2023;18(2):236–243. doi:10.1177/15589447211003175

10. Reese M, Mehta YA, Haupt MR, *et al.* Academic Influence and Industry Funding in Nerve Allograft Research: A Co-Authorship Network Analysis. *Plast Reconstr Surg.* Published online March 24, 2021:10.1097/PRS.0000000000011759. doi:10.1097/PRS.0000000000011759

11. Lans J, Eberlin KR, Evans PJ, Mercer D, Greenberg JA, Styron JF. A Systematic Review and Meta-Analysis of Nerve Gap Repair: Comparative Effectiveness of Allografts, Autografts, and Conduits. *Plast Reconstr Surg.* 2023;151(5):814e–827e. doi:10.1097/PRS.0000000000010088

12. Taylor R, Zhang, JK, Patterson JM, *et al.* A Video-Based Learning Module Is an Effective Way to Teach the Interpretation of Pre-Operative Electrodiagnostic Studies. *Plast Reconstr Surg.* 2024. Online ahead of print. doi: 10.1097/PRS.0000000000011907

13. Pripotnev S, Bucelli RC, Patterson JMM, Yee A, Pet MA, Mackinnon S. Interpreting Electrodiagnostic Studies for the Management of Nerve Injury. *J Hand Surg.* 2022;47(9):881–889. doi:10.1016/j.jhsa.2022.04.008

EDITOR COMMENTARY

This update is hot off the press from Professor MacKinnon's team. There is a comprehensive literature review with updated classifications (Sunderland 0-VI), the best use of electrodiagnostics, and current surgical approaches. The paper summarizes the latest thinking on grafts, transfers (including the variety of end-to-side connections), and allografts. These are important given the resurgence of nerve transfers, particularly in brachial plexus reconstruction, accompanied by a rise in innovative surgeries. The concept of the CPFR seems to offer an intuitive way to think about how nerve transfers, including SETS and STETS, can augment recovery.

Exploration (of the nerve) in an acute injury is not an emergency per se; having the appropriately experienced staff and other resources is more important as long as surgery is performed within 72 hours (after which intraoperative stimulation is not feasible). The initial management of closed injuries is generally conversative; electrodiagnostic tests are not needed until 3 months after the injury. Electrostimulation may enhance nerve regeneration.

Despite advances, what remains the most important factor influencing recovery is the time to reinnervation of the motor end plate/sensory receptors. When the nerve cannot be primarily repaired and there is a nerve gap, there are a variety of options discussed in the review.

CHAPTER 21

Toe Transplantation for Isolated Index Finger Amputations Distal to the Proximal Interphalangeal Joint

Demirkan F, Wei FC, Jeng SF, Cheng SL, Lin CH, Chuang DC.
Plast Reconstr Surg. 1999 Feb;103(2):499–507

AUTHOR COMMENTARY

Steven Lo and F.C. Wei

Study Design

In this study published in 1999, from Chang Gung Memorial Hospital, Linkou, Taiwan, a retrospective review was performed of 19 cases of isolated 2nd toe transfer to index finger amputations distal to the PIP joint, between May 1986 to August 1997.[1]

Follow-Up

Mean follow-up was 38 months (range 6 months to 9.5 years).

RESULTS

Similar to other studies of the era, outcome data was restricted to operative complications, clinicodemographic data, physical measurements including moving and static 2-point discrimination, grip strength, and unvalidated patient questionnaires. At this time, hand-specific patient-reported outcomes such as the Michigan Hand Questionnaire, which had only just been validated in 1998, were not in widespread use.[2] Results were documented as follows.

Operative Results

100% microsurgical success, with 16% re-exploration rate for arterial thrombosis. Secondary surgery included pulp-plasty in 11 patients and tenolysis in 2 patients.

Physical Measurements

Moving 2PD and static 2PD were a mean of 6 mm and 8 mm, respectively. Pinch grip (thumb to index) was reduced at 67.5% of the contralateral hand. The toe DIPJ had a relatively reduced range of motion of 19.5 degrees with 3 cases of DIPJ ankylosis.

DOI: 10.1201/9781003413738-21

Subjective Patient Outcomes

A total of 69% patients could use the toe-transfer-reconstructed digit in daily activities. Aesthetic donor site was rated as 74 out of 100, and functional ability rated as 70.5 out of 100 by patients. Physical examination revealed that fine manual dexterity was generally acceptable for tasks such as buttoning up a shirt, and using a computer keyboard, touchphone, or screwdriver. However, some activities requiring finer power control, such as picking up a coin, or proprioceptive feedback, such as touch typewriting (without looking at keyboard) were difficult, and the index finger was bypassed in favour of the middle finger.

STUDY LIMITATIONS

Limitations of this article may be considered in terms of study design, outcome measures, and comparator groups.

Study Design

This was a single retrospective group of toe transfers with a relatively low number of cases. All retrospective studies suffer from inherent selection bias in that patients who return for follow-up research studies may have better outcomes. A total of 10 of the 19 patients completed the follow-up patient questionnaire. No statistical analysis was performed in this study.

Outcome Measures

The importance of validated patient-reported outcome measures (PROMs) is a relatively recent concept. At the time of publication of this study, the DASH[3] and Michigan Hand Questionnaire (MHQ)[2] had been developed only in 1996 and 1998, respectively. Furthermore, the Minimal Clinically Important Difference (MCID) had also not yet been widely popularized, and it was not calculated for the MHQ until 2009.[4] PROMs allow validated comparisons across different medical centres and, more importantly, comparison between intervention and control groups. Additionally, they provide data that has undergone reliability and validity testing. This ensures that they measure what they are intended to measure, such as hand function, and that such results are repeatable. The MCID lets us know whether statistically significant differences are of relevance to patients and is of greater clinical significance than p values in isolation.

Comparator Groups

Stronger levels of evidence require comparison or control groups, as outcomes of the intervention group, such as toe-transfer-reconstructed hands, are difficult to interpret in isolation. The 1999 study only included one intervention group and therefore a direct comparison with results from a control group (such as replantation or revision amputation) were not possible.

With these study limitations in mind, we recently sought to evaluate a larger group of toe transfers with a comparator group of digital replantations, using validated reported outcomes, assessment of MCIDs, and with robust statistical methods. We discuss this study in brief later.

RELEVANT STUDIES

Microsurgical Reconstruction of Distal Digits Following Mutilating Hand Injuries: Results in 121 Patients (Wei FC et al., 1993)

A larger cohort of 152 microvascular partial toe transfers in 121 patients was described in 1993 at Chang Gung Memorial Hospital, Linkou, Taiwan, and at this time, partial toe transfers for minor defects were generally less accepted by the hand surgery community.[5] The partial toe transfers included modified great toe wraparound flap (42 cases), great toe pulp (10), partial 2nd toe (15), 2nd toe wraparound (20), toenail from 2nd toe donor (4), partial 3rd toe (7), 3rd toe pulp (6), and first webspace (20). A total of 98% were successful. 2PD varied from 5 to 15 mm with ROM 60% of normal at the PIP or IP joint. This landmark article demonstrated that minor toe transfers could be performed with extremely high success rates, but also that they could provide excellent recovery of function and aesthetics. This paper also challenged the traditional more conservative approach to finger reconstruction of the era.

The Indications for Toe Transfer after "Minor" Finger Injuries (Del Pinal F, 2004)

Management of "minor" finger defects with partial toe transfers was not restricted to Asian cultures, as demonstrated by Francisco Del Pinal in Santander, Spain, who described a series of single-digit distal amputations in 2004.[6] His preference was to reconstruct middle and ring digit amputations (rather than little and index finger), as amputated central digits were more aesthetically obvious, as they did not fit in with the finger cascade. Indications in this article for single toe transfer were non-smoker, < 40 years old, and manual workers (finding that they allowed better return to work outcomes). At the time, this was contrary to thinking of the majority of Western hand surgeons who would not consider toe transfers for minor defects, particularly in manual workers.

Recent Chang Gung Memorial Hospital Data (Lo and Wei 2024, Unpublished)

This cohort study (unpublished data) sought to assess whether toe transfers can match the function of replanted digits and address limitations of previous toe transfer studies that we have already alluded to. This study also assessed the variables that influenced functional outcomes of toe transfer reconstructed digits. A total of 75 patients with 126 toe transfers were compared with 52 patients with 96 digit replantations from the FRANCHISE study,[7] with both groups treated at Chang Gung Memorial Hospital, Linkou, Taiwan. Validated outcome measures included the Michigan Hand Questionnaire (MHQ) and 36-Item Short Form Health Survey (SF-36). Adjusted means revealed superior MHQ scores for toe transfers compared to replantation, with differences in MHQ scores exceeding the minimally important clinically difference – indicating that these differences were relevant to patients. Pairwise comparisons noted that these differences increased with increasing severity of injury; amputations involving two or more digits, irrespective of thumb inclusion, had significantly better

MHQ scores when treated with toe transfer. SF36 scores were higher for toe transfers than replantation. This study also looked at factors that influenced functional scores after toe transfer, using a multivariable regression approach. Moving 2-point discrimination, active range of motion, tripod grip, and SF36 scores contributed significantly to the MHQ score. These findings challenge current global approaches to digital amputation that focus on digit replantation to restore function. This is the first study in a large cohort of patients to demonstrate that toe transfers outperform equivalent digit replantations on validated PROMs. This data may transform future approaches to digit amputation and brings into question whether digit replantation is still the gold standard treatment after amputation.

STUDY IMPACTS

At the time of publication, this 1999 study was one of the first articles to challenge the accepted dogma that an isolated distal finger amputation, particularly of the index finger, was better served by revision amputation or ray amputation. However, toe and partial toe transfers for minor digital defects are still relatively limited worldwide, particularly in Western cultures. Study limitations relating to study design, patient-reported outcomes, and comparator groups may limit some of the applicability of this data in today's evidence-driven health frameworks. We hope that with our recent Chang Gung Memorial Hospital data – comparing toe transfer to digit replantation using validated patient-reported outcomes – that we will provide robust evidence that toe transfer provides superior functional outcomes to equivalent digit replantation. In doing so, we hope that we can produce another future landmark article that will transform global management of digital amputations.

REFERENCES

1. Demirkan, F. et al. (1999). Toe transplantation for isolated index finger amputations distal to the proximal interphalangeal joint. *Plast Reconstr Surg* 103, 499–507, doi:10.1097/00006534-199902000-00021.
2. Chung, K. C., Pillsbury, M. S., Walters, M. R. & Hayward, R. A. (1998). Reliability and validity testing of the michigan hand outcomes questionnaire. *J Hand Surg Am* 23, 575–587, doi:10.1016/s0363-5023(98)80042-7.
3. Hudak, P. L., Amadio, P. C. & Bombardier, C. (1996). Development of an upper extremity outcome measure: the DASH (disabilities of the arm, shoulder and hand) [corrected]. The Upper Extremity Collaborative Group (UECG). *Am J Ind Med* 29, 602–608, doi:10.1002/(sici)1097-0274(199606)29:6<602::Aid-ajim4>3.0.Co;2-l.
4. Shauver, M. J. & Chung, K. C. (2009). The minimal clinically important difference of the Michigan hand outcomes questionnaire. *J Hand Surg Am* 34, 509–514, doi:10.1016/j.jhsa.2008.11.001.
5. Wei, F. C., Epstein, M. D., Chen, H. C., Chuang, C. C. & Chen, H. T. (1993). Microsurgical reconstruction of distal digits following mutilating hand injuries: results in 121 patients. *Br J Plast Surg* 46, 181–186, doi:10.1016/0007-1226(93)90165-8.
6. del Piñal, F. (2004). The indications for toe transfer after "minor" finger injuries. *J Hand Surg Br* 29, 120–129, doi:10.1016/j.jhsb.2003.12.004.
7. Chung, K. C. *et al.* (2019). Patient-reported and functional outcomes after revision amputation and replantation of digit amputations: the FRANCHISE multicenter international retrospective cohort study. *JAMA Surg* 154, 637–646, doi:10.1001/jamasurg.2019.0418.

EDITOR COMMENTARY

It is often said that distal index finger amputations are well compensated for in functional terms and that complex reconstructions such as toe transfer are not indicated. These guidelines are usually based on some compromise between pragmatism, practicality, and use of resources. It usually takes advances in technique, skill, and philosophy from pioneers such as F.C. Wei to challenge the orthodoxy and change attitudes. There was a time when only loss of a thumb was considered an acceptable indication for toe transfer (Buncke HJ, 1973). F. del Pinal (2004) suggests that the basic aim should be to convert injured hands into "(near)normal" or "acceptable" ones, the latter being a three-fingered hand plus a thumb. The temptation to reconstruct every finger should be tempered by considerations such as the level of amputation, recognizing the inherent limitations of toes and aiming to produce a balanced hand. Koshima (2000) described a series of very distal finger defect reconstructions using partial toes, where the main indication was cosmesis.

The team at Chang Gung presents 19 cases of 2nd toe transfer for index reconstruction. The majority were for secondary reconstruction; only 5 had the transfer around the time of the injury, thus most patients had time to "live with" their deficit, which some surgeons regard as being helpful in tempering expectations. All flaps survived. At assessment at 6 months or more after surgery, all toes had reasonable sensory recovery – the average static 2-point discrimination was 8 mm. Regarding the concerns over the transplanted digit "getting in the way," they found involvement in daily activity score of 69% and functional score of 70.5%, testing activities such as buttons, keyboard, and phones. The major difficulties were with actions requiring fine control and intact proprioception. Reconstruction of those with an intact PIPJ will be much better than those without. Having said that, use of other reconstructive methods will likely result in poorer results and a lower usage rate compared to toe transfers.

Objective results seem to indicate that index reconstruction is worthwhile though the study lacks data from PROMs that would help to validate the approach with distal or "minor" injuries. The inclusion of pre-publication data whets the appetite for the full-published article.

REFERENCES

Buncke HJ, McLean DH, George PJ et al. Thumb replacement: great toe to hand transplantation by microvascular anastomosis. *British Journal of Plastic Surgery* 1973;26:194–201.

Koshima I, Inagawa K, Urushibara K, Okumoto K, and Moriguchi T. Fingertip reconstructions using partial-toe transfers. *Plastic and Reconstructive Surgery* 2000;105:1666–1674.

CHAPTER 22

Epinephrine in Local Anesthesia in Finger and Hand Surgery: The Case for Wide-Awake Anesthesia

Lalonde D, Martin A. *J Am Acad Orthop Surg.* 2013 Aug;21(8):443–447

EXPERT COMMENTARY

Wing-Lim Tse

This is an article summarizing the history of the revival in the use of epinephrine together with local anaesthetics in fingers, with a multitude of convincing evidence supporting the safety of this application, how to administer it, and the extended application of this concept to wide-awake local anaesthesia with no tourniquet (WALANT).

The authors explained that it was procaine (instead of epinephrine), with its acidity especially after prolonged storage, that was the cause of finger ischaemia following its injection with epinephrine. This was news to most surgeons, who had a strong belief that it was the epinephrine, which is known for vasoconstriction effect, that caused ischaemia. This observation is supported by numerous clinical studies that have proven the safety of coadministration of epinephrine with lidocaine. The authors also present evidence that finger ischaemia was not observed even with 100 times the strength of the currently used dilution of 1:100,000 epinephrine. These strongly support the safety of epinephrine. The authors also described the phenomenon of "white fingers," which is a scary sign after epinephrine plus lidocaine injection. The evidence is that despite blanching of finger, the SaO_2 of the finger (and thus a better indicator of tissue oxygenation) does not decrease significantly.

The recommended technique of anaesthetic injection was described in detail, including recommended sites and volumes. When there was doubt about tissue perfusion, more timely reversal of tissue blanching could be achieved with administration of phentolamine.

The clinical application of the extended use of WALANT surgery is also described with its distinctive usefulness in allowing more precise assessment of the tension required during tendon repair and tendon transfer. Traditionally these are mostly based on surgeon's experience, which one could argue was less objective. In my experience, the

DOI: 10.1201/9781003413738-22

use of WALANT enhances patient participation and satisfaction during the surgery, which, in turn, facilitates rehabilitation. The patient can visualize the outcome during the surgery, strengthening trust and rapport with the surgeon as he can witness that the surgery has been successfully executed.

Finally, the implication of expanding elective local anaesthesia surgery is discussed. This includes improving efficiency of patient turnover, with more cases being operated on at much less cost, less manpower, and less surgical equipment/disposables involved. There is also improved safety since patients do not need sedation, and a shorter period of postoperative monitoring is required.

This was a landmark development in hand and plastic surgery. Recent global economic changes due to multiple factors, including COVID-19, have greatly impacted medical systems all over the world. There are calls to reduce the cost of medical service while patient needs and expectations keep on rising. The wider application of surgery with epinephrine allows more complex upper limb surgeries to be performed with the patient kept wide awake [1–2], with reduced use of sedation, faster patient turnover, and executed in low-cost procedure rooms instead of operating theatres [3–4]. In my opinion, the popularization of this approach helps to maintain medical services during adverse economic times, and, most important, it enhances patient satisfaction [5–6] and possibly outcomes through participation during surgery. You can see the acceptance has increased exponentially over the past years, with more surgeries being performed under local anaesthesia; use has been expanding in hospitals and clinics all over the world.

REFERENCES

1. Lalonde DH. Conceptual origins, current practice, and views of wide awake hand surgery. *J Hand Surg Eur.* 2017;42(9):886–895.
2. Lalonde DH, Tang JB. How the wide awake tourniquet-free approach is changing hand surgery in most countries of the world. *Hand Clin.* 2019;35(1):xiii–xiv.
3. Tang JB, Xing SG, Ayhan E *et al.* Impact of wide-awake local anesthesia no tourniquet on departmental settings, cost, patient and surgeon satisfaction, and beyond. *Hand Clin.* 2019; 35(1):29–34.
4. Tang JB, Gong KT, Xing SG *et al.* Wide-awake hand surgery in two centers in China: experience in Nantong and Tianjin with 12,000 patients. *Hand Clin.* 2019;35(1):7–12.
5. Siu A, Wong RS, Ahmed Z, Talwar C, Nikkhah D. Patient satisfaction using Wide Awake Local Anaesthesia No Tourniquet (WALANT) in adults undergoing elective hand surgery: a systematic review and meta-analysis. *J Plast Reconstruct Aesthetic Surg.* 2024. doi: 10.1016/j.bjps.2024.10.027
6. Moscato L, Helmi A, Kouyoumdjian P, Lalonde D, Mares O. The impact of WALANT anesthesia and office-based settings on patient satisfaction after carpal tunnel release: A patient reported outcome study. *Orthop Traumatol Surg Res.* 2023;109(3):103134.

EDITOR COMMENTARY

Surgeons have long been warned about injecting adrenaline into the fingers (and other end-organs); the warning appeared in Bunnell's textbook in 1946. It has taken a great deal of evidence from Donald Lalonde (and others), and effort to overturn this fallacy, including work on "volunteers" to test out antidotes (Nodwell, 2003). The Dalhousie project found that the vasoconstriction with 1:100,000 adrenaline lasts for an average of 6 hours and 20 minutes; phentolamine rescue (1 mg/mL), when needed, e.g., accidental high dose (1:1,000) injection, reverses the effects by 1 hour and 25 minutes on average. Apparently, Lalonde has never had to use phentolamine in normal clinical practice. Busting the myths over the use of local anaesthesia with adrenaline by Lalonde led to development of protocols such as WALANT. This was a review paper that described the technique in detail without any comparisons or data per se.

The adrenaline reduces bleeding and supplements the effects of local anaesthesia, e.g., increase the maximum safe dose. The duration of anaesthesia with 5.4mL of 2% lignocaine with 1:100,000 adrenaline lasts for about 9 hours versus 4–5 hours for 1% lignocaine with 1:200,000 adrenaline versus 15 hours for 0.5% bupivacaine (BSSH Guidelines, 2020). The injection should be almost painless bar the first jab (use bicarbonate, 30G needle, inject slowly). This allows tourniquets to be avoided (though it may be prudent to apply one without inflating it) whilst providing adequate analgesia for patient comfort, allowing a variety of procedures to proceed, particularly those where a cooperative patient is useful – tendon surgery, e.g., repairs, transfers (Bezuhly et al., 2007), and tenolysis. Surgery no longer has to be a race against the (tourniquet) clock. This was a significant development, and it greatly improved results in tendon surgery (Lalonde, 2013). Lalonde commented (in Bezuhly et al., 2007) that cortical adaptation may be "immediate" because some transfers did not need to be "learned," though the reason for this was challenged. WALANT has been used for treatment of carpal tunnel syndrome, Dupuytren contracture, local flaps of the hand (Connors et al., 2023), etc. The list of reports gets longer and longer and boundaries are being pushed. WALANT is contraindicated in those with documented hypersensitivity to lignocaine and in peripheral vascular disease (as a very general category), whilst in those with cardiac disease, a very dilute concentration of adrenaline can be considered, e.g., 1:400,000. Other contraindications include children, those who are anxious/noncompliant, and those with active infection at or near proposed injection sites.

By avoiding general anaesthesia and intubation, the side effects and complications of these, such as nausea and vomiting, aspiration, etc. are eliminated. There were some concerns over field sterility and a possible increase in infections, but this seems to be minor as long as basic procedures/ precautions are followed. The surgeon has a chance to converse with the patient, giving them details of their injury, their surgery, and the rehabilitation. Patient satisfaction is high (McKnight et al., 2022). Bismil et al. (2012) demonstrated savings of 750,000GPD for the 1,000 cases (over 10 years) studied. The overall benefits were particularly obvious during the COVID-19 pandemic when general anaesthetic support was much restricted/limited. This greatly boosted the practice in the United Kingdom and in Hong Kong, in particular, with many units choosing to continue (at least in part) with WALANT for selected hand trauma surgery afterwards.

REFERENCES

Bezuhly M, Sparkes GL, Higgins A, Neumeister MW, Lalonde DH. Immediate thumb extension following extensor indicis proprius-to-extensor pollicis longus tendon transfer using the wide-awake approach. *Plast Reconstr Surg.* 2007 Apr 15;119(5):1507–1512. doi: 10.1097/01.prs.0000256071.00235.d0.

Bismil M, Bismil Q, Harding D, Harris P, Lamyman E, Sansby L. Transition to total one-stop wide-awake hand surgery service-audit: a retrospective review. *JRSM Short Rep.* 2012 Apr;3(4):23. doi: 10.1258/shorts.2012.012019.

Bunnell B. *Surgery of the Hand.* Philadelphia: J.B. Lippincott Publishers Company; 1944.

Connors KM, Kurtzman JS, Koehler SM. Successful use of WALANT in local and regional soft tissue flaps: a case series. *Plast Reconstr Surg Glob Open.* 2023 Jan 13;11(1):e4756. doi: 10.1097/GOX.0000000000004756.

Lalonde DH. How the wide awake approach is changing hand surgery and hand therapy: inaugural AAHS sponsored lecture at the ASHT meeting, San Diego, 2012. *J Hand Ther.* 2013;26:175–178.

Lalonde D, Bell M, Benoit P, Sparkes G, Denkler K, Chang P. A multicenter prospective study of 3,110 consecutive cases of elective epinephrine use in the fingers and hand: the Dalhousie project clinical phase. *J Hand Surg Am.* 2005 Sep;30(5):1061–1067. doi: 10.1016/j.jhsa.2005.05.006.

McKnight KN, Smith VJS, MacFadden LN, Chong ACM, Van Demark RE Jr. Wide-awake hand surgery has its benefits: a study of 1,011 patients. *J Hand Surg Glob Online.* 2022 Jun 17;4(6):394–398. doi: 10.1016/j.jhsg.2022.05.008.

Nodwell T, Lalonde D. How long does it take phentolamine to reverse adrenaline-induced vasoconstriction in the finger and hand? A prospective, randomized, blinded study: the Dalhousie project experimental phase. *Can J Plast Surg.* 2003;11:187–190.

CHAPTER 23

Algorithm for Free Perforator Flap Selection in Lower Extremity Reconstruction Based on 563 Cases

Abdelfattah U, Power HA, Song S, Min K, Suh HP, Hong JP. *Plast Reconstr Surg.* 2019 Nov;144(5):1202–1213 doi: 10.1097/PRS.0000000000006167. PMID: 31397793

EXPERT COMMENTARY

Marco Innocenti

Soft tissue reconstruction in the lower limb remains a controversial topic. New techniques have been added to the traditional armamentarium, largely to try to solve some of the known difficulties, including the shortage of local solutions in this anatomical region and the need for thin and pliable flaps in several areas like the knee, the foot, and the Achilles tendon region.

To our knowledge this is the only article in the international literature reporting a comprehensive retrospective review of a homogeneous series of perforator flaps used in a single institution for lower limb reconstruction with the aim of providing guidelines useful for the choice of the best option according to several parameters. The remarkable number of cases (563) meticulously recorded over a period of 7 years gives a lot of substance to this article and the conclusions reported by the authors are highly reliable.

Almost all the flaps were harvested above the deep fascia, providing thin or super-thin flaps with an average thickness of 6.2 mm. The most frequently used flaps were the SCIP flap (51.2%) and the ALT flap (33.2%). The value of thin perforator flaps in lower limb reconstruction in a variety of clinical conditions, including trauma, tumor resections, and osteomyelitis has been previously addressed by Koshima[7] and Nazerali,[19] and it is further endorsed in this article.

The operative algorithm suggested by the authors consider 5 variables as follows:

1. Patient position
2. Defect size
3. Flap thickness
4. Flap composition
5. Pedicle length required

 DOI: 10.1201/9781003413738-23

The first point is of paramount importance to simplify the OR setting and to avoid unnecessary turning of the patient intraoperatively and the donor site should be chosen accordingly. All the other variables are discussed in the text and the decision-making follows the attempt to satisfy as many of them as possible. The suggested algorithm provides a useful and straightforward guide in the choice of the best procedure in any single case. This article strongly supports the use of thin perforator flaps in the treatment of soft tissue defects in the lower limb in a variety of clinical conditions.

EDITOR COMMENTARY

The authors present results of a retrospective review of cases over a 7-year period performed at the Asian Medical Centre in Seoul. Among the 9 different flaps documented, they mostly used SCIP and ALT flaps. The PIOP and SCIP flaps have particularly short pedicles, but otherwise they offer good thin pliable skin. The authors offer a potentially useful algorithm to guide flap selection for lower limb defects based on patient position, defect size, flap thickness, flap composition, and pedicle length required. The recipient site/anastomosis was placed out of the zone of injury where possible and end-to-side anastomoses were preferred to preserve distal vascularity. They do not mention the profunda femoris artery perforator flap, which seems to be having a bit of a moment.

The primary indications for reconstruction in this cohort were traumatic and diabetic leg/feet wounds. The last group is particularly significant as the condition was often regarded as not being particularly conducive to microvascular reconstruction due to the perceived microvessel disease. Yet overall success rate was 96.2% despite the relatively large number of diabetic limb salvage cases (almost a quarter of this cohort). J.P. Hong probably has the largest experience in diabetic foot reconstruction, built up over many years, and he follows a very exacting protocol. Most other reconstructive surgeons are unlikely to come across even a tiny fraction of such cases and are even more unlikely to get similar results.

This study busts the "myth" that muscle flaps, which had long been the mainstay of lower limb reconstruction, were the first/best choice for these types of wounds. This paper shows that fasciocutaneous perforator flaps can fulfil the same roles and successfully treat challenging cases, such as osteomyelitis wounds, and salvage diabetic limbs, whilst also offering a thinner flap with better contour and potentially allow patients to wear standard footwear. Perforator flaps also offer a simpler path should revision surgery be required, e.g., to underlying bones/fractures. In a follow-up paper of sorts, the same center reported that perforators could be reliably used as recipient vessels for free flap reconstruction of the lower extremity (Power et al., 2022). The posterior interosseus perforator flap is an extremely elegant flap in their hands, providing an almost ideal flap for some of their diabetic cases.

The authors did not address outcomes apart from flap survival, stating that this would come in a separate article, which I am unable to find. They make very convincing points based on very sound principles. An amazing amount of work has been put into formulating an algorithm, and there is probably nothing better out there to guide the thinking processes of a reconstructive surgeon as they tailor it to their own patient mix and their own surgical expertise. It would have been the icing on the cake if there had been more objective quantitative data or statistics to support their claims/suggestions.

REFERENCE

Power HA, Cho J, Kwon JG, Abdelfattah U, Pak CJ, Suh HP, Hong JP. Are Perforators Reliable as Recipient Arteries in Lower Extremity Reconstruction? Analysis of 423 Free Perforator Flaps. *Plast Reconstr Surg*. 2022 Mar 1;149(3):750–760. doi: 10.1097/PRS.0000000000008873.

CHAPTER 24

Corneal Neurotization: A Novel Solution to Neurotrophic Keratopathy

Terzis JK, Dryer MM, Bodner BI. *Plast Reconstr Surg.* 2009 Jan;123(1):112–120
doi: 10.1097/PRS.0b013e3181904d3a PMID: 19116544

EXPERT COMMENTARY

Jordan R. Crabtree, Gregory H. Borschel, and Asim Ali

Research Question/Objective

Neurotrophic keratopathy (NK) is a rare but important cause of reduced visual acuity, corneal ulceration, and blindness. NK is caused by deficient innervation of the cornea by branches of the trigeminal nerve, leading to corneal anesthesia and loss of corneal epithelial integrity. This study introduced a novel method of correcting this deficit by the transfer of contralateral divisions of the ophthalmic nerve – the supraorbital and supratrochlear nerves – to the perilimbal region of the anesthetic eye as sensory donors.

Study Design

Retrospective chart review

Follow-Up

At the time of publication, the average postoperative follow-up was 16. 3 ± 2.42 years. In addition to objective evaluation of corneal sensation by Cochet-Bonnet aesthesiometry, a follow-up questionnaire was employed for subjective assessment of corneal health and psychosocial impacts of corneal neurotization (CN).

RESULTS

Patients reported the presence of subjective corneal sensation between 6 months and 1 year, and the average time to objective sensation was 2.80 ± 2.17 years. Cochet-Bonnet evaluation yielded a reported improvement for all patients from a mean value of 2.00 ± 4.47 mm to 278.00 ± 226.00 mm (p < 0.016) following CN. The postoperative value is erroneous as the Cochet Bonnet scale ranges from 0 mm to 60 mm. We presume that the authors meant 27.8 ± 22 mm, but this is unclear because one patient was tested with a different device (von Frey hair), which measures in mBar, and how multiple postop readings for the same patient were handled was not clarified in the manuscript.

All six eyes exhibited improvements in corneal health, reduction in corneal opacification, and best corrected visual acuity. Two complications (1 subgaleal hematoma and 1 neuroma) were reported, both of which did not require intervention.

Study Limitations

This study was limited by a relatively small sample size of 6 eyes and noted infrequent follow-up as a barrier to obtaining more accurate assessments of sensation and the recovery timeline following CN. The study was also limited in NK etiology, as 4 patients had developed NK following removal of an acoustic neuroma, 1 patient from removal of a meningioma, and 1 patient from trauma.

Study Impacts

Though descriptions of CN can be found as early as 1981 by Samii,[1] this study was the first to offer CN as a definitive solution to NK, and it is often recognized for introducing CN as a modern technique. This spurred a series of innovations in donor nerve selection, surgical approach, and methods of joining sensory donor nerves with the anesthetic cornea for the surgical treatment of NK.

The tunneling method used in the Terzis et al. study is a major contributor to its landmark significance, as prior attempts at CN required invasive approaches to the ciliary nerves and, at its inception, craniotomy.[1] In contrast, transferring the contralateral branches of the trigeminal nerve required a bicoronal incision and tunneling to an incision along the upper lid crease of the anesthetic eye. In recent years, the use of autologous nerve grafts from donor sites, such as the sural nerve, expanded the effective range of available donors outside of the periocular region and allowed for less invasive approaches.[2]

As CN has been popularized, numerous sensory source nerves have been explored as reliable sensory donor options. In addition to the ipsilateral and contralateral supratrochlear and supraorbital nerves, the ipsilateral infraorbital[3] and ipsilateral great auricular nerves[4] have been reliably employed. Neurotization from dual sensory donors, bilateral neurotization using a single donor nerve, and the use of end-to-side approaches in joining the sensory nerve and anesthetic cornea are among other variations of neurotization recorded.[5]

Though initially applied in adult patients with acquired NK, CN has emerged as a treatment for all ages. This includes developmental etiologies in pediatric patients. NK has been described to treat congenital corneal anesthesia associated with Stuve–Wiedemann syndrome,[6] Ramos–Arroyo syndrome,[7] cerebellar hypoplasia,[2] pontine tegmental cap dysplasia,[8] and several other undetermined developmental causes of NK. Interestingly, despite being insensate since birth, these patients often develop appropriate protective pain responses and reflexes, perhaps reflecting the plasticity of the developing nervous system. Provided that sensation can be elicited by monofilament testing, light touch (e.g., "Ten test"), or pain from pinching the dermatomal distribution of a local sensory nerve, it has the potential to serve as a donor to an anesthetic cornea. Promising additional options include the occipital and supraclavicular nerves when the entire trigeminal nerve distribution is not available.

Outcomes of CN to date have shown it to be a safe and effective treatment for NK, with several studies pointing to similar outcomes as those seen by Terzis et al. in 2009. The majority of patients experience stable or improved visual acuity, protection from the recurrence of epithelial defects, and objective improvement in corneal sensibility.[9,10] A recent meta-analysis of CN studies through 2020 found significant improvements in visual acuity in 70% of cases, stability in 24%, and worsening in 6%. The same study reported that the Mackie stage (which categorizes ocular surface health) improved in 81% of cases and was unchanged in 19%. All patients included in the meta-analysis exhibited improvements in corneal sensation. A notable difference between these more recent studies and the initial Terzis study is a shorter reported time to reinnervation, with an overall time of 9 months to return of sensation. This may be explained by the noted difference in median reinnervation time between congenital/developmental (6 months) and acquired (14 months) etiologies, and the fact that the Terzis et al. study included only adult patients with acquired NK, finding an average time to reinnervation of 2.8 years.

Notably, since the publication of the Terzis study, NK management has gained a promising non-surgical treatment in topical recombinant human NGF (rhNGF) (cenegermin, Oxervate, Dompé farmaceutici S.p.A., Milan, Italy). Though CN remains the only definitive treatment of the cause of NK – insufficient corneal innervation – the coadministration of rhNGF pre-, peri-, or postoperatively in patients undergoing CN may further enhance patient outcomes.

In a long-term outcome study in 2022, Woo et al. noted that innervation continues to improve beyond 12 months. They also noted that patients who achieved higher levels of sensory recovery were significantly protected from future epithelial defects, in effect noting a dose-response effect between innervation and ocular surface protection.[11]

It is important to warn patients that their ocular surfaces remain vulnerable for months after CN, and they must, therefore, continue protective measures until innervation becomes robust. Further, they should be counseled that once nerve fibers connect with the ocular surface, they may feel discomfort if the integrity of the ocular surface is impaired.

Summary

Corneal neurotization, by leveraging fundamental principles of nerve transfers, has emerged as a reliable, safe treatment for neurotrophic keratopathy. Indications presently include all forms of NK, provided patients possess functioning regional sensory nerves that can be directed into the denervated cornea.

REFERENCES

1. Samii M. Reconstruction of the trigeminal nerve. In: Samii M, Jannetta PJ, eds. *The Cranial Nerves: Anatomy Pathology Pathophysiology Diagnosis Treatment*. Springer Berlin Heidelberg; 1981:352–358.

2. Elbaz U, Bains R, Zuker RM, Borschel GH, Ali A. Restoration of corneal sensation with regional nerve transfers and nerve grafts: a new approach to a difficult problem. *JAMA Ophthalmol.* Nov 2014;132(11):1289–1295. doi:10.1001/jamaophthalmol.2014.2316.

3. Gennaro P, Gabriele G, Aboh IV, *et al.* The second division of trigeminal nerve for corneal neurotization: a novel one-stage technique in combination with facial reanimation. *J Craniofac Surg.* Jun 2019;30(4):1252–1254. doi:10.1097/scs.0000000000005483.

4. Gross JN, Bhagat N, Tran K, *et al.* Minimally invasive corneal neurotization: 10-year update in technique including novel donor transfer of the great auricular nerve. *Plast Reconstruct Surg.* 2024;154(4):795e–798e. doi:10.1097/prs.0000000000011250.

5. Crabtree JR, Mulenga C, Tran K, *et al.* Corneal neurotization: essentials for the facial paralysis surgeon. *Facial Plast Surg.* 2024 Aug;40(4):424–432. doi: 10.1055/a-2272-6077. Epub 2024 Feb 20. PMID: 38378042.

6. Wiebe JE, Rowe LW, Boente CS, Borschel GH. Single-stage bilateral corneal neurotization for neurotrophic keratopathy in Stüve-Wiedemann syndrome: a case report and literature review. *J Pediatr Ophthalmol Strabismus.* Sep–Oct 2024;61(5):e54–e58. doi:10.3928/01913913-20240807-04.

7. Rowe LW, Berns J, Boente CS, Borschel GH. Bilateral corneal neurotization for ramos-arroyo syndrome and developmental neurotrophic keratopathy: case report and literature review. *Cornea.* Mar 1 2023;42(3):369–371. doi:10.1097/ICO.0000000000003143.

8. Lau N, Osborne SF, Vasquez-Perez A, Wilde CL, Manisali M, Jayaram R. Corneal neurotization using the great auricular nerve for bilateral congenital trigeminal anesthesia. *Cornea.* May 1 2022;41(5):654–657. doi:10.1097/ico.0000000000002951.

9. Wisely CE, Rafailov L, Cypen S, Proia AD, Boehlke CS, Leyngold IM. Clinical and morphologic outcomes of minimally invasive direct corneal neurotization. *Ophthalmic Plast Reconstr Surg.* 2020;36(5):451–457. doi:10.1097/iop.0000000000001586.

10. Catapano J, Fung SSM, Halliday W, *et al.* Treatment of neurotrophic keratopathy with minimally invasive corneal neurotisation: long-term clinical outcomes and evidence of corneal reinnervation. *Br J Ophthalmol.* Dec 2019;103(12):1724–1731. doi:10.1136/bjophthalmol-2018-313042.

11. Woo JH, Daeschler SC, Mireskandari K, Borschel GH, Ali A. Minimally invasive corneal neurotization provides sensory function, protects against recurrent ulceration, and improves visual acuity. *Am J Ophthalmol.* Sep 2022;241:179–189. doi:10.1016/j.ajo.2022.04.013.

EDITOR COMMENTARY

At a meeting in Broomfield where I first met J. Terzis, I heard G. Borschel give a lecture on the topic of CN; I was fascinated and have been trying to establish this in HK ever since. That was 10 years ago, and I am still waiting on my ophthalmological colleagues.

It is somewhat ironic that, in general, plastic surgeons seem a great deal keener than Ophthalmologists on CN. The results in terms of return of objective sensation, clearing and healing of cornea seem to speak for themselves; the presence of nerve fibers in patients after CN has been documented using in vivo confocal microscopy (Fung et al., 2018).

The use of a bicoronal incision in this original paper limited the wider uptake of CN but Elbaz et al. (2014) described a much less invasive technique with sub-brow incision and end-to-side sural nerve grafts. Improvement in corneal sensation was noted as early as 3 months in some – this may be related to the younger patients studied but may represent the more robust nerves used instead of the "wispy" ends of the distal supratrochlear/ supraorbital nerves. More recently, surgeons have leaned toward even more "minimally invasive" approaches using endoscopic assistance (Leyngold et al., 2018) and nerve allografts. There are currently many variants with little research comparing these in meaningful ways.

REFERENCES

Elbaz U, Bains R, Zuker RM, Borschel GH, Ali A. Restoration of Corneal Sensation with Regional Nerve Transfers and Nerve Grafts: A New Approach to a Difficult Problem. JAMA Ophthalmol. 2014 Nov;132(11):1289-95. doi: 10.1001/jamaophthalmol.2014.2316. PMID: 25010775.

Fung SSM, Catapano J, Elbaz U, Zuker RM, Borschel GH, Ali A. In Vivo Confocal Microscopy Reveals Corneal Reinnervation after Treatment of Neurotrophic Keratopathy with Corneal Neurotization. Cornea. 2018 Jan;37(1):109-112. doi: 10.1097/ICO.0000000000001315. PMID: 29053558.

Leyngold I, Weller C, Leyngold M, Espana E, Black KD, Hall KL, Tabor M. Endoscopic Corneal Neurotization: Cadaver Feasibility Study. Ophthalmic Plast Reconstr Surg. 2018 May/Jun;34(3):213-216. doi: 10.1097/IOP.0000000000000913. PMID: 28472009.

CHAPTER 25

The Most Current Algorithms for the Treatment and Prevention of Hypertrophic Scars and Keloids: A 2020 Update of the Algorithms Published 10 Years Ago

Ogawa R. *Plast Reconstr Surg.* 2022 Jan 1;149(1):79e–94e

AUTHOR COMMENTARY

Rei Ogawa

Study Design

This study[1] updates the treatment and prevention algorithms for hypertrophic scars and keloids initially introduced in a comprehensive review in 2010.[2] Over the past decade, substantial advancements have been made in understanding the pathogenesis and management of these scars. This study integrates findings from recent randomized controlled trials, systematic reviews, meta-analyses, and clinical guidelines to refine the original algorithms. It emphasizes the identification of risk factors. including local, systemic, genetic, and lifestyle influences, that contribute to scar formation and progression.

A systematic approach was employed to assess the methodological quality of each included study and to extract key data on patient characteristics, interventions, and outcomes. This rigorous methodology ensures that the updated algorithms are evidence-based and aligned with the latest high-quality research. The aim is to equip clinicians with optimized scar management strategies tailored to the specific characteristics of each patient's hypertrophic scars or keloids.

RESULTS

The updated treatment algorithms for hypertrophic scars and keloids differentiate between mild and severe scar contractures. For hypertrophic scars, surgical intervention is recommended in cases of severe contracture, while non-surgical conservative therapies are advised for milder cases. Keloid management is determined based on the size and number of keloids: small, single keloids respond well to surgery combined with adjuvant

DOI: 10.1201/9781003413738-25

therapy, such as radiotherapy or multimodal conservative approaches, whereas large or multiple keloids are better managed with volume-reducing surgery.

Regardless of the treatment chosen, the algorithms emphasize the importance of long-term follow-up to monitor recurrence risk in all patients. The study also underscores the growth in randomized controlled trials over the past decade, which has expanded the understanding of hypertrophic scar and keloid management. This includes advancements in treatments such as silicone gel sheets, steroid plasters, radiotherapy, and systemic therapies, including oral agents.

STUDY LIMITATIONS

Despite the significant advancements outlined in this study, several limitations remain. The evidence supporting many treatment modalities, particularly non-invasive options like gel sheets and steroid injections, is still limited due to the quality of existing trials, many of which lack long-term follow-up and are constrained by small sample sizes. Furthermore, while the algorithms are largely based on randomized controlled trials, these often focus on highly specific patient populations that may not fully represent broader clinical scenarios.

Another limitation is the regional variation in scar prevalence, especially the genetic predisposition to keloids in certain ethnic groups, which may impact the generalizability of these algorithms across diverse populations. Additionally, the algorithms emphasize physical interventions but give less attention to psychological factors and patient-reported outcomes related to scar treatment. The study recommends that future research should address these gaps by conducting more higher-quality, longer-term studies with larger, more diverse patient populations.

STUDY IMPACTS

A key strength of this study is its comprehensive, up-to-date synthesis of the latest evidence-based approaches for the treatment and prevention of hypertrophic scars and keloids. By incorporating findings from numerous randomized controlled trials, systematic reviews, and meta-analyses from the past decade, the study provides an authoritative update to previously established treatment algorithms.

Another notable strength is the clear differentiation in management strategies for hypertrophic scars and keloids, acknowledging their distinct pathophysiology and clinical behavior. The tailored approach, which considers the severity of scar contracture for hypertrophic scars and the size and number of keloids, enhances the applicability of the algorithms in clinical practice. Additionally, the study emphasizes the importance of long-term follow-up and offers practical, multimodal treatment options – ranging from surgery to non-invasive therapies – to ensure comprehensive patient care.

The inclusion of details on newer modalities, such as advanced steroid plasters and refined postoperative radiotherapy protocols, underscores the study's commitment to optimizing patient outcomes while minimizing complications. Supported by high-quality evidence, these treatment strategies enhance the study's reliability and solidify its value as a practical resource for clinicians. In particular, substantial advancements have been made over the past decade in understanding the efficacy of steroid tapes and plasters. Notably, keloids that were previously challenging to treat have shown promising responses to Eclar plaster, a deprodone propionate formulation, as demonstrated in separate case reports.[3] Although various steroid tapes are available globally, the author's experience indicates that deprodone propionate formulations – available only in Japan – have shown the highest efficacy. This non-halogenated steroid, with moderate potency, provides a gradual anti-inflammatory effect, resulting in significantly fewer side effects than other steroid tapes, making it suitable for long-term use. In Japan, where Eclar plaster is most widely utilized, it is increasingly applied postoperatively to prevent the formation of keloids and hypertrophic scars, highlighting its utility not only as a therapeutic option but also as a potential preventive measure.

Currently, the primary treatment for severe keloids involves surgery followed by postoperative radiation therapy.[4] Advances in radiation therapy protocols have enhanced both the safety and the effectiveness of this approach. Nevertheless, despite these improvements in radiation therapy protocols, they cannot fully eliminate the risk of long-term side effects, such as carcinogenesis. Therefore, it remains essential to investigate the underlying causes of keloids and hypertrophic scars and to prioritize the development of molecular-targeted therapies and new treatment agents.

It is crucial for researchers to recognize that keloids and hypertrophic scars are fundamentally inflammatory conditions rather than fibroblast-driven tumors like desmoid tumors.[5] Fibroblast proliferation in these scars is secondary and non-tumorigenic, arising as a result of persistent tissue inflammation, which subsequently leads to fibroblast activity and fibrous tissue production. Future research should thus concentrate on blood vessels, which play a central role in the inflammatory process, to enhance understanding of the root causes and develop targeted interventions for these conditions.

REFERENCES

1. Ogawa R. The most current algorithms for the treatment and prevention of hypertrophic scars and keloids: a 2020 update of the algorithms published 10 years ago. *Plast Reconstr Surg.* 2022 Jan 1;149(1):79e–94e.
2. Ogawa R. The most current algorithms for the treatment and prevention of hypertrophic scars and keloids. *Plast Reconstr Surg.* 2010 Feb;125(2):557–568.
3. Ogawa R, Quong WL. Effective treatment of an aggressive chest wall keloid in a woman using deprodone propionate plaster without surgery, radiotherapy, or injection. *Plast Reconstr Surg Glob Open.* 2024 Sep 3;12(9):e6117.
4. Ogawa R, Tosa M, Dohi T, Akaishi S, Kuribayashi S. Surgical excision and postoperative radiotherapy for keloids. *Scars Burn Heal.* 2019 Dec 10;5:2059513119891113.
5. Ogawa R. Keloid and hypertrophic scars are the result of chronic inflammation in the reticular dermis. *Int J Mol Sci.* 2017 Mar 10;18(3):606.

EDITOR COMMENTARY

Professor Rei Ogawa is probably the world authority on scar and keloid management, particularly in Asians, who are much more prone to problematic scarring. He offers a compelling framework to understanding and managing HTS and keloids through exhaustive review of the literature. This is certainly the reference work when it comes to practical scar management.

This is an update of the 2010 guidelines by the same author, incorporating findings from recent studies and reviews. Tension is highlighted as a risk/aetiological factor; inflammation and endothelial dysfunction is also implicated. Intralesional injections such as steroids (high-concentration tapes are also effective) and 5-FU are still the mainstay for smaller scars. There is an emphasis on surgery and radiotherapy for keloids. There have been a handful of reports of cancer after radiotherapy for keloids, but the association is not clear cut in most cases. More than 90% of radiation oncologists accept that keloid treatment is a valid indication for radiation treatment.

A few small case series have looked at the potential role of fat/ adipose derived stem cell injection in scar treatment particularly for softening wider areas of scarring after burn injuries/grafting. The effect seems to be mainly an improvement of the contour and pliability of mature scars rather than changing hypertrophic/keloid scars per se, which can be regarded as "persistent immature" scars.

CHAPTER 26

Comparison of Clinical and Functional Outcomes and Hospital Costs Following Pharyngoesophageal Reconstruction with the Anterolateral Thigh Free Flap versus the Jejunal Flap

Yu P, Lewin JS, Reece GP, Robb GL. *Plast Reconstr Surg.* 2006 Mar;117(3):968–974

EXPERT COMMENTARY

Velda Chow

Study Design

Retrospective comparative study of patients who underwent free anterolateral thigh flap (ALT) and free jejunal flap (FJ) for circumferential pharyngoesophageal (PE) reconstruction over a 6-year period in a single centre. Patient demographics, perioperative outcomes, functional outcomes, and hospital costs were analyzed and compared.

Follow-Up

FJ flap had been the work-horse flap for PE reconstruction in the study unit, whereas use of the free ALT flap for PE reconstruction started more recently in 2001, a few years before publication. Mean follow-up was 25.9 (1.0–73.0) months and 13.7 (3.0–25.0) months for FJ and free ALT flaps, respectively.

RESULTS

Between 1998 and 2004, 57 patients who underwent circumferential PE reconstruction with free ALT flap (n = 26) and FJ flap (n = 31) were included. Free ALT and FJ flaps included in this study were performed by 1 surgeon and 6 surgeons, respectively.

There was no significant difference in patient demographics and medical comorbidities between the two groups. There were no operative mortalities. Total flap loss was noted in 3 patients (ALT n = 1, 3.8%; FJ n = 2, 6.5%). There was no significant difference in

DOI: 10.1201/9781003413738-26

anastomotic dehiscence (ALT n = 1, 3.8% vs FJ n = 1, 3.2%), pharyngocutaneous fistula (ALT n = 2, 7.7% vs FJ n = 1, 3.2%, p = 0.59), and stricture rates (ALT n = 4, 15.4% vs FJ n = 6, 19.4%, p = 0.47) between the two groups. Post-reconstructive radiotherapy did not have a significant effect on stricture rates (p = 0.2).

Spasticity causing dysphagia was noted in 3 FJ patients. The majority of patients undergoing free ALT flap reconstruction were able to resume full oral diet (ALT 95% vs FJ 65%, p = 0.01). Speech outcome was assessed only in those who opted for tracheoesophageal speech (ALT n = 9 and FJ n = 9). Fluent tracheoesophageal speech was noted in 88.9% and 22.2% free ALT and FJ patients, respectively (p = 0.01).

Ventilator support, ICU stay, and hospital stay were significantly shorter for patients undergoing free ALT flap reconstruction (p = 0.01), resulting in significantly lower hospital charges (p = 0.02).

Study Limitations

This was a retrospective study comparing a single surgeon's outcome versus that of multiple surgeons in a small sample.

The shorter follow-up time in the free ALT group might have underestimated long-term stricture rate and associated adverse swallowing and speech outcomes.

Tracheoesophageal speech is not the only speech modality available for post-laryngectomy patients. In fact, less than half of the patients in each arm opted for tracheoesophageal speech rehabilitation. A more objective speech assessment of all modalities would give a better reflection and comparison of speech outcomes in these two groups of patients.

Relevant Studies and Study Impacts

PE defects are frequently the result of ablative surgery for malignant diseases involving the hypopharynx and/or the cervical oesophagus. The aims of reconstruction are to restore alimentary tract integrity, form, and function (swallowing and speech) in a single-stage operation with minimal donor site morbidities and short hospital stay, as well as to facilitate early commencement of adjuvant treatment. The choice of reconstruction depends on several factors: length of the defect and the site of the distal anastomosis, history of previous surgery and/or radiotherapy, availability of suitable recipient vessels, medical comorbidities, and the availability of surgical expertise. Various fasciocutaneous flaps and visceral flaps have been described for PE reconstruction, most notably the free ALT flap and FJ flap. There is currently no prospective randomised controlled trial comparing the outcomes of these two reconstructive options (Bouhadana, 2021).

The free ALT flap is a versatile flap which enables great flexibility in terms of design and tissue composition. The flap can be harvested with a lengthy pedicle, which, in turn, increases reach when performing microvascular anastomosis in the neck and in the superior mediastinum, e.g., the internal mammary vessels in case of tumours involving the cervical oesophagus. As the authors have demonstrated, donor site morbidities are seldom life-threatening, nor do they warrant re-operation, prolonged ventilator support, or prolonged intensive care unit and hospital stay. The ALT flap may be tubed to reconstruct the tubular PE conduit. However, tubing a cutaneous flap would necessitate two T-junctions – one at the oropharynx above and another at the oesophagus below. These two T-junctions together with the longitudinal suture line in between increases the risk of anastomotic leakage, fistulation, and stricture in the long term. Furthermore, a bulky ALT flap and size discrepancy with the small calibre oesophagus below would increase the risk of leakage, mediastinitis, and mortality. Instead of tubing the ALT flap, insetting the ALT skin island against the prevertebral fascia in a "horseshoe" manner, and interdigitating cutaneous and mucosal surfaces can be adopted to reduce leakage and stricture rates.

The free jejunal flap, being an intrinsically tubular structure, results in lower anastomotic leakage, pharyngocutaneous fistulation, and anastomotic stricture rates compared with its fasciocutaneous flap counterparts. It has a good size match with the oesophagus below, rendering a lower leakage and mediastinitis rate. Size discrepancy at the oropharynx can be catered for by primarily closing and sizing down the oropharynx and splitting the FJ flap along the anti-mesenteric border prior to anastomosis. A lower leakage, fistulation, and stricture rate results in superior swallowing outcomes (Costantino, 2022). Speech outcomes are also better as the free jejunal flap luminal thickness resembles the natural thickness of the pharyngeal wall the most. Although donor site morbidities can potentially be life-threatening, with appropriate expertise donor site morbidity is low. Intensive care unit stay is not routine, and hospital stay is not significantly prolonged as a result of using the FJ flap. This is particularly true in Asian publications, which may be due to the difference in patient demographics, body build, and medical comorbidities.

Regardless of choice of PE reconstruction, early detection and management of anastomotic leakage can sometimes help to prevent progression to dehiscence, infection, infection-induced flap vascular compromise, fistulation, mediastinitis, and blowout complications. As a result, patients can commence adjuvant therapies early for optimal oncological control. Prolonged leakage and inflammation can increase scarring and anastomotic stricture rates in the long term, thereby causing swallowing and speech disturbances. Interesting to note, given comparable anastomotic leakage rates, scarring and stricture appears to be more severe with fasciocutaneous flap reconstruction in non-Caucasian populations. This may be related to the increased tendency of hypertrophic scarring in those with darker Fitzpatrick skin types. Although not shown to be significant in this study, reports have shown that primary tracheoesophageal puncture and adjuvant radiotherapy are also associated with higher leakage and stricture rates (Chan, 2011; Koh, 2019).

Swallowing problems frequently encountered by those who have undergone FJ for PE reconstruction include nasal regurgitation of food boluses, most notably when drinking thin fluids; and increased food bolus transit time, requiring repeated swallowing for food bolus clearance. Video-fluoroscopic swallowing studies and high-resolution manometry studies demonstrated asynchronous contractions along the segment of transferred jejunum which was out of phase with those of the oesophagus below. Sub-adventitial

Botox injection along the anti-mesenteric border of the transferred jejunum during the index operation has been shown to decrease asynchronous contractions, thereby significantly reducing regurgitation and food bolus transit times (Chow, 2020). MDADI score was also significantly higher for those who have undergone Botox injection. In view of decreased contractions and faster transit times of accumulated secretions, speech quality was less watery compared to those without Botox injection.

BIBLIOGRAPHY

Bouhadana G, Azzi AJ, Gilardino MS. The ideal flap for reconstruction of circumferential pharyngeal defects: a systematic review and meta-analysis of surgical outcomes. *J Plast Reconstr Aesthet Surg.* 2021 Aug;74(8):1779–1790. doi: 10.1016/j.bjps.2021.03.042.

Chan YW, Ng RW, Liu LH, Chung HP, Wei WI. Reconstruction of circumferential pharyngeal defects after tumour resection: reference or preference. *J Plast Reconstr Aesthet Surg.* 2011 Aug;64(8):1022–1028. doi: 10.1016/j.bjps.2011.03.021.

Chow VL, Chan JY, Cheng IK, Chan KM. Swallowing disorders following free jejunal flap reconstruction of circumferential pharyngeal defect: does Botox help? *Oral Oncol.* 2020 May;104:104612. doi: 10.1016/j.oraloncology.2020.104612.

Costantino A, Festa BM, Ferreli F, Russo E, Malvezzi L, Giannitto C, Spriano G, Mercante G, De Virgilio A. Circumferential pharyngeal reconstruction after total laryngopharyngectomy: A systematic review and network meta-analysis. *Oral Oncol.* 2022 Apr;127:105809. doi: 10.1016/j.oraloncology.2022.105809.

Koh HK, Tan NC, Tan BK, Ooi ASH. Comparison of outcomes of fasciocutaneous free flaps and jejunal free flaps in pharyngolaryngoesophageal reconstruction: A systematic review and meta-analysis. *Ann Plast Surg.* 2019 Jun;82(6):646–652. doi: 10.1097/SAP.0000000000001776.

EDITOR COMMENTARY

The reconstruction of a circumferential pharyngeal defect is a particular challenge. The common choices are free jejunal flap or a free tubularised anterolateral thigh flap (9–10 cm for a 3 cm diameter tube). I prefer to use the ALT flap largely because I do not know how to harvest a FJ (said partly in jest). I find it easy to adjust the versatile ALT flap design to accommodate the different diameters of the upper and lower anastomoses. A separate skin island on a separate perforator can be used for neck skin if needed, and, if not, a little nubbin of muscle supplied by a separate distal perforator can be used to fashion a mini-chimeric flap that can be used for monitoring of the buried component. I agree that "fatter" ALT flaps may be more prone to fistulae and this may underlie some of the experiences in Western countries compared to Asia, particularly where results with six patients were so bad (3 had to be replaced by FJ) that they went back to FJ exclusively (Parmar et al., 2014).

One should be wary of drawing too many conclusions from small studies like this; meta-analyses or systematic reviews of similarly small and often heterogeneous studies may also be of limited value. Reviews that do exist (Tan NC et al., 2015; Koh HK et al., 2019) generally demonstrate little functional difference (speech and diet) between the different options. HRQOL studies for head and neck reconstruction have consistently shown that the "trauma" associated with resection usually overshadows any subtle differences between reconstruction options.

The experience of the team with their preferred technique is probably more important that the inherent (dis)advantages of the flap chosen.

REFERENCES

Koh HK, Tan NC, Tan BK, Ooi ASH. Comparison of outcomes of fasciocutaneous free flaps and jejunal free flaps in pharyngolaryngoesophageal reconstruction: a systematic review and meta-analysis. *Ann Plast Surg.* 2019 Jun;82(6):646–652. doi: 10.1097/SAP.0000000000001776. Erratum in: *Ann Plast Surg.* 2019 Sep;83(3):369. doi: 10.1097/SAP.0000000000002073.

Parmar S, Al Asaadi Z, Martin T, Jennings C, Pracy P. The anterolateral fasciocutaneous thigh flap for circumferential pharyngeal defects: can it really replace the jejunum? *Br J Oral Maxillofac Surg.* 2014 Mar;52(3):247–250. doi: 10.1016/j.bjoms.2013.12.008.

Tan NC, Lin PY, Kuo PJ, Tsai YT, Chen YC, Nguyen KT, Kuo YR. An objective comparison regarding rate of fistula and stricture among anterolateral thigh, radial forearm, and jejunal free tissue transfers in circumferential pharyngo-esophageal reconstruction. *Microsurgery.* 2015 Jul;35(5):345–349. doi: 10.1002/micr.22359.

CHAPTER 27

Have We Found an Ideal Soft-Tissue Flap? An Experience with 672 Anterolateral Thigh Flaps

Wei FC, Jain V, Celik N, Chen HC, Chuang DC, Lin CH.
Plast Reconstr Surg. 2002 Jun;109(7):2219–2226

AUTHOR COMMENTARY

Luccie M. Wo and Fu-Chan Wei

Summary

This commentary reviews the landmark paper "Have we found an ideal soft-tissue flap? An experience with 672 anterolateral thigh flaps" originally published in 2002, and it has since been cited over 1,600 times in the literature.[1] The anterolateral thigh (ALT) flap is a workhorse flap with numerous applications in microsurgical coverage and soft tissue reconstruction. In the following, we will review the highlights of the landmark article, trace evolutions of the ALT flap since 2002, and discuss some of the new applications and innovations.

INTRODUCTION

The ALT flap was first described by Song et al. in 1984.[2] Adoption of the ALT flap was slow initially because it was raised only when a septocutaneous vessel to the skin was encountered. However, Wei FC et al. (2002) described the feasibility and reliability of elevating an ALT with either septocutaneous vessels or musculocutaneous perforators, with the latter anatomy being much more common and thereby opening the door for wider applications of the ALT flap as a reliable soft tissue option for head and neck, lower extremity, upper extremity, and trunk reconstruction.[1]

Summarized nicely in the original article, the authors identified that the ALT was the "ideal" soft tissue free flap because it can have potentially large dimensions with tailorable thickness, a long vascular pedicle, could be elevated as a sensate and/or flow through flap, and is conveniently located to allow for a two-team approach. Furthermore, the ALT flap had minimal donor site morbidity as most defects can be closed primarily, especially when the width of the donor defect was under 9 cm.

Study Design and Results

This was a retrospective study looking at 660 consecutive patients who underwent reconstruction with ALT flaps over the course of 4 years (between June 1996 and August 2000) at a single institute. The total number of flaps reviewed was 672. Variables analyzed included patient demographics, indications for reconstruction, details regarding the ALT flap and its anatomy, management of donor site, and immediate surgical complications.

In this cohort, the overall success rate for microvascular transfer of ALT flap was 95.7% with a 1.8% incidence of total flap loss and 2.5% incidence of partial flap loss. The majority of flaps were used for head and neck reconstruction (70.7%), 18% were used for lower extremity reconstruction, 8.6% for upper extremity reconstruction, and 1.3% for trunk reconstruction.

The ALT flap was most commonly elevated as a fasciocutaneous flap (52%), the second most common plane was the cutaneous flap with elevation in the suprafascial plane (22.9%). The pedicle length ranged from 8 to 16 cm and pedicle vessel diameter was greater than 2 mm at its origin from the source artery. The authors noted that the majority of the skin vessels for the ALT flap can be found within 3 cm of the midpoint of a line between the anterior superior iliac spine and the superolateral corner of the patella. A total of 87.1% of the vessels to the skin were musculocutaneous perforators and 12.9% were septocutaneous vessels.

There were 63 chimeric flaps in the series, demonstrating that chimerism was possible with rectus femoris muscle, vastus lateralis muscle, tensor fascia lata, anteromedial thigh flaps, and a combination thereof. Finally, all donor sites less than 9 cm in width were closed primarily and the remainder closed with skin grafts.

The Evolution

This was the first paper to establish the ALT flap as a fundamental tool in a reconstructive surgeon's armamentarium. The paper covered an incredible breadth of indications and versatility.[1–5] In 2004, Yu et al. elaborated on the ALT skin vessel anatomy, identifying that the ALT flap typically had one to three skin vessels and established a classification depending on where the source vessels are from: descending, transverse branch of the lateral circumflex femoral artery, or the profunda femoris artery.[3] Wong et al. identified an additional oblique branch from the lateral circumflex femoral artery as a source vessel for the ALT flap.[4] Ultimately, the ease of harvesting the ALT flap is directly related to the presence of a septocutaneous skin vessel or musculocutaneous perforator and the length of a perforator's intramuscular course.[3,4]

The 2002 article also demonstrated that in 1% of cases, no sizable skin vessels are encountered in the ALT flap despite reassuring preoperative Doppler signals. In that scenario, the flap can be salvaged by converting to a myocutaneous flap by including the underlying vastus lateralis muscle or shifting to tensor fascia lata flap or anteromedial thigh flap from the same donor wound.[6–9] Yu found an inverse relationship between the presence of ALT skin vessels and AMT skin vessels where patients with one or fewer ALT skin vessels are four times more likely to have skin vessels from the AMT system though the quality of the evidence is not high.[9]

Over time, the applications and indications for the ALT flap have expanded. Preserving the distal runoff allows it to be used as a flow through flap, to facilitate reconstructing extensive, multiple subunit defects which require double free flaps. The ALT flap can also be used as a pedicled flap for knee, lower abdomen, and pelvis, including external genitalia and urinary bladder.[10,11]

As reconstructive surgeons became more adept with microsurgical techniques, the need to adhere to named flaps with named pedicle vessels diminished. As long as a skin vessel can be identified in the supra- or subfascial plane, and the surgeon is able to complete an intramuscular dissection to retrogradely trace the skin vessels to its originating vessel, a free flap can be harvested from any part of the body. This concept of free style flap was first introduced in thigh-based skin flaps by Wei and Mardini in 2003 as the next evolution from ALT free flaps.[12]

Current Innovations

Reconstructive microsurgery continues to pursue ever higher free flap survival and reliability, despite being already 97%–98% in major medical centers globally. Innovations in imaging are being utilized to replace some of the guesswork and uncertainty in microsurgery. One such innovation that is particularly noteworthy is ultra-high-frequency ultrasound. With linear probes emitting 48 and 70mHz waves, surgeons can visualize vessels as small as 30 micrometers to allow preoperative vessel selection for raising thin and ultra-thin ALT flaps.[13,14] Another technology is the use of indocyanine green and fluorescence imaging to perform real-time objective measurements of tissue perfusion,[15] as well as to detect vasculature less than 0.2 in diameter.[15]

CONCLUSION

The most valuable part of this landmark paper "Have we found an ideal soft-tissue flap? An experience with 672 anterolateral thigh flaps" was laying the groundwork for establishing ALT flap as the primary workhorse flap, transforming microsurgical coverage and soft tissue reconstruction in recent decades.

REFERENCES

1. Wei F Chan, Jain V, Celik N, Chen H Chi, Chuang DCC, Lin C Hung. Have we found an ideal soft-tissue flap? An experience with 672 anterolateral thigh flaps. *Plast Reconstr Surg.* 2002;109(7):2219–2226; discussion 2227–2230. doi:10.1097/00006534-200206000-00007.
2. Song Y Guang, Chen G Zhang, Song Y Liang. The free thigh flap: a new free flap concept based on the septocutaneous artery. *Br J Plast Surg.* 1984;37(2):149–159. doi:10.1016/0007-1226(84)90002-X.
3. Yu P. Characteristics of the anterolateral thigh flap in a Western population and its application in head and neck reconstruction. *Head Neck.* 2004;26(9):759–769. doi:10.1002/hed.20050.

4. Wong CH, Wei FC, Fu B, Chen YA, Lin JY. Alternative vascular pedicle of the anterolateral thigh flap: the oblique branch of the lateral circumflex femoral artery. *Plast Reconstr Surg.* 2009;123(2):571. doi:10.1097/PRS.0b013e318195658f.
5. Lakhiani C, Lee MR, Saint-Cyr M. Vascular anatomy of the anterolateral thigh flap: a systematic review. *Plast Reconstr Surg.* 2012;130(6):1254–1268. doi:10.1097/PRS.0b013e31826d1662.
6. Hsieh CH, Yang JCS, Chen CC, Kuo YR, Jeng SF. Alternative reconstructive choices for anterolateral thigh flap dissection in cases in which no sizable skin perforator is available. *Head Neck.* 2009;31(5):571–575. doi:10.1002/hed.20995.
7. Contedini F, Negosanti L, Pinto V, *et al.* Tensor fascia latae perforator flap: an alternative reconstructive choice for anterolateral thigh flap when no sizable skin perforator is available. *Indian J Plast Surg.* 2013;46(1):55–58. doi:10.4103/0970-0358.113707.
8. Namgoong S, Yoon YD, Yoo KH, Han SK, Kim WK, Dhong ES. Alternative choices for anterolateral thigh flaps lacking suitable perforators: a systematic review. *J Reconstr Microsurg.* 2018;34(7):465–471. doi:10.1055/s-0038-1639366.
9. Yu P. Inverse relationship of the anterolateral and anteromedial thigh flap perforator anatomy. *J Reconstr Microsurg.* 2014;30(7):463–468. doi:10.1055/s-0034-1370361.
10. Gravvanis AI, Tsoutsos DA, Karakitsos D, *et al.* Application of the pedicled anterolateral thigh flap to defects from the pelvis to the knee. *Microsurgery.* 2006;26(6):432–438. doi:10.1002/micr.20267.
11. Felici N, Felici A. A new phalloplasty technique: the free anterolateral thigh flap phalloplasty. *J Plast Reconstruct Aesthet Surg.* 2006;59(2):153–157. doi:10.1016/j.bjps.2005.05.016.
12. Mardini S, Tsai FC, Wei FC. The thigh as a model for free style free flaps. *Clin Plast Surg.* 2003;30(3):473–480. doi:10.1016/S0094-1298(03)00047-6.
13. Visconti G, Bianchi A, Hayashi A, Salgarello M. Pure skin perforator flap direct elevation above the subdermal plane using preoperative ultra-high frequency ultrasound planning: A proof of concept. *J Plast Reconstruct Aesthet Surg.* 2019;72(10):1700–1738. doi:10.1016/j.bjps.2019.06.016.
14. Yoshimatsu H, Hayashi A, Yamamoto T, *et al.* Visualization of the "intradermal plexus" using ultrasonography in the dermis flap: a step beyond perforator flaps. *Plast Reconstr Surg Glob Open.* 2019;7(11):e2411. doi:10.1097/GOX.0000000000002411.
15. Ludolph I, Horch RE, Arkudas A, Schmitz M. Enhancing safety in reconstructive microsurgery using intraoperative indocyanine green angiography. *Frontiers in Surgery.* 2019;6:39. Accessed January 14, 2024. https://www.frontiersin.org/articles/10.3389/fsurg.2019.00039. PMID: 31334246; PMCID: PMC6614526.

EXPERT COMMENTARY

Lianne N.Y. Leung

Objective of Study

Review the Advantages and Versatility of Anterolateral Thigh (ALT) Flap for Soft Tissue Reconstruction and to Describe the Anatomy and Techniques for ALT Flap Harvest

Study Design

Retrospective cohort from a single institution.

Sample Size

- 672 ALT flaps in 660 patients

Results

- *Flap type*: 439 musculocutaneous perforator flaps, 58 septocutaneous perforator flaps, 95 musculocutaneous flaps, 63 chimeric flaps.

- *Region of reconstruction*: 484 head and neck, 58 upper extremity, 121 lower extremity, 9 trunk.

- *Flap survival*: Total flap failure in 12 patients (1.79%), partial flap failure in 17 patients (2.53%). Overall flap success rate of 95.68%. The only other outcome measure was donor site healing/closure.

The anterolateral thigh flap was first described by Song et al.[1] in 1984 and subsequently its clinical applications were further promoted by Koshima et al. in 1993.[2] Song described the flap harvested based on septocutaneous perforators arising from a point where the rectus femoris, vastus lateralis, and tensor fascia lata meet. However, subsequent studies illustrated that septocutaneous perforators are relatively uncommon compared with musculocutaneous perforators.[3] Due to the perceived wide range of anatomical variation of the perforators and the possibility of absence of perforators, this flap had not gained widespread popularity at the time this study was published. In this study there were only 6 cases with no perforators identified (<1%) and musculocutaneous perforators were found in 87.1% with only 12.9 % being septocutaneous perforators. At the present time, anxiety over the inability to identify perforators intraoperatively has been ameliorated by collective experience and can be further reduced by advancements in preoperative imaging, such as CT angiogram (CTA) and color Doppler ultrasound (CDU). The use of preoperative CDU to locate fasciocutaneous perforators was first described by Hallock in 1994.[4] Recent meta-analysis including 23 studies of perforator localization in ALT flaps found that CDU has a perforator localization sensitivity of 95.3%, compared to 90.4% with CTA.[5]

This paper discusses the anatomy of the ALT flap and describes the harvest techniques with different thicknesses (suprafascial, fasciocutaneous, myocutaneous), chimeric, and as a flow through flap. This series found that the anatomy of the main pedicle – the descending branch of lateral circumflex femoral artery – is consistently located in intermuscular space between the rectus femoris and vastus lateralis along with the nerve to vastus lateralis. This pedicle is usually 8–16 cm, consists of an artery accompanied by two venae comitantes, and has a vessel diameter >2 mm. The authors advocate using surface landmark of a midpoint between a line drawn from ASIS to the superolateral corner of the patella. When a circle with radius 3 cm is drawn around the midpoint, most skin perforators are found located in the lateral and inferior quadrant of this circle. More recent clinical and cadaveric studies of ALT perforators have found the mean number of perforators to range from 1.15 to 4.26 per thigh.[6] Although the majority of perforators arise from the descending branch of the lateral circumflex femoral artery (LCFA), they can also originate from the transverse branch of the LCFA, the LCFA proper, the profunda femoris, or directly from the femoral artery. Variability of perforator location also exists within the same individual between the left and right thighs.

Various advantages of the ALT flap for soft tissue reconstruction include a large volume of tissue available with minimal donor morbidity, long pedicle with sizable vessel diameters, ease of harvest in the supine position (amenable to a two-team approach), and the general versatility of this flap. Flap thickness can be tailored to the recipient site by harvesting suprafascially, as a fasciocutaneous flap, or as a (chimeric) myocutaneous flap if bulk or other components are needed. Further evolution of thin ALT harvest have been described, such as the superthin and ultrathin ALT flap when harvested at the superficial fascia or through the superficial fat.[7]

The donor site can often be closed primarily; partial-thickness skin grafts (PTSG) could be performed for larger defects as described in this paper. Further efforts to avoid the poor cosmesis of PTSG can be achieved by using the KISS flap technique described by Zhang where multiple small skin paddles are raised on individual perforators and then inset side by side to cover a large wide defect whilst allowing direct closure of their individual donor sites.[8] Other methods include using a retrograde or anterograde pedicle flap based on a proximal or distal perforator to close the donor site in a VY advancement pattern.[9] Keystone flaps have also been used.

In this paper the ALT flap was most commonly used to reconstruct head and neck defects. Its versatile design as a potential chimeric flap allows it to be customized to many different defects. Multiple perforators allow for an ALT flap to be harvested as multiple separate skin islands. This is useful in complex head and neck defects requiring internal mucosal lining and external skin reconstruction. Vastus lateralis muscle or rectus femoris muscle can be harvested in chimeric fashion to obliterate cavities whilst the cutaneous islands resurface the cheek skin and or oral mucosal surfaces. ALT flaps with innervated vastus lateralis muscle can be used in dynamic tongue reconstruction for subtotal/total glossectomy defects or facial reanimation in advanced parotidectomy malignancies. ALT flaps with vascularized motor nerve and fascia lata chimeric flaps has been used for facial nerve reconstruction with a static sling to the oral commissure.

Extremity reconstruction often involves defects with tendon, nerve, or vascular injury, and reconstructions over the distal extremity should be sensate for maximal function. The lateral femoral cutaneous nerve can be included to give a sensate flap. Chimeric fascia lata ALT flaps can reconstruct tendon gaps whilst also providing soft tissue cover, such as hand dorsum extensor tendon reconstruction and Achilles tendon reconstruction.[10] As a flow through flap, it is superior to other options when a large defect with a long vascular gap needs to be reconstructed.

Of the 672 ALT flaps in this paper, only 9 were used in trunk reconstruction. This reflects the fact that other flaps, such as deep inferior epigastric perforator flap, superior epigastric artery perforator flap, internal mammary artery perforator flap, or thoracodorsal artery perforator flap (TDAP) remain popular choices in this region.

The TDAP and its chimeric combinations using the subscapular system have similar versatility to the ALT flap. Their main disadvantage is the position change required when reconstructing defects in the supine position. They can be successfully harvested in the (modified) supine position, but this necessitates a greater learning curve.

As we gain more understanding of perforator angiosomes and vascular supply, there has been a paradigm shift where perforator flaps have become the preferred method of reconstruction. A reliable perforator flap is characterized as consistently having at least one good perforator with a diameter more than 0.5 mm and with a predictable and consistent pedicle anatomy and reasonable pedicle length.[11] The ALT perforator flap fulfills these criteria and is an essential addition to a reconstructive surgeon's armamentarium. With the skills to harvest an ALT flap, a surgeon can deal with the majority of soft tissue defects that may be encountered. Over the past 20 years, this flap is certainly one the most popular soft tissue free flaps for head and neck reconstruction. With advances in oncological treatment, patients are enjoying longer survival and are demanding more for function and/or cosmesis. Many secondary procedures are being performed after remission to replace the initial free flap with a combination of local flaps and tissue expansion techniques. Furthermore, it is not uncommon for patients to survive through two to three recurrences in which both ALT flaps have been exhausted, and, hence demands are made that reconstructive surgeons be equipped with ability to harvest diverse range of perforator flaps and even freestyle perforator flaps.

REFERENCES

1. Song, Y., Chen, G., & Song, Y. (1984). The free thigh flap: A new free flap concept based on the septocutaneous artery. *British Journal of Plastic Surgery, 37*(2), 149–159. https://doi.org/10.1016/0007-1226(84)90002-x.
2. Koshima, I., Fukuda, H., Yamamoto, H., Moriguchi, T., Soeda, S., & Ohta, S. (1993). Free anterolateral thigh flaps for reconstruction of head and neck defects. *Plastic and Reconstructive Surgery, 92*(3), 421–428. https://doi.org/10.1097/00006534-199309000-00005.
3. Kimata, Y., Uchiyama, K., Ebihara, S., Nakatsuka, T., & Harii, K. (1998). Anatomic variations and technical problems of the anterolateral thigh flap: A report of 74 cases. *Plastic and Reconstructive Surgery, 102*(5), 1517–1523. https://doi.org/10.1097/00006534-199810000-00026.
4. Hallock, G. G. (1994). Evaluation of fasciocutaneous perforators using color duplex imaging. *Plastic and Reconstructive Surgery, 94*(5), 644–651. https://doi.org/10.1097/00006534-199410000-00012.
5. Moore, R., Mullner, D., Nichols, G., Scomacao, I., & Herrera, F. (2021). Color Doppler ultrasound versus computed tomography angiography for preoperative anterolateral thigh flap perforator imaging: A systematic review and meta-analysis. *Journal of Reconstructive Microsurgery, 38*(07), 563–570. https://doi.org/10.1055/s-0041-1740958.
6. Smith, R. K., Wykes, J., Martin, D. T., & Niles, N. (2017). Perforator variability in the Anterolateral Thigh Free Flap: A systematic review. *Surgical and Radiologic Anatomy, 39*(7), 779–789. https://doi.org/10.1007/s00276-016-1802-y.
7. Cha, H. G., Hur, J., Ahn, C., Hong, J. P., & Suh, H. P. (2023). Ultra-thin anterolateral thigh free flap: An adipocutaneous flap with the most superficial elevation plane. *Plastic & Reconstructive Surgery. 152*(4), 718e–723e. https://doi.org/10.1097/prs.0000000000010295. Epub 2023 Feb 14. PMID: 36780355.
8. Zhang, Y. X., Hayakawa, T. J., Levin, L. S., Hallock, G. G., & Lazzeri, D. (2016). The economy in autologous tissue transfer. *Plastic and Reconstructive Surgery, 137*(3), 1018–1030. https://doi.org/10.1097/01.prs.0000479971.99309.21.

9. Pachón Suárez, J. E., Sadigh, P. L., Shih, H.-S., Hsieh, C.-H., & Jeng, S. F. (2014). Achieving direct closure of the anterolateral thigh flap donor site—an algorithmic approach. *Plastic and Reconstructive Surgery Global Open*, 2(10), e232. https://doi.org/10.1097/gox.0000000000000205. PMID: 25426349; PMCID: PMC4236377.

10. Sơn, T. T., Dung, P. T., Thúy, T. T., Nghĩa, P. T., & Chiến, V. H. (2024). Using free chimeric anterolateral thigh flap for reconstruction of composite dorsal hand defect. *JPRAS Open*, 39, 106–113. https://doi.org/10.1016/j.jpra.2023.11.011.

11. Choi, J.-W., Alshomer, F., & Kim, Y.-C. (2022). Current status and evolution of microsurgical tongue reconstructions, part I. *Archives of Craniofacial Surgery*, 23(4), 139–151. https://doi.org/10.7181/acfs.2022.00654.

EDITOR COMMENTARY

I think every microsurgeon has read this paper. The number of flaps is staggering for a single team in just over 4 years.

I remember assisting in the elevation of what was then the first ALT flap in HK. We had a printout of this paper to guide us. We were so nervous about cutting these "perforators" that it took hours. Remarkably, it has become the workhorse flap in head and neck reconstruction in my practice. Most often localizing the perforators with a handheld Doppler (HHD) suffices as long as you are aware that there is a significant false-positive rate and often the position where the perforator goes to skin is a little off. Some suggest that even HHD is not needed, relying simply on the landmark (a 3 cm radius circle at the midpoint of a line from ASIS to the superolateral patella), but this seems to be taking things a bit too far; after all, the HHD is cheap and quick to use. It is preferable to have a better idea of perforator position when harvesting smaller flaps or multiple skin islands. There was a vogue for these small thermal cameras that connect to smartphones, but their utility over a HHD is limited – when used in a dynamic thermography fashion with a "cold challenge" they allow you to guesstimate perforator positions in a no-touch manner without disturbing your sterile field, which is useful when you do not have access to the sterile intraoperative Doppler probes.

Certainly, unlike the DIEP flap, CTA/MRA preoperative perforator mapping is less useful for the ALT flap, except perhaps in cases after trauma/prior surgery. The septocutaneous vs musculocutaneous question becomes less important as you become more adept with the flap – finding a septocutaneous perforator just becomes a "nice surprise." What I have encountered on occasion are instances where the descending branch is wholly embedded in the vastus lateralis, something I sometimes call the "wholly intramuscular perforator," but it has no significance except for a more tedious dissection.

The pedicled ALT has emerged as a decent second choice flap for phalloplasty in gender affirming surgery, though a separate strategy for the urethra is often needed as the bulk often precludes a "Chang" tube-in-tube design and the presence of hairs is not desirable.

CHAPTER 28

Effects of Cutting Planes on Costal Cartilage Warping

Ratanapoompinyo S, Kiranantawat K. *Plast Reconstr Surg.*
2024 Dec 1;154(6):1219–1228

AUTHOR COMMENTARY

Kidakorn Kiranantawat and Sanathorn Ratanapoompinyo

Why do we think that this study is important to read?

Warping of harvested costal cartilage has long posed a challenge for plastic surgeons performing rhinoplasty. Many surgeons have proposed various methods to minimize this warping effect, such as irradiation,[1] K-wire fixation,[2] etc. From our experience, we have observed that slicing the cartilage in specific planes, regardless of whether they come from the central or peripheral portions of the ribs, is associated with less warping. This approach introduces a new principle that helps surgeons to minimize costal cartilage warping while reducing costal cartilage discard.

This study is an experimental investigation conducted on fresh cadavers. Costal cartilage grafts were obtained by slicing the harvested costal cartilage along 3 primary planes: cephalocaudal, anteroposterior, and parallel to the synchondrosis plane. Each group corresponding to these main planes was further subdivided into grafts taken from the central and peripheral portions. These subgroups were further categorized into three thicknesses: 1 mm, 2 mm, and 3 mm. In total, 207 cartilage grafts were prepared, with approximately 10 pieces per subgroup. All grafts were photographed at the following time intervals: immediate, 30 minutes, 1 hour, 1 day, 1 week, and 1 month. The angle of warping was subsequently measured using Adobe Photoshop (Adobe Inc., San Jose, California, USA).

Follow-Up

All grafts were stored in a normal saline solution at a temperature of 5°C . Photos were taken by the same operator using consistent settings and distances at the following intervals: immediate, 30 minutes, 1 hour, 1 day, 1 week, and 1 month. To find warping angles, all photographs were analyzed using Foulad's method[1] by the same operator.

Inclusion/Exclusion

Inclusion criteria comprised cadavers aged between 18 and 65 years, no known chest wall pathology, and a time of death not exceeding 48 hours. We believe that costal cartilage harvested in this manner resembles the real scenario of rhinoplasty using costal cartilage. Therefore, the results of the study are likely to be applicable to the surgeons' daily practice.

RESULTS

The study demonstrates that grafts exhibited their maximum changes 30 minutes after being cut. All cartilage grafts showed significantly greater warping when cut in the cephalocaudal plane compared to the anteroposterior ($p < 0.001$) and synchondrosis planes ($p < 0.001$) in all thicknesses. Regardless of the cutting plane, the central group generally exhibited less warping than the peripheral group, but this difference was not statistically significant.

Limitations

This study was conducted in vitro. Warping of the cartilage slices was observed with storage at 5°C in a normal saline solution, which is, of course, not the same as the conditions inside the human body. Therefore, the warping effect might be different from that of a real rhinoplasty. However, based on the senior author's experience – having performed structural rhinoplasty using anteroposterior cuts of costal cartilage for internal grafts (including caudal septal extension grafts, spreader grafts, columella strut grafts, and more) for over 10 years – there have been no warping issues or undesirable outcomes associated with using these principles in patients.

An ideal in vivo study could involve cutting costal cartilage grafts and placing them inside the human body, followed by later harvesting to assess warping. However, such an approach would raise ethical concerns and not be practical.

Relevant Study

In the past, studies on cartilage warping have primarily focused on the concepts of "balanced cross-sectional carving" or "concentric vs eccentric carving." It has been found that cartilage grafts carved symmetrically from the central part of the ribs exhibit the least warping. This principle was first introduced by Gibson and Davis,[3] who noted that superficial cuts in cartilage tend to bow toward the perichondrium, while deeper cuts do not. Harris found that cartilage cut peripherally warped twice as much as cartilage cut centrally.[4]

Numerous surgeons and colleagues have reported results consistent with the "balanced cross-sectional carving" principle.[1] For example, Kim et al. discovered that eccentric dorsal onlay grafts warped more than concentric dorsal onlay grafts.[5] Lopez confirmed that central grafts exhibited significantly less warping than peripheral grafts in an in vivo study conducted with live pigs.[6] Similarly, Safvet found that central grafts with thicknesses of 1–3 mm warped less than peripheral grafts, while grafts thicker than 4 mm did not show the same trend.[7]

Recently, more studies have focused on cutting planes. One study by Fargas and his team compared the anteroposterior and cephalocaudal planes.[8] However, both groups used the balanced cross-section technique, and no statistically significant differences were found. The study had a low sample size of grafts and cadavers. Moreover, the study did not address whether age differences among cadavers were significant or not.

Teshima TL et al. introduced a new method of cutting grafts called "transverse junctional sliced grafts." The study compared three methods – transverse junctional sliced grafts, concentric, and eccentric – and found that the newly proposed method exhibited the least warping. However, the literature did not clearly differentiate between the concentric and transverse junctional sliced methods.[9]

Eren Tastan et al. proposed the "oblique split method," which involves cutting costal cartilage at a 45-degree angle to the long axis of the rib to minimize warping and maximize graft length. However, results were based solely on patient satisfaction.[10] Wilson et al. later compared grafts cut using the oblique split technique at a 30° angle to the long axis with concentric anteroposterior cut grafts, finding no statistically significant difference between the two groups.[11]

A review of past literature reveals that many studies lack clear definitions of cutting planes. Comparisons often mix cutting plane methodologies with concentric/eccentric concepts. We believe that the terms "concentric/eccentric" (or "central/peripheral") should be distinctly separated from cutting planes, which have clearer definitions in a three-dimensional perspective.

This study combines these two principles: concentric versus eccentric carving and comparisons of cutting planes – an approach not previously addressed in existing literature. It demonstrates that central (concentric) and peripheral (eccentric) graft warping are not significantly different. This helps to minimize cartilage waste, allowing surgeons to utilize all available graft material effectively. Additionally, this study encompasses the largest sample size of subgroups within the plane categories (anteroposterior, cephalocaudal, and parallel to synchondrosis), each containing 30 samples. Each subgroup was further divided into central and peripheral groups, categorized by thickness (1–3 mm).

Study Impact

This study enhances our understanding of the nature of warping in costal cartilage grafts. The principle of balanced cross-sectional carving may limit surgeons to focusing solely on grafts sliced from the central part, leading to the wasting of the remaining material. A better understanding of the planes can help surgeons save time and optimize the use of costal cartilage. In this study, grafts from the central group exhibited less warping than those from the peripheral group, but the difference was not significant. We believe this study has the largest sample size of cartilage from the central part (n = 98) compared to the peripheral part (n = 109). Furthermore, subgroups from the peripheral anteroposterior and synchondrosis groups showed less warping than the central cephalocaudal group.

Upon detailed analysis, the plane parallel to the synchondrosis is another variation of the anteroposterior plane, as both cuts are made perpendicular to the cephalocaudal plane of the rib. The oblique split method[10,11] is also categorized as a variation of the anteroposterior approach. From the result of this study, cutting cartilage in anteroposterior and synchondrosis planes demonstrated minimal warping compared to significant warping of the cartilage cut in the cephalocaudal plane. Even though the anteroposterior plane shows slightly less warping than the synchondrosis plane, this difference is not statistically significant. Therefore, surgeons can choose any of these anteroposterior cut variations to obtain straight cartilage slices.

In our practice, after slicing the cartilage grafts in the desired plane, most of the peripheral area can still be utilized without additional warping effects. Only two thin outermost peripheral slices of the anteroposterior cut are discarded. At least 75% of the cartilage volume can be used to obtain the straight slices. Moreover, the peripheral part of each slice is also usable without the need to remove it. However, the complete elimination of warping is impossible to achieve. We recommend that surgeons should additionally employ double-opposing techniques to minimize the warping effect. Notably, the maximum warping observed in this study occurred within 30 minutes, aligning with findings from Rod Rohrich's previous research.[12] Therefore, we advise surgeons to place grafts in a normal saline solution and allow the maximum warping to occur at least 30 minutes after the last cut. For dorsal onlay grafts, a wider cartilage piece is necessary. When cutting in the anteroposterior plane, the width might be insufficient, necessitating cuts in the cephalocaudal plane instead. We recommend using the central portion of the cartilage when cutting in the cephalocaudal plane, and ensuring that the grafts are thicker than 3 mm to mitigate warping effects. If this cannot be done, other techniques, such as laminated dorsal onlay graft or diced cartilage, must be considered to minimize cartilage warping.

REFERENCES

1. Foulad A, Ghasri P, Garg R, Wong B. Stabilization of costal cartilage graft warping using infrared laser irradiation in a porcine model. *Arch Facial Plast Surg.* 2010;12(6):405–411.
2. Gunter JP, Clark CP, Friedman RM. Internal stabilization of autogenous rib cartilage grafts in rhinoplasty: A barrier to cartilage warping. *Plast Reconstr Surg.* 1997;100(1):161–169.
3. Gibson T, Davis WB. The distortion of autogenous cartilage grafts: Its cause and prevention. *Br J Plast Surg.* 1958;10:257–274.
4. Harris S, Pan Y, Peterson R, Stal S, Spira M. Cartilage warping: An experimental model. *Plast Reconstr Surg.* 1993;92(5):912–915.
5. Kim DW, Shah AR, Toriumi DM. Concentric and eccentric carved costal cartilage: A comparison of warping. *Arch Facial Plast Surg.* 2006;8(1):42–46.
6. Lopez MA, Shah AR, Westine JG, O'Grady K, Toriumi DM. Analysis of the physical properties of costal cartilage in a porcine model. *Arch Facial Plast Surg.* 2007;9(1):35–39.
7. Ors S. Measurement of warping angle in human rib graft: An experimental study. *Plast Reconstr Surg.* 2018;141(5):1147–1157.

8. Farkas JP, Lee MR, Lakianhi C, Rohrich RJ. Effects of carving plane, level of harvest, and oppositional suturing techniques on costal cartilage warping. *Plast Reconstr Surg.* 2013;132(2):319–325.
9. Teshima TL, Cheng H, Pakdel A, Kiss A, Fialkov JA. Transverse slicing of the sixth-seventh costal cartilaginous junction: A novel technique to prevent warping in nasal surgery. *J Craniofac Surg.* 2016;27(1):e50–e55.
10. Taştan E, Yücel ÖT, Aydın E, Aydoğan F, Beriat K, Ulusoy MG. The oblique split method. *JAMA Facial Plast Surg.* 2013;15(3):198.
11. Wilson GC, Dias L, Faris C. A comparison of costal cartilage warping using oblique split vs concentric carving methods. *JAMA Facial Plast Surg.* 2017;19(6):484–489.
12. Adams WP, Rohrich RJ, Gunter J, Clark C, Robinson J. The rate of warping in irradiated and nonirradiated homograft rib cartilage: a controlled comparison and clinical implications. *Plast Reconstr Surg.* 1999;103(1):265–270.

EDITOR COMMENTARY

The authors detailed the warping of autologous rib grafts in a systematic manner although it is not exactly news to experienced surgeons routinely harvesting rib cartilage (Farkas et al. 2013) who have already formulated their own favorite ways of cutting the cartilage (Tastan et al. 2013). It does provide some decent basic research into how rib cartilage from different regions and cut in different planes warp. Wider clinical adoption will show in the long term how valid the principles are; a better understanding of the behavior of rib cartilage will allow more effective and efficient use. What is missing is offering some sort of explanation for the phenomenon.

Similar work should probably be done on fresh frozen costal cartilage (FFCC), which is increasing in use in the United States. Like the 30-minute wait advocated by the authors, FFCC should fully thawed for at least 1 hour before being placed in the nose – the frozen cartilage is always straight but can later warp on thawing. Straight thawed pieces can be selected or carved from thawed curved FFCC. FFCC does not respond to scoring, unlike septal cartilage.

The take-home message seems to be that central segments of cartilage cut in an AP direction seem least likely to warp. However, delayed warping 1 month after insertion has still been described. Paired bilateral grafts can have a greater tolerance for some degree of warping if the warped pieces can be placed symmetrically.

CHAPTER 29

Early Nerve Grafting for Facial Paralysis after Cerebellopontine Angle Tumor Resection with Preserved Facial Nerve Continuity

Albathi M, Oyer S, Ishii LE, Byrne P, Ishii M, Boahene KO.
JAMA Facial Plast Surg. 2016 Jan–Feb;18(1):54–60

EXPERT COMMENTARY

Alp Ercan and Wei Wang

Research Objective

Objectively investigate how long surgeons need to wait before intervening in patients with uninterrupted facial nerves after CPA tumor excision and not showing any meaningful signs of recovery.

Study Design

A prospective study where patients with an uninterrupted cranial nerve VII after CPA tumor resection at The Johns Hopkins Hospital who subsequently developed significant facial paralysis were followed up to assess whether there is a suitable time limit to wait to allow for viable spontaneous recovery and a date to move forward for facial reanimation surgery when there is no meaningful chance for recovery. Patients who showed no clinical recovery after the first 6 postoperative months were counselled for early facial nerve exploration and nerve transfer with a masseteric or hypoglossal nerve transfer. Patients who agreed to early intervention proceeded to surgery by 12 months after CPA tumor resection. Those who declined early intervention were further observed. A subset of patients with no spontaneous recovery subsequently agreed to intervention and underwent nerve grafting after 12 months.

Sample Size

The study cohort included 62 patients with uninterrupted facial nerves but who developed facial paralysis after CPA tumor resection between January 1, 2009 and March 31, 2015.

DOI: 10.1201/9781003413738-29

Inclusion/Exclusion Criteria

Patients who developed significant facial paralysis (HB grade IV-V-VI) after CPA tumor resection despite having full uninterrupted continuity of facial nerve were recruited for the study. A total of 27 patients showing no meaningful signs of recovery at the 6th month mark were included in the study

Follow-Up

Patients (n = 62) with no signs of recovery who agreed to nerve transfer surgery at various times after 6 months were followed up for a mean of 12 months. Patients who declined nerve transfer surgery despite showing no signs of meaningful recovery were followed up without intervention for a mean time of 20 months.

Results

A total of 35 patients showed spontaneous recovery before the 6th month mark, and, out of the remaining 27, 10 patients underwent nerve grafting by 12 months, 9 patients received grafting after 12 months, and 8 patients had no intervention. In all patients who underwent nerve grafting (19 in total), there were no detectable facial muscle movements or electromyographic (EMG) responses to direct facial nerve stimulation. During surgeries either the masseteric nerve or the hypoglosssal nerve was used as the donor nerve (single source innervation) and when these two sources were compared, masseteric nerve transfer was associated with earlier recovery compared to hypoglossal nerve transfer (5.6 vs 10.8 months, p = .005). Patients who showed no signs of recovery by 6 months after CPA surgery but declined facial reanimation surgery demonstrated, at best, HB grade V recovery after 18 months of observation.

Study Limitations

Like most prospective studies investigating the effect of interventions on a small group of potential patients, a greater sample size would offer further validity to these results. Additionally, as the investigators stressed, a larger cohort in which all patients undergo the same intervention at the same time is needed to more accurately evaluate outcomes after facial reanimation surgery.

Relevant Studies

In 1999, Axon and Ramsden evaluated 184 patients with facial paralysis after vestibular schwannoma resection and concluded that the severity of immediate postoperative clinical facial function was the most accurate predictor of long-term outcomes.[1] The same Johns Hopkins group of investigators who performed this study reported in 2011 that for patients starting with HB grade V or VI function after vestibular schwannoma resection, the postoperative rate of recovery was the most reliable predictor of poor outcome after 1 year.[2]

Study Impacts

When dealing with a post-CPA tumor resection patient with a documented uninterrupted facial nerve but significant facial paralysis, the most vital question for both facial reanimation surgeon and patient is when to intervene.[3-5] In facial reanimation, making the decision if and when to intervene can be very complicated.[6] It is a difficult decision to call time on the spontaneous recovery of a facial nerve in continuum and then potentially disrupt this recovery by opting for another source, whether a different nerve on the same side or contralateral facial nerve; thus, the only feasible option is often just to wait.[7] However, often we do not know for how long we should wait before making a concrete decision. There is a lack of studies with large patient numbers that objectively compared patients operated on after variable intervals after the initial nerve insult, so decisions have been usually based on anecdotal data and the subjective experience of the practitioner.[8]

This prospective study is the first of its kind by setting a deadline to move forward with nerve transfer surgery in the patient not showing significant recovery after the 6-month mark. A period of 6 months affords ample time to salvage the mimetic muscles with a nerve transfer whilst avoiding inadvertently jeopardizing spontaneous recovery of the native facial nerve, which was proven by this study to be very unlikely at this stage.

There are multiple angles to consider when constructing a treatment plan for these patients. The most important ones are:

- The best source of innervation for facial reanimation is the native facial nerve, if there is a chance of an adequately functioning facial nerve then that chance should be taken as it provides the best possible outcome.[9]

- Every second counts. Even though facial reanimation can be delayed up to 2 years in theory, the transition from the recoverable functional muscle tissue to non-functional fibro-fatty tissue does not happen overnight. Therefore, the later re-innervation happens, the lower the chance of adequate recovery than can be possible only with restoring a meaningful mass of contracting muscle.[10,11]

- If there is a point of no (or low chance) return, that can be a proper milestone to move forward with nerve transfer, nerve graft, or a combination of both.

Up until this article, there had been a lack of prospective studies that could give us a projection for a patient at the 6-month mark with no meaningful sign of recovery. The finding that none of the (8) patients who chose not to have surgery achieved any functional recovery is immensely helpful in making an informed decision for both parties involved, the surgeon and the patient. Research has not demonstrated any difference in functional recovery between hypoglossal and masseteric transfer, albeit recovery with a masseteric transfer was usually a tad faster. In our experience, use of the masseteric nerve has significant advantages over the hypoglossal as a donor nerve because it is easier to control and has a lower risk of causing a functional deformity.[12,13] Difficulty in articulation and problems with manipulating food intraorally are unwanted but possible risks of hypoglossal transfer due to weakening of the tongue.[14,15] However, it is still a widely used and viable option. There was a subgroup of patients who elected to have their surgery after the 12th month and thus had a nerve transfer later than remaining patients in the intervention group. No differences were found between two subgroups in the study with the only downside being having to live longer with facial palsy. We believe a larger cohort would show a better recovery in patients who are treated earlier rather than later as they would, in theory, have more muscle mass recovery.

In conclusion, the recovery pattern in the first 6 postoperative months among patients who develop facial paralysis after CPA tumor resection can be a very useful clinical selection tool in deciding to offer facial reanimation surgery or not, because this study demonstrates that occult re-innervation is unlikely when there is no clinical improvement in paralysis after 6 months. That is, the patients who show no clinical signs of improvement over the first 6 postoperative months are unlikely to regain satisfactory facial function without surgical intervention, even though the facial nerve is grossly intact. Therefore, earlier nerve re-routing options will shorten the total duration of paralysis and possibly may result in better recovery compared to intervention at a later stage. With this information, patients can be offered counseling about the prognosis of their facial recovery and can have potentially better outcomes with timely intervention.

REFERENCES

1. Axon PR, Ramsden RT. Intraoperative electromyography for predicting facial function in vestibular schwannoma surgery. *Laryngoscope.* 1999;109(6):922–926.
2. Rivas A, Boahene KD, Bravo HC, Tan M, Tamargo RJ, Francis HW. A model for early prediction of facial nerve recovery after vestibular schwannoma surgery. *Otol Neurotol.* 2011;32(5):826–833.
3. Falcioni M, Fois P, Taibah A, Sanna M. Facial nerve function after vestibular schwannoma surgery. *J Neurosurg.* 2011;115(4):820–826.
4. Isaacson B, Kileny PR, El-Kashlan HK. Prediction of long-term facial nerve outcomes with intraoperative nerve monitoring. *Otol Neurotol.* 2005;26(2):270–273.
5. Boahene K. Facial reanimation after acoustic neuroma resection: options and timing of intervention. *Facial Plast Surg.* 2015;31(2):103–109.
6. Samii M, Matthies C. Management of 1000 vestibular schwannomas (acoustic neuromas): the facial nerve–preservation and restitution of function. *Neurosurgery.* 1997;40(4):684–694.
7. Tos T, Caye-Thomasen P, Stangerup SE, Thomsen J, Tos M. Need for facial reanimation after operations for vestibular schwannoma: patients perspective. *Scand J Plast Reconstr Surg Hand Surg.* 2003;37(2):75–80.
8. Terzis JK, Konofaos P. Experience with 60 adult patients with facial paralysis secondary to tumor extirpation. *Plast Reconstr Surg.* 2012;130:51e–66e.
9. Terzis JK, Tzafetta K. The "babysitter" procedure: minihypoglossal to facial nerve transfer and cross-facial nerve grafting. *Plast Reconstr Surg.* 2009;123:865–876.
10. Kobayashi J, Mackinnon SE, Watanabe O, *et al.* The effect of duration of muscle denervation on functional recovery in the rat model. *Muscle Nerve.* 1997;20:858–866.
11. Carraro U, Catani C, Dalla Libera L. Myosin light and heavy chains in rat gastrocnemius and diaphragm muscles after chronic denervation or reinnervation. *Exp Neurol.* 1981;72:401–412.
12. Harris BN, Tollefson TT. Facial reanimation. *Curr Opin Otolaryngol Head Neck Surg.* 2015;23(5):399–406.
13. Cheng A, Audolfsson T, Rodriguez-Lorenzo A, Wong C, Rozen S. A reliable anatomic approach for identification of the masseteric nerve. *J Plast Reconstr Aesthet Surg.* 2013;66(10):1438–1440.
14. Kalantarian B, Rice DC, Tiangco DA, Terzis JK. Gains and losses of the XII-VII component of the "baby-sitter" procedure: a morphometric analysis. *J Reconstr Microsurg.* 1998;14:459–471.
15. Mersa B, Tiangco DA, Terzis JK. Efficacy of the "baby-sitter" procedure after prolonged denervation. *J Reconstr Microsurg.* 2000;16:27–35.

EDITOR COMMENTARY

The "watch and wait" strategy has been likened to purgatory for patients with facial palsy, particularly children. The authors of this study found that 6 months was a workable time to make a judgment on the likelihood of spontaneous recovery. A prior model from the same institution had estimated that at this point, the chance that ultimately there would be no recovery (i.e., "futile" waiting) could be predicted with 97% specificity and sensitivity (Rivas A et al., 2011). A mixed retrospective study from Michigan (Luryi AL et al., 2020) found that at 180 days, 83.7% had achieved their final level of facial nerve function. In this study, cases that opted for early surgery showed no evidence of "occult recovery" upon intraoperative EMG at the time of surgery whilst cases that declined surgery showed more limited recovery (HB V).

Whilst it is unclear if earlier intervention would yield better results (and there are good theoretical advantages to earlier reinnervation), there is no point (beyond the 3% chance) in waiting longer, and the patient can be spared 6 months or more of extra pointless waiting.

The option of the masseteric nerve is also a convenient and relatively simple alternative to the hypoglossal nerve (Wang W et al., 2014).

REFERENCES

Luryi AL, Babu S, Michaelides EM, Bojrab DI, Kveton JF, Hong RS, Jacob JT, Schutt CA. Natural history of facial weakness following surgery of the cerebellopontine angle: a tertiary care cohort. *Otol Neurotol.* 2020;41(10):e1284–e1289. doi: 10.1097/MAO.0000000000002427

Rivas A, Boahene KD, Bravo HC, Tan M, Tamargo RJ, Francis HW. A model for early prediction of facial nerve recovery after vestibular schwannoma surgery. *Otol Neurotol.* 2011 Jul;32(5):826–833. doi: 10.1097/MAO.0b013e31821b0afd.

Wang W, Yang C, Li Q, Li W, Yang X, Zhang YX. Masseter-to-facial nerve transfer: a highly effective technique for facial reanimation after acoustic neuroma resection. *Ann Plast Surg.* 2014 Sep;73 Suppl 1:S63–S69. doi: 10.1097/SAP.0000000000000246.

CHAPTER 30

Developmental Biology and Classification of Congenital Anomalies of the Hand and Upper Extremity

Oberg KC, Feenstra JM, Manske PR, Tonkin MA.
J Hand Surg Am. 2010 Dec;35(12):2066–2076

EXPERT COMMENTARY

Jeannette Ting

In 1964, Alfred Swanson published a paper in *Bulletin: Academy of Medicine of New Jersey* describing a classification for congenital malformations of the hand.[1] He addressed the need to clearly classify conditions that affected one or more units of the upper limb. This became known as the Swanson classification of congenital hand anomalies. It was a groundbreaking paper and was published just as one of the most devastating medical disasters was unfolding – the use of thalidomide in pregnant women. Thalidomide was thought to have been responsible for thousands of miscarriages and many cases of phocomelia. This classification facilitated communication between health professionals and allowed for a more accurate collection of data for research, follow-up, and audit. In 1974, the International Federation of Society for Surgery of the Hand (IFSSH) adopted this as the classification system, known then simply as the Swanson classification, for congenital anomalies, and it was used almost universally.

For over 50 years the Swanson classification was "the" classification for congenital hand anomalies. It was easy to use as it was based predominantly on the phenotypical appearance of the anomaly as well as on some developmental assumptions. However, it was criticized for not having a true embryological basis. In addition, there was overlap of several presentations whilst some conditions, such as constriction band syndrome, were added almost as an after-thought. Some conditions were excluded with failure to recognize some developmentally related anomalies, e.g., patients with cleft hands. It was difficult to classify them properly, resulting in a modified classification proposed by Ogino in 1996,[2] which was adopted by the Japanese Society of Hand Surgery.

In 2010, Oberg, Feenstra, Manske, and Tonkin published this paper, which has changed the way we think about and, therefore, classify congenital limb anomalies. Over time, their classification became known as the OMT classification named after the 3 main authors. Interestingly, the authors came together from different backgrounds and

DOI: 10.1201/9781003413738-30

different countries. Kerby Oberg is currently a Professor of Anatomy, a paediatric pathologist, and a developmental biologist who has a special interest in congenital variations. He runs the Molecular Embryopathy Research Laboratory at Loma Linda University in the United States. Paul Manske, who passed away soon after this paper appeared in 2011, was an orthopedic surgeon who mainly worked at St. Louis Children's Hospital and Shriner's Hospital for Children also at St. Louis. He was the longest serving editor in chief of the *Journal of Hand Surgery*. Michael Tonkin is an orthopedic surgeon and a professor working at Royal North Shore Hospital in Australia and was a past president of the International Federation of Societies for Surgery of the Hand (IFSSH, 2013–2016).

In 2014, the IFSSH Committee on Congenital Conditions officially adopted the "OMT" classification as the official classification system for congenital anomalies of the hand and upper limb. The main advantages of the OMT classification are that it considers the anomaly based on the variation to growth according to its underlying embryological variation. It also classifies the anomaly based on how much of the upper limb is involved whilst using widely used terms which surgeons are familiar with. Another advantage of the classification system is that it allows for classification of more than one diagnosis, including syndromes.

This landmark paper published in 2010 followed on from an earlier paper by Manske and Oberg a year before which had proposed modifications to the Swanson classification.[3] This current paper is divided into several sections. Following the introduction, it details the normal embryology of limb development. This is followed by a description of the embryology of the anomalies according to disruption of various axis of growth, abnormality in hand plate formation and differentiation, and deficiencies in differentiation of soft tissue and skeletal elements of the upper limb. The remaining pages subsequently explain the shortcomings of the Swanson classification and justify the need for their new classification system.

Swanson initially classified upper limb anomalies into 7 categories, namely failure of formation, failure of differentiation, duplication, overgrowth, undergrowth, constriction band syndrome and generalized skeletal disorder. The OMT classification in this paper named their categories as malformations, deformations, and dysplasia. Interestingly, the two classification systems share the same name for the first item, "malformation," but, on closer examination, they are quite different. The new OMT system defined the anomaly based on whether there was a failure of axis formation/differentiation in whole upper limb or hand plate in known axis and failure of hand plate formation/differentiation in an unspecified axis. (This can be quite confusing.) There are no other similarities in the subsequent subclassification to this and therefore significantly changes the way we think about congenital upper limb anomalies.

The OMT classification has itself undergone significant changes since this particular paper. Whilst the last official update was in in 2020,[4] the most recent IFFSH report was submitted in July 2024.[5] Some of the changes over the years include the simplification of handplate anomalies into one category. The term "failure of" has been replaced by "abnormal" in the category of malformations. Arthrogryposis, classified in this paper as a deformation, is now classified as a malformation involving the entire upper limb. There was also no classification of "Syndromes" in this version of OMT. The paper stated: "it has become less meaningful to separate these into a separate category rather than the presenting limb morphologies." The updated versions of the OMT classification have included 50 syndromes, recognizing that patients could be classified by more than one category and that the syndromes often affect the child's development as a whole person. Patients with trigger digits, obstetric brachial nerve palsy, and cerebral palsy have been excluded from this classification. These conditions are present at birth but are not congenital in origin. These patients require the same skill set and expertise of surgeons and therapists who deal with truly "congenital" anomalies. Implications of this include potential exclusion of funding and research for these patients who nevertheless attend congenital upper limb anomalies clinics. The numbering system – a mixture of numbers, Roman numerals, and capital and small letters can be confusing. Lastly, there are still recognized classification controversies that remained unresolved in the last official OMT update in 2020.[4]

By no means is our understanding of upper limb embryology complete and by no means is this classification system perfect. IFSSH has suggested the need to revisit and appraise the system on a 3-yearly basis. This effort to ensure that the classification keeps up with our increased understanding of upper limb embryology is commendable. However, it does mean that it could be difficult for readers to keep abreast of its changes. This landmark paper in congenital upper limb anomalies has incited discussion amongst hand surgeons and has been pivotal in promoting increased interest in formation of registries[6] and, therefore, advancing improved patient care in the long term.

REFERENCES

1. Swanson AB. A classification for congenital malformations of the hand. *NJ Bull Acad Med.* 1964 Oct;10:166–169.
2. Ogino T. Modified IFSSH classification. *J Japan Soc Surg Hand.* 2000;17:353–365.
3. Manske PR, Oberg KC. Classification and developmental biology of congenital anomalies of the hand and upper extremity. *J Bone Jt Surg.* 2009;91(Suppl. 4):3–18.
4. Goldfarb CA, Ezaki M, Wall LB, Lam WL, Oberg KC. The Oberg-Manske-Tonkin (OMT) classification of congenital upper extremities: update for 2020. *J Hand Surg Am.* [Internet]. 2020;45(6):542–547. Available from: https://www.sciencedirect.com/science/article/pii/S0363502320300071
5. Lam W, Goldfarb C, Huelsemann W, Mccombe D, Wall L. IFSSH Scientific Committee on Congenital Hand Conditions. 2024.
6. Ho PC, Tse WL, Mak M, Koo SCJ, Ting J. The first congenital upper limb anomalies (CULA) database in Hong Kong: registry of CULA in Prince of Wales Hospital. Health and Medical Research Fund. Hong Kong, Oct 2019.

EDITOR COMMENTARY

Classification is necessary to cultivate a common language when dealing with the complex area of congenital hand anomalies. An update/alternative to the Swanson/ IFSSH classification is described in this paper. The Oberg modification that became known as the OMT system incorporates recent advances in understanding, in particular separating malformations from deformations and dysplasia. In simple terms, malformations are abnormalities of formation and/or differentiation of tissues. Deformations are abnormalities that occur after tissue is formed. Dysplasias are abnormalities resulting from a lack of normal organization of cells into tissue. It has been continually refined and expanded. Sletten et al. (2022) found that the OMT classification demonstrates acceptable inter- and intra-observer reliability.

There have been a variety of criticisms (Lowry RB et al., 2017 etc.), particularly with the issue of symbrachydactyly (Goldfarb CA, 2015). The most recent update came in 2020 (Goldfarb CA et al., 2020). An international survey in 2023 (Goldfarb CA et al., 2023) found that over half of the respondents were using the OMT in their daily practice. The reasons given for not using it included the belief that it did not help with patient management and that it took too long to complete, whilst 15% said there were too many problems with the classification itself – the Swanson classification, in their view, was easier to conceptualize.

REFERENCES

Charles A. Goldfarb, Lindley B. Wall, David McCombe, Wiebke Huelsemann, Wee Lam. An international survey on the adoption and practicality of the Oberg, Manske, Tonkin classification. *J Hand Surg Eur.* 2023;48:1233–1236.
Goldfarb CA, Ezaki M, Wall LB, Lam WL, Oberg KC. The Oberg-Manske-Tonkin (OMT) classification of congenital upper extremities: update for 2020. *J Hand Surg Am.* 2020 Jun;45(6):542–547. doi: 10.1016/j.jhsa.2020.01.002. Erratum in: *J Hand Surg Am.* 2020 Aug;45(8):771–772. doi: 10.1016/j.jhsa.2020.06.004.
Goldfarb CA, Wall LB, Bohn DC, Moen P, Van Heest AE. Epidemiology of congenital upper limb anomalies in a midwest United States population: an assessment using the Oberg, Manske, and Tonkin classification. *J Hand Surg Am.* 2015 Jan;40(1):127–132.e1-2. doi: 10.1016/j.jhsa.2014.10.038.
Lowry RB, Bedard T, Kiefer GN, Sass KR. Views on the Oberg-Manske-Tonkin classification system for congenital anomalies of the hand and upper limb. *J Hand Surg Am.* 2017 May;42(5):378–381. doi: 10.1016/j.jhsa.2017.02.018.
Sletten IN, Winge MI, Hülsemann W, Arner M, Hansen KL, Jokihaara J. Inter- and intra-rater reliability of the Oberg-Manske-Tonkin classification of congenital upper limb anomalies. *J Hand Surg Eur Vol.* 2022 Nov;47(10):1016–1024. doi: 10.1177/17531934221107264.

CHAPTER 31

A New Method of Total Reconstruction of the Auricle for Microtia

Nagata Satoru. *Plast Reconstr Surg.* 1993 Aug;92(2):187–201

EXPERT COMMENTARY

Valerie Ho Wai Yee

Ear reconstruction is an art; it is an interplay between the skin envelope and the ear framework. Ideally speaking, the skin envelope should be as thin and natural looking as the native auricular skin with mobility over the framework, while the framework has to be symmetrical to the normal contralateral side if present, durable with time yet also possessing elasticity.

Professor Nagata Satoru modified the traditional methods of ear reconstruction from Tanzer's six-staged approach reported in 1959,[1] Brent's four-stage approach in 1980,[2] to the two-stage approach in this article. A total of 36 patients were included with the longest follow-up at 7 years. The results were satisfactory, consistent, and reproducible. The techniques were described in great detail with clear step-by-step illustrations drawn by the author. The first stage involved fabrication of the three-dimensional framework from the sixth to ninth costal cartilages and, then, after careful planning of skin incisions, meticulous skin flap elevation. After at least 6 months, the second stage would involve elevation of the framework by fixing a semilunar cartilage block between the posterior surface of the reconstructed auricle and mastoid surface. The cartilage over the posterior surface would then be completely covered by the temporoparietal fascial flap, followed by a piece of extremely thin split-thickness skin graft harvested from the scalp secured by a tie-over dressing.

There were no complications of wire penetration or extrusion, no deformation or irregularities of the grafted frame, and no infections or cartilage exposure reported in the series. Nagata's two-stage technique has since become popular among plastic surgeons worldwide.

Generally speaking, microtia has been graded according to severity by Marx,[3] Roger, and Tanzer, into the following grades:

- Marx Grade I
  - Slightly smaller ear than normal
  - All structures are identifiable and essentially normal

DOI: 10.1201/9781003413738-31

- Marx Grade II
  - Small
  - Some features are abnormal while others are recognizable
- Marx Grade III
  - Absence of the external ear with a small deformed vestigial structure with no recognizable features.
  - Often associated with aural atresia
- Marx Grade IV / Anotia
  - Complete absence of the external ear

As microtia is a spectrum of congenital anomalies, no single microtia deformity looks exactly the same as another, and, hence, surgeons need to be well-equipped with various technical approaches to tackle different situations. In view of this, after being inspired by Professor Nagata, Françoise Firmin modified her technical approaches and proposed a surgical classification system, which is summarized as follows[4]:

- *Skin Approach Classification*
  - Type 1: Z-plasty
  - Type 2: Transfixation incision with adhesion
  - Type 3a: Skin-only incision (One stage)
  - Type 3b: Skin-only incision (Two stage)
- *Framework Classification*
  - Type I: Complete framework
  - Type II: Complete framework without a tragus
  - Type III: Complete Framework without a tragus and antitragus
- *Projection Piece Classification*
  - PI: Beneath the root of helix and tragus
  - PII: Beneath the antihelix
  - PIII: Beneath the antitragus and lobule

Firmin has also listed "The 10 Commandments" in Ear Reconstruction Principles for guiding ear reconstructive surgeons-in-training[5]:

1. When analyzing an auricular defect, the first step is always to make a model of the normal ear and place it in the ideal position on the affected side.
2. The auricular skin is the best for reconstructing an ear; fascia flaps should be used only when auricular skin is not available.
3. Skin-only flaps without support cannot reproduce the complex contours of an ear, and the best support currently is autologous cartilage.
4. Conchal cartilage can be used only when the size of the defect is no more than a quarter of the ear and involves no more than two planes; otherwise, costal cartilage must be used.
5. When harvesting conchal cartilage, the entire floor of the conchal bowl must be harvested leaving intact the root of the helix to prevent a visible ear deformity.
6. Once the three-dimensional contours of the ear are understood and after training, sculpting should become the routine part of the surgery and management of the skin the difficult part.

7. Everything will be visible under the very thin auricular skin; therefore, no compromise with the shape of the framework is acceptable.
8. In choosing a skin approach, surgeons should always consider the existing scars and the position of the remnants.
9. Never elevate an ear whose contours are unsatisfactory after the first stage.
10. For consistent results, surgeons must perform ear reconstruction procedures frequently.

The above-mentioned served as the quintessence in ear reconstruction. Notwithstanding that all these are followed, surgeons should always watch out for any potential complications, e.g., skin necrosis, incisural inflammation, haematoma or seroma, scar alopecia, extrusion of wire sutures, keloid, sulcus retraction, infection, cartilage exposure, fracture or cartilage resorption of the framework, fascial flap or skin graft failure, or facial nerve palsy, and they should manage the complications promptly. Finally, the drawbacks of harvesting costal cartilage include pneumothorax, atelectasis, chest wall deformity, pain and hypertrophic scarring, etc.

In autologous reconstruction, the chest wall comorbidities are inevitable. In addition, patients must wait until the cartilage stock is adequate before reconstruction is possible. And even then, the quality of the cartilage may not be optimal if calcification is present. The associated psychological morbidity that young patients face should never be underestimated. Furthermore, the learning curve is steep.

Surgeons have explored many different alloplastic materials for ear reconstruction so that patients can have a new auricle at a younger age regardless of chest wall growth. The use of various materials has been reported since the early 20th century, such as silicone, celluloid, tantalum wire cage, nylon mesh, polyethylene, and acrylic.[6–8] Among these, high-density porous polyethylene produced markedly superior results as the porous structure allows tissue ingrowth and, hence, a more secure integration to the soft tissue over the mastoid region.

John F. Reinisch and Sheryl Lewin clearly described the technique of ear reconstruction using a porous polyethylene framework and coverage by temporoparietal fascia flap and skin grafts in 2009.[9] A total of 786 ear reconstructions were performed over an 18-year period and the complications were closely examined. Complications were common in the initial phase, especially implant fractures (25%) and exposures (44%). With improved implant design and complete coverage of the implant by the temporoparietal fascial flap and the subgaleal fascia, the complication of rim fracture (2.7%) and implant exposure (7.3%) dropped significantly over a follow-up of 12 years. The learning curve was also shorter than that needed for the cartilage method.

The success of porous implant ear reconstruction relies on prevention of complications and an ability to manage the complications promptly should they occur. This was thoroughly reviewed by Lewin in 2015.[10] In 2013, Lewin modified the implant from a two-piece into a one-piece implant, hence eliminating the weak point in the two-piece implant, which was often the culprit for implant fracture.

Mastering and reproducing the harmonious three-dimensional structure of the ear is a prerequisite for the surgeon.[11] Three-dimensional stereo-photogrammetry can provide a mirror image of the normal contralateral ear and aid surgical planning. Chen et al. advocated for this technology and demonstrated that the precision of 3dMD was better than direct measurement. The application is diverse and has extended beyond template production not only in soft tissue analysis to improve surgical outcomes, but also in preoperative counselling and education of patients and parents.[12,13] Patient-specific porous polyethylene implants should offer a better solution for patients in experienced hands. 3D printed bio-scaffolds using synthetic polymer have also been reported in a case series with a follow-up period of 1 year.[14] Longer-term follow-up would be necessary to assess the outcomes and to observe for complications if any.

Finally, reconstructive surgeons should always cooperate closely with otologists on formulating a plan for hearing restoration. HEAR MAPS is a classification for congenital microtia/atresia based on evaluation of 742 patients in a study led by Joseph B. Roberson Jr. and John F. Reinisch.[15] This classification system can help to enhance multidisciplinary communication and hence better coordination of care. Simultaneous auricular reconstruction with a hearing restoration procedure has been shown to be feasible and safe in carefully selected patients.[16]

The current article was selected as one of the *50 Landmark Papers every Plastic Surgeon Should Know* in memory of Satoru Nagata (1950–2022) for his unprecedented revolutions and contributions made in the history of ear reconstruction.

REFERENCES

1. Tanzer RC. Total reconstruction of the external ear. *Plast Reconstr Surg Transplant Bull.* 1959;23:115.
2. Brent B. The correction of microtia with autogenous cartilage grafts: I. The classic deformity? *Plast Reconstr Surg.* 1980;66:112.
3. Marx H. Die Missbildungen des Ohres. In: Henke F, Lubarsh O, eds. *Handbuch der Spez Path Anatomie Histologie.* Berlin, Germany: Springer; 1926:620–625.
4. Firmin F. Ear reconstruction in cases of typical microtia: personal experience based on 352 microtic ear corrections. *Scand J Plast Reconstr Surg Hand Surg.* 1998;32:3547.
5. Firmin F, Dusseldorp JR, Marchac A. *Auricular Reconstruction,* 1st edn. New York: Thieme; 2016.
6. Greeley PW. Reconstructive otoplasty; further observations; utilization of tantalum wire mesh support. *Arch Surg.* 1946;53:24–31.
7. Rubin LR, Robertson GW, Shapiro RN. Polyethelene in reconstructive surgery. *Plast Reconstr Surg (1946).* 1948;3:586–593.
8. Macomber DW. Plastic mesh as a supporting medium in ear reconstruction. *Plast Reconstr Surg Transplant Bull.* 1960;25:248–252.
9. Reinisch JF, Lewin S. Ear reconstruction using a porous polyethylene framework and temporoparietal fascia flap. *Facial Plast Surg.* 2009;25(3):181–189.
10. Lewin S. Complications after total porous implant ear reconstruction and their management. *Facial Plast Surg.* 2015;31(6):617–625.
11. Reinisch J, Tahiri Y. Polyethylene ear reconstruction: a state-of-the-art surgical journey. *Plast Reconstr Surg.* 2018 Feb;141(2):461–470.
12. Chen Z-C, Albdour M, Lizardo J, Chen Y-A, Chen P. Precision of three dimensional stereo-photogrammetry (3dMD™) in anthropometry of the auricle and its application in microtia reconstruction. *J Plast Reconstr Aesthet Surg.* 2015;68:622–631. doi: 10.1016/j.bjps.2015.02.020. Epub 2015 Mar 9. PMID: 25892285.

13. Chen H-Y, Ng L-S, Chang C-S, Lu TC, Chen N-H, Chen Z-C. Pursuing mirror image reconstruction in unilateral microtia: customizing auricular framework by application of three-dimensional imaging and three-dimensional printing. *Plast Reconstr Surg*. 2017;139:1433–1443.
14. Kim M, Kim YJ, Kim YS, Roh TS, Lee EJ, Shim JH, Kang EH, Kim MJ, Yun IS. One-year results of ear reconstruction with 3D printed implants. *Yonsei Med J*. 2024 Aug;65(8):456–462.
15. Roberson JB Jr, Goldsztein H, Balaker A, Schendel SA, Reinisch JF. HEAR MAPS a classification for congenital microtia/atresia based on the evaluation of 742 patients. *Int J Pediatr Otorhinolaryngol*. 2013 Sep;77(9):1551–1554. doi: 10.1016/j.ijporl.2013.07.002.
16. Chan KC, Ho VWY, Chen ZC, *et al*. Simultaneous auricular reconstruction and transcutaneous bone conduction device implantation in patients with microtia. *J Formos Med Assoc*. 2019 Aug;118(8):1202–1210.

EDITOR COMMENTARY

The use of autologous rib cartilage (Tanzer RC, 1959) was a major turning point in modern ear reconstruction. Brent (1980) further advanced reconstruction to the next level 20 years or so later with his safe step-by-step 4-stage technique. He dealt with one of the major issues with previous techniques by moving the lobule in a second stage using a 4-level framework that increased projection whilst the use of suction drainage improved contours and reduced collections and secondary fibrosis. Whilst this technique was capable of consistently delivering what would be regarded as "satisfactory" results, common criticisms included the imperfect contour, particularly around the tragal area, with a tendency for late skin retraction reducing projection.

Nagata describes how he does it in two stages in this paper (1993), effectively condensing the first three Brent stages into one step whilst solving some of the main criticisms of the Brent technique. The major innovations included transposing lobule during first surgery, constructing a framework that includes a tragus whilst constructing the posterior wall of the concha during the second stage. The framework is elevated with additional cartilage to increase projection with coverage by a galeal flap and scalp SSG. The more complete framework requires more cartilage – 4 rib segments – yet there is often less chest deformity due to the preservation of perichondrium. Wire sutures are used to fix the framework with the aim of making it look as though it was made in one piece. The Nagata technique requires particular attention to the blood supply of the flaps, and partial necrosis of the posterior flap is a specific complication of the first stage that needs to be (pro-actively) avoided. The price of these advantages (better appearance, fewer stages) is that it is more challenging. Firmin suggested a training device to specifically practice carving. Poor surgery with the Nagata technique is more likely to give bad results. A further very detailed three paper series appeared during the following year.

Firmin (1998) compared the Brent and Nagata techniques in detail. Her modified Nagata technique with its own improvements is often referred to as the Firmin technique (2010).

REFERENCES

Firmin F. Ear reconstruction in cases of typical microtia. Personal experience based on 352 microtic ear corrections. *Scand J Plast Reconstr Surg Hand Surg*. 1998 Mar;32(1):35–47. doi: 10.1080/02844319850158930.

Firmin F, Marchac A. A novel algorithm for autologous ear reconstruction. *Semin Plast Surg*. 2011 Nov;25(4):257–264. doi: 10.1055/s-0031-1288917.

Nagata S. Modification of the stages in total reconstruction of the auricle: Part I. Grafting the three-dimensional costal cartilage framework for lobule-type microtia. *Plast Reconstr Surg*. 1994 Feb;93(2):221–230.

Nagata S. Modification of the stages in total reconstruction of the auricle: Part II. Grafting the three-dimensional costal cartilage framework for concha-type microtia. *Plast Reconstr Surg*. 1994 Feb;93(2):231–242.

Nagata S. Modification of the stages in total reconstruction of the auricle: Part III. Grafting the three-dimensional costal cartilage framework for small concha-type microtia. *Plast Reconstr Surg*. 1994 Feb;93(2):243–253.

CHAPTER 32

Robotic Davydov Peritoneal Flap Vaginoplasty for Augmentation of Vaginal Depth in Feminizing Vaginoplasty

Jacoby A, Maliha S, Granieri MA, Cohen O, Dy GW, Bluebond-Langner R, Zhao LC. *J Urol.* 2019 Jun;201(6):1171–1176

AUTHOR COMMENTARY

Isabel S. Robinson and Rachel Bluebond-Langner

Study Design

The authors conducted a retrospective review of their experience with gender affirming vaginoplasty using robotically harvested peritoneal flaps to line a portion of the vaginal canal. The da Vinci Xi robot was used in all cases. Chart review collected data on patient demographics, medical comorbidities, preoperative physical exam, intraoperative details, complications, and postoperative vaginal depth and width determined by surgeon-administered dilation exams. Patients' most recent recorded dilation measurements were reported. Patient-reported outcomes measured were not included.

FOLLOW-UP

The average follow-up was 114 ± 79 days after surgery. Patients were evaluated in the office at 2, 3, 4, 6, and 12 weeks, 6 months, and then annually postoperatively. Speculum exams were performed and dilation depth was recorded at each of these visits.

RESULTS

A total of 41 patients were included in this study. Average preoperative penile length was 8.7 ± 2.5 cm. Average age was 34 ± 14 years and the cohort was relatively healthy, although granular data on medical comorbidities is not reported. Average operative time was 262 ± 35 minutes. There were no complications related to peritoneal flap harvest. A total of 20% of patients were noted to have either granulation tissue within the canal or delayed wound healing at the introitus, both of which were managed in the outpatient setting. All patients reported erogenous sensation. At most recent follow-up, average vaginal canal depth was 14.2 ± 0.7 cm and average vaginal canal width was 3.6 ± 0.2 cm.

DOI: 10.1201/9781003413738-32

STUDY LIMITATIONS

This study is limited by its small sample size, relatively short follow-up time, and retrospective single surgical team design. As a preliminary technique paper, there is limited granularity in the reporting of medical history, including puberty blockade, preoperative physical exam measurements other than penile length, and postoperative outcomes including aesthetic satisfaction and patient-reported outcomes. The authors have addressed most of these limitations in subsequent publications.

RELEVANT STUDIES

The use of peritoneal flaps for vaginal canal lining in cases of vaginal agenesis was first described by Davydov in 1965.[2] Prior to the report by Jacoby et al., options for vaginal canal lining in penile inversion vaginoplasty techniques included inverted penile skin flaps, skin grafts harvested from the scrotum or extra-genital donor sites, and acellular dermal matrices.[3]

Since their initial technique description the authors have transitioned from using the da Vinci Xi robot, which is a four-armed system using four to five port sites, to the da Vinci Single Port (SP) system, which uses a single access port for control of three multi-jointed surgical instruments plus a second laparoscopic assistant port.[4,5] In a retrospective comparison of their experience with the two systems, the authors found that the SP system reduced operative time by approximately 30 minutes without a difference in vaginal depth or complication rates.[4]

The use of peritoneal flaps for vaginal canal lining increases the amount of penoscrotal tissue available for vulvoplasty. Vulvar aesthetic complaints are a common indication for revision following vaginoplasty, particularly effacement of the labia minora.[11] The peritoneal flap technique allows the majority of the penile skin to be used for formation of the vulvar subunits rather than canal lining.[12] Long-term studies are needed to determine whether this translates to a quantifiable improvement in vulvar aesthetics.

An important indication for peritoneal flaps is in patients with insufficient penoscrotal tissue for conventional penile inversion vaginoplasty. Prior to this technique the only option for patients with very limited genital tissue was enteric vaginoplasty, which is associated with a significant complication profile.[10] The authors reviewed their outcomes following peritoneal flap vaginoplasty in patients with genital hypoplasia, defined as stretched penile length <7 cm, compared to randomly selected controls with stretched penile lengths ≥7 cm. At 1-year follow-up there were no differences in average vaginal depth or width between the two groups, and no difference in complication rates.

The authors have also described the application of peritoneal flap vaginoplasty to revision vaginoplasty in cases of severe canal stenosis.[6] In a series of 24 patients undergoing vaginal canal revision following standard penile inversion vaginoplasty, average vaginal depth and width were 13.6 cm and 3.6 cm, respectively, at a mean follow-up of 410 days.

While rare, intra-abdominal complications following peritoneal flap harvest have been reported. In their first 274 peritoneal flap vaginoplasties, the authors observed 6 intra-abdominal complications (2.2%), including 2 internal hernias, 2 intra-abdominal abscesses, 1 intra-abdominal hematoma, and 1 patient with recurrent small bowel obstructions without hernia.[7]

STUDY IMPACTS

This is the first report on the use of Davydov peritoneal flaps to line a portion of the vaginal canal in gender affirming vaginoplasty. Since its publication, the use of robotically harvested peritoneal flaps for canal lining in primary and revision vaginoplasty has been adopted by multiple high-volume centers.[8,9] Benefits of the robotically assisted technique include improved visualization during canal dissection, shorter operative times owing to the two-team approach, and decreased reliance on natal penoscrotal tissue, as well as potentially improved long-term aesthetic outcomes.

REFERENCES

1. Jacoby A, Maliha S, Granieri MA, et al. Robotic davydov peritoneal flap vaginoplasty for augmentation of vaginal depth in feminizing vaginoplasty. *J Urol.* 2019;201:1171–1176.
2. Davydov SN. Colpoiesis from the peritoneum of the urorectal space. *Akush Ginek (Moskva).* 1965;45:55–57.
3. Salibian AA, Schechter LS, Kuzon WM, *et al.* Vaginal canal reconstruction in penile inversion vaginoplasty with flaps, peritoneum, or skin grafts: Where is the evidence? *Plast Reconstr Surg.* 2021;147:634e–643e.
4. Dy GW, Jun MS, Blasdel G, Bluebond-Langner R, Zhao LC. Outcomes of gender affirming peritoneal flap vaginoplasty using the da vinci single port versus xi robotic systems. *Eur Urol.* 2021;79:676–683.
5. Robinson IS, Zhao LC, Bluebond-Langner R. Robotics in gender affirming surgery: Current applications and future directions. *Semin Plast Surg.* 2023;37:193–198.
6. Dy GW, Blasdel G, Shakir NA, Bluebond-Langner R, Zhao LC. Robotic peritoneal flap revision of gender affirming vaginoplasty: A novel technique for treating neovaginal stenosis. *Urology.* 2021;154:308–314.
7. Robinson IS, Blasdel G, Bluebond-Langner R, Zhao LC. The management of intra-abdominal complications following peritoneal flap vaginoplasty. *Urology.* 2022;164:278–285.
8. Peters BR, Martin LH, Butler C, Dugi D, Dy GW. Robotic peritoneal flap vs. Perineal penile inversion techniques for gender-affirming vaginoplasty. *Curr Urol Rep.* 2022;23:211–218.
9. Jun MS, Gonzalez E, Zhao LC, Bluebond-Langner R. Penile inversion vaginoplasty with robotically assisted peritoneal flaps. *Plast Reconstr Surg.* 2021;148:439–442.
10. Robinson IS, Cripps CN, Bluebond-Langner R, Zhao LC. Operative management of complications following intestinal vaginoplasty: A case series and systematic review. *Urology.* 2023;180:105–112.
11. Dy GW, Salibian AA, Blasdel G, Zhao LC, Bluebond-Langner R. External genital revisions after gender-affirming penile inversion vaginoplasty: Surgical assessment, techniques, and outcomes. *Plast Reconstr Surg.* 2022;149:1429–1438.
12. Dy GW, Dugi DD, Peters BR. Skin management during robotic peritoneal flap vaginoplasty for penoscrotal hypoplasia secondary to pubertal suppression. *Urology.* 2023 Mar;173:226–227. doi: 10.1016/j.urology.2022.12.020. Epub 2022 Dec 30. PMID: 36592702.

EDITOR COMMENTARY

Gender-affirming surgery has many benefits for those with gender dysphoria and is becoming a larger part of a reconstructive surgery service. Penile inversion vaginoplasty has long been the gold standard for construction of a vagina in transwomen. However, one of the main issues is the inadequate depth due to a shortage of penile skin (average 8.7 cm in this study), exacerbated by the effects of exogenous hormones or previous surgery. The trend for earlier use of puberty blockers is likely to have an impact on the availability of penile skin for vaginoplasty; the advantages of a robotic Davydov technique may be most evident here.

The robot is used to assist in the difficult vaginal canal dissection – with experience in open perineal prostatectomies being lost, this may be another particularly useful feature of using the robot especially in cases of revisional surgery. The average cavity created was 14.2 cm. Patients can usually be discharged on day 5. There are significant additional costs involved, but it is on the cutting edge as demand for GAS is growing. In experienced hands, the operating time does not seem to be extended as the harvest can be done concurrent with the external surgery (vulvoplasty) (Peters et al., 2022). Severe obesity with the attendant risks with pneumoperitoneum and surgical positioning is probably a relative contraindication for robotic surgery.

The Vecchietti technique is another alternative increasing in popularity, particularly for Mayer–Rokitansky–Kuster–Hauser syndrome; Yang (2021) reported on a "simpler" modification with some "home-grown" solutions.

REFERENCES

Peters BR, Martin LH, Butler C, et al. Robotic peritoneal flap vs. perineal penile inversion techniques for gender-affirming vaginoplasty. *Curr Urol Rep.* 2022;23:211–218. doi: 10.1007/s11934-022-01106-9

Yang X, Liang J, Li W, Chen B, Sun X, Xie Z. Modified Vecchietti vaginoplasty using self-made single-port laparoscopy in Mayer-Rokitansky-Küster-Hauser syndrome. *Fertil Steril.* 2021 Jul;116(1):266–268. doi: 10.1016/j.fertnstert.2020.10.001.

CHAPTER 33

The Superficial Musculo-Aponeurotic System (SMAS) in the Parotid and Cheek Area

Mitz V, Peyronie M. *Plast Reconstr Surg.* 1976;58(1):80–88

EXPERT COMMENTARY

Sophie Ricketts

Introduction

Subcutaneous rhytidectomy (the skin only facelift) had been the procedure of choice for facial rejuvenation since its inception sometime in the early 1900s. It became apparent that the undermining, redraping, and excision of skin alone resulted in short-lived surgical outcomes. Tord Skoog, a Swedish plastic surgeon, in 1968 developed a flap to elevate the platysma muscle of the neck and lower part of the face without detaching the skin. Manipulation of these deeper structures of the face was a significant innovation in facelift surgery. Skoog first published his work in his textbook in 1974 (Skoog, 1974 [1]). It was not until 1976 that Vladmir Mitz and Martine Peyronie (Mitz and Peyronie, 1976 [2]), working under the tutelage of Paul Tessier, formally described the anatomical superficial musculo-aponeurotic system (SMAS). The concept and utilization of the SMAS layer in facelifting was a significant paradigm shift and still forms the basis of most techniques that are utilized today.

SUMMARY

Described as the "anatomic basis of the modern facelift," in their groundbreaking 1976 study, Mitz and Peyronie introduced the concept of the SMAS. They described the SMAS in the cheek and parotidomasseteric region as a distinct, fibrous layer that connects the muscles of the face with the dermis. This anatomical layer was characterized by its continuity with the platysma in the neck and the temporoparietal fascia and frontalis muscle in the upper face. They utilized 15 cadaveric dissections, using imaging and histological sectioning to describe this layer. It was found to be thick overlying the parotidomasseteric fascia and thin and discontinuous in the cheek area. The paper describes the anatomical relationships of the SMAS with the facial nerve lying deep to the SMAS along with the facial artery and vein. Overlying the parotid

DOI: 10.1201/9781003413738-33

region, the SMAS can be safely elevated without risk to the facial nerve. Further anterior beyond the parotid, the facial nerve lies relatively unprotected deep to the SMAS. The SMAS was noted to play a significant role in the dynamic movement of facial tissues, providing structural support and a framework for soft tissue manipulation. The dissection studies demonstrated that the SMAS could be mobilized and repositioned independently of the skin, a finding that had profound implications for surgical practice, particularly in achieving longer-lasting facelift outcomes.

IMPLICATIONS FOR THE EVOLUTION OF SURGICAL TECHNIQUES IN FACELIFT

A Paradigm Shift in Facelift Surgery

Prior to the identification of the SMAS, facelifts primarily targeted the skin, resulting in tension-based techniques that often led to unnatural appearances and limited longevity. Mitz and Peyronie's work facilitated better understanding of facial anatomy, enabling surgeons to achieve more effective and longer lasting results by manipulation of the SMAS layer. Many modifications of techniques utilizing this layer were to follow.

Key Advancements Enabled by the SMAS

1. **SMAS Elevation and Plication**: The discovery of the SMAS introduced the concept of plicating to lift, or elevating and repositioning this layer independently of the skin. This innovation allowed for tension redistribution, reducing reliance on skin tightening and yielding more natural outcomes (Baker, 1997 [3]).
2. **Deep-Plane Facelift**: Hamra's deep-plane facelift, developed in the 1990s, capitalized on SMAS manipulation by dissecting below the layer to release the retaining ligaments of the face to allow more extensive repositioning of the soft tissues (Hamra, 1990 [4]). The technique, which elevates a thick musculocutaneous layer comprising skin, subcutaneous fat and the platysma muscle, is described in detail along with possible complications and touts improved appearance of the nasolabial fold, jawline, and neckline.
3. **Composite Facelift**: Building on the deep plane concept, composite facelifts incorporated adjacent structures, such as the orbicularis oculi muscle, to improve not only the midface (elevation of cheek fat) and jawline (platysma muscle elevation) but also the upper facial region (Hamra, 1992 [5]).
4. **Extended and High SMAS Facelift**: The extended and high SMAS technique extended dissection of the SMAS above the zygomatic arch, allowing for enhanced correction of malar fat pad descent and midface volume loss (Stuzin et al., 1995 [7]; Barton, 2002 [8]).
5. **Minimally Invasive Techniques**: Procedures like the minimal access cranial suspension (MACS) lift utilized vertical suspension sutures anchored to the SMAS to achieve facial rejuvenation whilst boasting smaller incisions, with less risk to the facial nerve and quicker recovery times (Tonnard, 2002 [8]).

6. **Extended Deep-Plane Technique**: This technique described by Andrew Jacono extends the sub-SMAS dissection below the mandibular angle allowing for more movement of the deeper structures of the neck as an alternative to the corset platysmaplasty (Jacono, 2011 [9]).

CONCLUSION

The discovery of the SMAS by Mitz and Peyronie marked a turning point in facial plastic surgery. It provided a critical anatomical insight that allowed surgeons to advance beyond skin-only techniques and address the deeper structures responsible for aging. Furthermore, the foundational work by Mitz and Peyronie paved the way for continued innovations in both surgical and non-surgical facial rejuvenation modalities. The SMAS continues to serve as a cornerstone for modern facelift procedures.

REFERENCES

1. Skoog, T. *Plastic Surgery: New Methods and Refinements*. Philadelphia: Saunders; 1974.
2. Mitz V, Peyronie M. The superficial musculosaponeurotic system (SMAS) in the parotid and cheek area. *Plast Reconstr Surg.* 1976;58(1):80–88.
3. Baker DC. Lateral SMASectomy. *Plast Reconstr Surg.* 1997;100(2):509–513.
4. Hamra ST. The deep-plane rhytidectomy. *Plast Reconstr Surg.* 1990;86(1):53–61.
5. Hamra ST. Composite rhytidectomy. *Plast Reconstr Surg.* 1992;90(1):1–13.
6. Stuzin JM, Baker TJ, Gordon HL. Extended SMAS dissection as an approach to midface rejuvenation. *Clin Plast Surg.* 1995;22(2):295–311.
7. Barton FE. The "high SMAS" face lift technique. *Aesthetic Surg J.* 2002;22:481–486
8. Tonnard P, Verpaele A. The MACS-lift: a minimal access cranial suspension lift. *Plast Reconstr Surg.* 2002;109(6):2285–2298.
9. Jacono AA, Parikh SS. The minimal access deep plane extended vertical facelift. *Aesthet Surg J.* 2011;31(8):874–890.

EDITOR COMMENTARY

It seems somewhat amusing that the elucidation of this somewhat bland simplistic anatomical feature is often heralded as one of the greatest advances that resulted in a major paradigm shift in facelift surgery. It is a condensed layer that is distinct from the parotid fascia that sometimes has muscle fibres, thus "musculoaponeurotic." In the parotid area, only sensory nerves lie above the SMAS (and pierce it), whilst the facial nerve lies protected in the parotid gland.

First, Skoog realized that manipulation of this deeper "buccal fascia" (besides the skin only) led to improved fascial contours and longer-lasting results. Several years later in 1974, Mitz and Peyronie presented their work at the French Society of Plastic Surgeons. They provided a great deal of anatomical details, including the relationship of the SMAS to nearby structures, such as nerves, vessels, parotid gland, and muscles. They go on to argue that mobilization of the SMAS is safe and results in a more effective lift compared to only undermining the skin. However, there were no clinical outcomes reported in their paper.

Others built further on this work. Sam Hamra described a deep-plane lift in conjunction with a "Skoog-type sub-SMAS dissection" to correct the nasolabial folds and jaw/neckline. Certainly elucidation of the SMAS has proved to be the foundation of modern facelifts.

CHAPTER 34

Fifteen-Year Survey of One-Stage Latissimus Dorsi Muscle Transfer for Treatment of Longstanding Facial Paralysis

Takushima A, Harii K, Asato H, Kurita M, Shiraishi T.
J Plast Reconstr Aesthet Surg. 2013 Jan;66(1):29–36

AUTHOR COMMENTARY

Akihiko Takushima

Since the first development of free muscle transfer for facial reanimation, selection of donor muscle and motor source has been a controversial matter. The two-stage operation combining the cross-facial nerve graft with the free-muscle transfer is still a standard option. However, the long recovery period associated with this strategy may dissuade patients from engaging in this therapy. To overcome this problem, one-stage latissimus dorsi muscle transfer was described by Wang (1989) and Harii (1998) but did not see much use. This paper proved the versatility and usefulness of this method by describing the results of 344 LD muscle transfer.

EDITOR COMMENTARY

This paper comes from the same unit that pioneered the wider use of the free gracilis flap in facial reanimation (Harii, 1976). In this paper, the authors, including Harii himself, present long-term results of one-stage reanimation of patients with established facial palsy.

This was a retrospective review of 344 patients undergoing one stage latissimus dorsi (LD) transfer in the unit at Kyorin University, Tokyo, from 1993 to 2008. Patients were evaluated with a combination of clinical and electromyographic investigations; the investigators examined various aspects, including the duration from operation to neuromuscular recovery and found that those who showed signs of recovery earlier tended to have better results overall. One of the major limitations of the study is the lack of a control population, for example, a comparison with patients who had CFNG and gracilis transfer would have been very enlightening.

DOI: 10.1201/9781003413738-34

The single-stage LD (SSLD) for reanimation was first described by Wang Wei in the Chinese-language literature in 1989, designing the TD nerve harvest as a vascularized nerve of sorts. The muscle is harvested at the same time as the face is prepared; the patient is positioned "semi-supine" with the harvest side (usually also the paralyzed side) propped up. Specific donor site issues include local pain and effects on shoulder mobility; the muscle also tends to be bulkier than the gracilis.

The thoracodorsal pedicle splits into medial and lateral branches; they divide further especially the lateral branch to form 4–6 distinct segmental neurovascular units. The applied anatomy of the SSLD was elegantly elucidated by Ferguson et al. (2011), showing the pedicle is 10–14 cm long to where it enters the muscle; intramuscular dissection can isolate smaller chimeric segments with their own defined neurovascular supply and effectively lengthen the pedicle by a modest amount.

The SSLD technique is very exacting – a partial latissimus dorsi muscle flap is harvested with nerve "elongation" by careful dissection of the nerve close to its origin from the posterior cord of the brachial plexus and dissection of the first lateral branch of the TDN whilst avoiding significant intramuscular dissection. Disposable staplers as used in gut surgery are used to divide the muscle neatly and help to provide anchor points for sutures. The additional nerve length allows the nerve to cross to the contralateral facial stumps, potentially avoiding a two-stage CFNG and offering faster recovery of function. The ipsilateral masseteric nerve (MN) can be used as an alternative/additional motor source, but the results are often described less "natural." Park et al. (2022) evaluated the difference between single nerve LD (MN) versus double nerve (ipsilateral MN and contralateral buccal branch of facial nerve) and found the latter often produced better spontaneous smiles.

The LD has straight muscle fibres like the gracilis, but the latter has longer excursion in practice and, thus, could be regarded as the first choice for a muscle flap. However, the need for 2 nerve coaptations reduces the number of axons innervating the muscle and, overall, the results of 2 stage versus 1 stage are largely similar (though controlled comparative studies are lacking). The authors agree that the gracilis can give better results than the LD and it is their flap of choice if the ipsilateral stump is available. However, when it comes to the contralateral stump, they believe that using the LD to avoid the second suture line is a worthwhile compromise. There are those who believe that only the CFNG can restore spontaneous smiles, but many (Manktelow et al., 2006) have shown successful smile restoration with the ipsilateral MN, presumably due to cortical adapation and the high axonal load.

One particular issue with the SSLD is that the strength of contraction can be inconsistent due to axonal loss along the long thoracodorsal nerve (with all branches cut). There has been a trend for dual innervation of muscle flaps for facial reanimation. Okazaki recommends this strategy for those prone to achieving weaker muscle action with SSLD, i.e., middle-aged male patients with fat-heavy cheeks; the MN is used for restoring voluntary smiling, whilst a CFNG is used to reinnervate a separate LD segment. The drawback is that unconscious movements caused by the ipsilateral MN during clenching might remain even after CFNG has made spontaneous smiling possible. This usually resolves with time; otherwise, the muscle supplied by the MN can be debulked. Other variants on this dual innervation method have been described by Watanabe et al. (2009) and Biglioli et al. (2012).

REFERENCES

Biglioli F, Colombo V, Tarabbia F, Pedrazzoli M, Battista V, Giovanditto F, Dalla Toffola E, Lozza A, Frigerio A. Double innervation in free-flap surgery for long-standing facial paralysis. *J Plast Reconstr Aesthet Surg.* 2012 Oct;65(10):1343–1349. doi: 10.1016/j.bjps.2012.04.030.

Ferguson LD, Paterson T, Ramsay F, Arrol K, Dabernig J, Shaw-Dunn J, Morley S. Applied anatomy of the latissimus dorsi free flap for refinement in one-stage facial reanimation. *J Plast Reconstr Aesthet Surg.* 2011 Nov;64(11):1417–1423. doi: 10.1016/j.bjps.2011.06.013.

Harii K, Asato H, Yoshimura K, Sugawara Y, Nakatsuka T, Ueda K. One-stage transfer of the latissimus dorsi muscle for reanimation of a paralyzed face: A new alternative. *Plast Reconstr Surg.* 1998;102:941–951.

Harii K, Ohmori K, Torii S. Free gracilis muscle transplantation, with microneurovascular anastomoses for the treatment of facial paralysis. A preliminary report. *Plast Reconstr Surg.* 1976 Feb;57(2):133–143. doi: 10.1097/00006534-197602000-00001.

Manktelow RT, Tomat LR, Zuker RM, Chang M. Smile reconstruction in adults with free muscle transfer innervated by the masseter motor nerve: effectiveness and cerebral adaptation. *Plast Reconstr Surg.* 2006;118:885–899.

Okazaki M, Kentaro T, Noriko U, Satoshi U, Tsutomu H, Alisa O, Mayuko H, Hiroki M. One-stage dual latissimus dorsi muscle flap transfer with a pair of vascular anastomoses and double nerve suturing for long-standing facial paralysis. *J Plast Reconstr Aesthet Surg.* 2015 Jun;68(6):e113–e119.

Park JH, Park SO, Chang H. Facial reanimation using free partial latissimus dorsi muscle transfer: single versus dual innervation method. *J Cranio-Maxillo-Facial Surg.* 2022;50:778–784.

Wang W, Chang T, Yang C. Cross-face neurovascular latissimus dorsi for facial reanimating in one stage. *Chin J Microsurg.* 1989; 12:155

Watanabe Y, Akizuki T, Ozawa T, Yoshimura K, Agawa K, Ota T. Dual innervation method using one-stage reconstruction with free latissimus dorsi muscle transfer for re-animation of established facial paralysis: simultaneous reinnervation of the ipsilateral masseter motor nerve and the contralateral facial nerve to improve the quality of smile and emotional facial expressions. *J Plast Reconstr Aesthet Surg.* 2009 Dec;62(12):1589–1597. doi: 10.1016/j.bjps.2008.07.025.

CHAPTER 35

Burn Resuscitation Practices in North America: Results of the Acute Burn ResUscitation Multicentre Prospective Trial (ABRUPT)

Greenhalgh DG, Cartotto R, Taylor SL, Fine JR, Lewis GM, Smith DJ Jr, Marano MA, Gibson A, Wibbenmeyer LA, Holmes JH, Rizzo JA, Foster KN, Khandelwal A, Fischer S, Hemmila MR, Hill D, Aballay AM, Tredget EE, Goverman J, Phelan H, Jimenez CJ, Baldea A, Sood R. *Ann Surg.* 2023 Mar 1;277(3):512–519. doi: 10.1097/SLA.0000000000005166

EXPERT COMMENTARY

Francois Stapelberg

An ode to the randomized clinical trial and better trial design.

In clinical medicine formula are to be regarded only as guides; some formula are, of course, better than others. One such example is, of course, the Parkland formula formulated by the seminal work of Charlie Baxter done 60 years ago, which has become the most widely known burn formula and is used to calculate fluid requirements during burn resuscitation.

Arguably the nomination for landmark paper should go to Dr. Baxter for any one of the series of 9 papers that he published over 50 years ago, with very much mixed methodology that includes animal studies in primates, but which still informs our practice. A key finding that Baxter pointed out at the time was that 3.7 to 4.3 mL/kg/TBSA% would be predictive of crystalloid resuscitation volume requirements in the first 24 hours for 70% of patients but that 12% of patients would need more fluid and 18% of patients less crystalloid. Burn depth variability and the fluid requirements of individual patients meant that the formula can be used only as a guideline and not as the ultimate volume for every patient.

Using the same formula 50 years later, fluid resuscitation volumes regularly exceed the predicted volumes and the term "fluid creep" has become well known over the last 25 years, leading to complications, including abdominal compartment syndrome, pleural and pericardial effusions, as well as ocular compartment syndrome.

DOI: 10.1201/9781003413738-35

Strategies to reduce excessive fluid volumes include the current approaches by both ABLS and EMSB courses that the Parkland formula should be used only to calculate a starting rate and should be adjusted according to urine output. Early use of albumin in larger and deeper burns to reduce fluid requirements and resulting oedema have become regular occurrences, supported by evidence that it rapidly lowers the input-output ratio whilst increasing urine output. Evidence about the reduction in fluid requirements is less convincing with some studies showing a trend in reduction only.

Most of the evidence available to date has come from smaller trials, reflecting the difficulty in recruiting enough subjects to detect meaningful effects. The ABRUPT trial set out to study the efficacy of albumin in moderating fluid resuscitation volumes, designed as a prospective, multicentre observational trial with a sample size adequate to detect a 1 mL/kg/TBSA% burn difference at 48 hours if albumin was used, which required enrollment of 400 subjects to ensure the calculated sample size of 183 subjects per group was reached. Over a 38-month period, 21 sites contributed to enrollment of 400 subjects, with 21 exclusions. Data collection was done using REDCap technology, which is a secure, web-based application that supports data capture and data management for research studies, thus enabling more sites to participate in multicentre trials.

The main findings were that 24-hour fluid requirements, as guided by urine output, were 4.6 mL/kg/TBSA%, with a higher requirement in the albumin group with total volume of 5.2 mL/kg/TBSA%, which was ascribed to larger and deeper burns in older patients. Urine output remained within 0.5–1 mL/kg/hour range, which was reassuring, confirming to some extent that urine output remains a good indicator of hourly resuscitation adequacy.

Subjects who required mechanical ventilation received 1.32 mL/kg/TBSA% more fluids over 48 hours compared to those who were not ventilated, explained by intrathoracic pressure changes requiring increased preload, as well as the vasodilation of sedative or anxiolytic agents used. Completion of resuscitation was defined as resuscitation volumes decreased to match calculated basal and evaporative losses being reached at 24 hours for all subjects in the crystalloid only group and at 48 hours for the albumin group.

The findings of ABRUPT were then used to design a prospective, randomized trial (ABRUPT 2) where the intervention consisted of a ratio of one-third 5% albumin to two-thirds crystalloid started within 12 hours. The control would be crystalloid only. The inclusion criteria were changed to larger burn sizes >25% TBSA or >20% full thickness, a good example of trial enrichment.

At the time of writing in 2024, ABRUPT 2 [https://clinicaltrials.gov/study/ NCT04356859] is underway and recruiting at 26 sites in the United States and Canada. Whether investigator equipoise exists might be a challenge for the study, with many clinicians already opting for early use of albumin in larger burns. Other interventions also being considered are fresh frozen plasma to address the possibility of preserving or restoring the endothelial glycocalyx earlier, leading to reduced fluid requirements, [https://clinicaltrials.gov/study/NCT05069922], as well as the PROpOLIS study investigating the use of modern pathogen-reduced plasma PRP in lyophilized plasma [https://clinicaltrials.gov/study/NCT04681638].

The real importance of ABRUPT in the investigation of albumin lies in focusing our collective minds on the role of multicentre trials to demand trials that are designed to deliver valid conclusions that are replicable in other centres "in the real world." Valid conclusions can be reached only from trials with adequate sample sizes, a difficult prospect when studying major burns. There are opportunities to use newer trial design methodology, including prognostic and predictive enrichment, where subjects who are more likely to benefit from the intervention are enrolled; platform trials, where more than one intervention can be trialled; or adaptive trials, where the study design can be changed based on the interim results from an ongoing trial. Using registry-based outcome data is another method to consider, which will increase the use of patient specific outcome measures, considering that most of the acute care trials in burn cases use surrogate outcome measures.

EDITOR COMMENTARY

The ABRUPT trial was a prospective observational (non-interventional) study of resuscitation protocols at 21 North American burn centres; ABRUPT 2 will compare crystalloid only to a colloid-crystalloid mix with primary completion in September 2025. The Parkland formula is the most used resuscitation formula, with the Modified Brooke formula being the most common alternative. There is a much more variable practice in the use of colloids. Colloids were the "original" resuscitation fluid, but cost, concerns over exacerbating oedema and the findings of the Cochrane study led to a switch to crystalloid formulae. These, in turn, probably contributed to the phenomenon of fluid creep. Current practice seems to follow more conservative crystalloid volumes in combination with judicious but early use of colloid. The current EMSB guidelines use 3× instead of 4× as the multiplier in the Parkland formula. In this study, patients who had colloid (albumin) were older, had larger and deeper burns, more inhalational injury, and more organ failure. Dr. Stapelberg makes very astute comments about the design and conduct of trials.

CHAPTER 36

Cell Therapies and Its Derivatives as Immunomodulators in Vascularized Composite Allotransplantation

Huang CH, Chen WY, Chen RF, Ramachandran S, Liu KF,
Kuo YR. *Asian J Surg.* 2024 Oct;47(10):4251–4259

AUTHOR COMMENTARY

Chao-Hsin Huang, Chia-Chun Lee, and Yur-Ren Kuo

Background

Advancements in immunosuppression have significantly improved outcomes in solid organ transplantation, including kidney, liver, heart, and lung transplants. This progress has been further supported by advancements in microsurgical techniques. Autologous tissue transfers have been the primary approach for reconstruction. However, their usefulness is limited in cases involving extensive composite defects, such as those caused by severe trauma or tumor resection where allografts or allotransplants have emerged as a viable alternative. With improved flap transfer reliability and the development of advanced immunotherapy protocols, vascularized composite tissue allotransplantation (VCA) has become a promising option "replacing like with like" in aesthetic and functional reconstructions.

Over 250 cases of VCA have been reported worldwide (Figure 36.1). The earliest recorded attempt at a VCA took place in 1964, when an Ecuadorian team conducted a forearm transplant that was technically successful but rejected 21 days later.[1] The first successful human hand transplant came in 1998 by Dubernard,[2] followed by the first facial transplant (Devauchelle et al., 2006).[3] Other cases of VCA, including abdominal wall uterus, penis, and larynx transplants, have also been reported worldwide (Figures 36.2 and 36.3). VCA has the potential to improve quality of life and offer solutions for injuries that are difficult if not impossible to address with conventional methods. Notably, uterine VCA also provides a unique solution for infertility.

UPPER EXTREMITIES VCA

Upper extremity transplants are the most frequently performed VCA procedure. Since Dubernard, over 100 have been performed worldwide.[1,4] For patients with severe upper

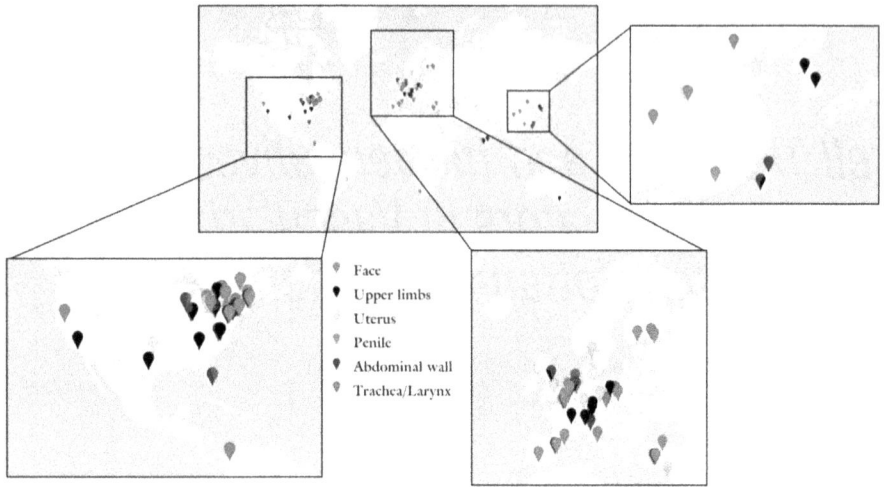

Figure 36.1 Graphical representation of VCAs performed in the world. The cities that had performed VCA operations are marked.

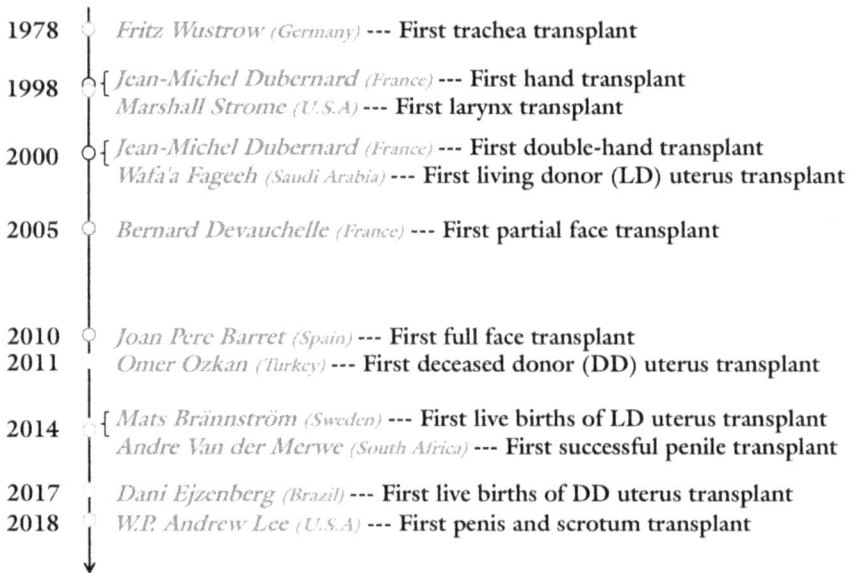

1978	*Fritz Wustrow (Germany)* --- **First trachea transplant**	
1998	*Jean-Michel Dubernard (France)* --- **First hand transplant**	
	Marshall Strome (U.S.A) --- **First larynx transplant**	
2000	*Jean-Michel Dubernard (France)* --- **First double-hand transplant**	
	Wafa'a Fageeh (Saudi Arabia) --- **First living donor (LD) uterus transplant**	
2005	*Bernard Devauchelle (France)* --- **First partial face transplant**	
2010	*Joan Pere Barret (Spain)* --- **First full face transplant**	
2011	*Omer Ozkan (Turkey)* --- **First deceased donor (DD) uterus transplant**	
2014	*Mats Brännström (Sweden)* --- **First live births of LD uterus transplant**	
	Andre Van der Merwe (South Africa) --- **First successful penile transplant**	
2017	*Dani Ejzenberg (Brazil)* --- **First live births of DD uterus transplant**	
2018	*W.P. Andrew Lee (U.S.A)* --- **First penis and scrotum transplant**	

Figure 36.2 Important milestones in VCA history.

limb loss, upper limb VCA offers the potential to restore function, sensation, and aesthetic appearance. The transfers have been performed at various levels, from the shoulder to the wrist. Preoperative preparation is essential, including matching the donor and recipient by skin color, limb and bone size, and joint mobility.[5]

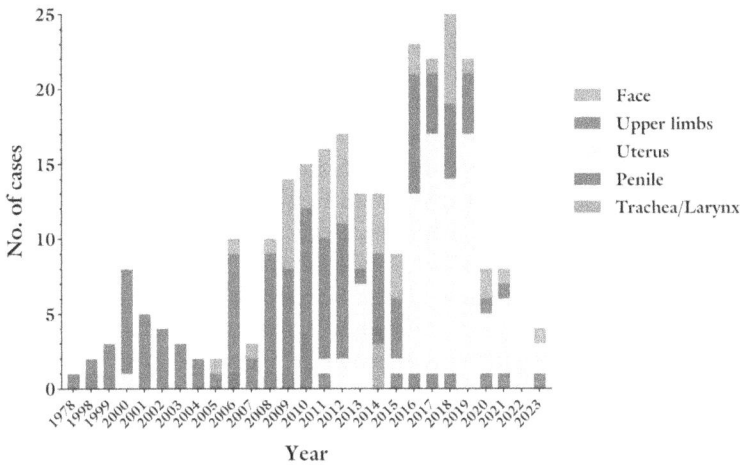

Figure 36.3   Annual volume of VCA operations between 1979 and 2023.

The surgical procedure involves sequential osteosynthesis, vascular anastomosis, muscle and tendon repair, and, finally, nerve repair. Postoperative rehabilitation is crucial, beginning with range-of-motion exercises within the first week, supported by physical and occupational therapy. This rehabilitation program typically extends for over a year. Functional outcomes are assessed using tools such as the Carroll test, the Sollerman hand function test, and the Disabilities of the Arm, Shoulder, and Hand (DASH) questionnaire.[5,6] Sensory recovery is evaluated through the Semmes–Weinstein (SW) test and the 2-point discrimination test. The more distal the level of the transplant, the shorter the recovery time for motor and sensory function.[7] The motor recovery is detected in proximal to distal, extrinsic to intrinsic order. Sensibility continues to recover years after the operation, and over 80% of the cases experienced recovery of discriminative sensibility and tactile sensibility.[6] Patients with more distal transplants demonstrated the best overall function, whereas those with proximal or bilateral transplants showed the most significant functional improvements.[8] To date, the earlier overall success rate exceeds 90% in patients with upper limb VCAs.[8]

FACE VCA

Since the first facial transplant in Amiens in 2005, more than 48 cases have been reported worldwide.[3,9] Facial transplantation, either partial or total, is a viable option for patients with extensive facial deformities resulting from trauma (particularly gunshot wounds), animal attacks, or burns, particularly chemical assault.[10] Careful classification of soft tissue and skeletal defects is essential to guide the reconstruction of both functional and aesthetic facial structures.[11] Computer-aided surgical planning with customized cutting guides is recommended to achieve precise osteotomies in both the graft and the recipient.

The primary arterial pedicles used are the external carotid and facial arteries, with the maxillary artery recommended for midface vascularization.[12] Venous anastomosis is performed end to end between the internal jugular veins of the donor and the recipient. Coaptation of the facial nerves is critical for restoring facial expression.[10] Sensory recovery, including light touch and temperature sensation, is typically observed between 3 months and 1-year postoperatively, whereas motor recovery occurs more slowly, ranging from 6 months to several years.[13] Evaluations of functional outcomes include the assessment of olfaction, oral intake, respiration, speech, and facial expressions.[9,14] In facial transplant cases, the 5-year and 10-year survival rates are 85% and 74%, respectively.[15] The main cause of allograft loss was chronic immunological rejection, occurring after a median of 7.5 years.[16] Research indicates that 85% of VCA recipients, including face transplant patients, experienced acute rejection episodes within the first year, with 77% also developing opportunistic infections.[7]

LARYNX VCA

The first total laryngeal transplant was performed in 1998 on a 40-year-old male with traumatic laryngeal loss.[17] The anatomical components of the transplanted larynx included the thyroid gland, a segment of the trachea, the larynx, and the pharynx. Vascular anastomoses were established between the donor and the recipient's superior thyroid arteries and between the internal jugular veins of both. Nerve coaptation involved the superior and recurrent laryngeal nerves. Notably, perfusion of the donor graft was reestablished prior to the excision of the recipient's larynx.[17] Outcomes of laryngeal transplantation are evaluated based on parameters such as voice quality, respiratory function, and swallowing ability.[17–20] In patients with head and neck cancer, laryngeal transplantation poses ethical considerations due to the potential for an increased risk of cancer recurrence associated with immunosuppressant therapy.

ABDOMINAL WALL VCA

Abdominal wall transplantation was first proposed by Levi et al. in 2003.[21] The concept of abdominal wall transplantation emerged when surgeons observed that intestinal transplantation failures were often related to the inadequate abdominal space leading to pressure following primary closure of the abdomen. Thus, abdominal wall transplantation has often been performed in conjunction with multivisceral transplantation in cases where primary abdominal closure is not achievable. This approach provides adequate coverage without requiring additional immunosuppression. The perfusion territories and anatomy of the abdominal wall were described by Light et al.[22] The maximum potential size of the flap can encompass the area bordered by the pubic symphysis, the fusion of the false ribs, the bilateral anterior superior iliac spine, and the xiphoid process, covering approximately 870 cm^2.[22] Harvested muscle components include the external oblique, internal oblique, and transversus abdominis. The vascular supply is predominantly supported by the iliofemoral system, originating from the deep inferior epigastric vessels in continuity with the iliac and femoral vessels.[22,23]

Extended cold ischemia time and prior allocation of visceral organ transplants present significant challenges for abdominal wall transplantation. Thus, strategies such as arteriovenous loops[23] and forearm banking[24] have been proposed. To date, approximately 40 cases of full-thickness vascularized abdominal wall transplants have been reported worldwide.[24] Rejection was noted around 25% cases,[24] and other complications such as infection, and hernia, thrombosis were observed.[25]

UTERUS VCA

Uterus transplantation has emerged as a fertility option for those who were diagnosed with absolute uterine factor infertility (AUFI), which may be due to uterine agenesis/hypoplasia or status post-hysterectomy.[26] Women with AUFI have traditionally had to seek surrogacy or adoption, both of which have their own potential religious or legal issues.[27] VCA of the uterus offers the hope of carrying and giving birth to their own children. The first uterine transplant was performed at King Fahad Hospital and Research Center in Saudi Arabia in 2000.[28] Unfortunately, the patient developed acute vascular thrombosis 3 months after the transplant.[28] The second uterine transplant case was performed in Turkey in 2011,[29] and, although pregnancy attempts resulted in miscarriages, this was the first case of a heartbeating fetus in a transplanted uterus.[30] The first uterine transplantation leading to the birth of the first baby from a transplanted uterus took place in Sweden in 2014.[27]

The surgical procedure begins by positioning the donor uterus in the recipient's pelvis. The vascular anastomosis involves connecting the donor's uterine vessels to the recipient's external iliac vessels artery.[27] Complications include vessel thrombosis, vaginal stricture, and infection, all of which can lead to graft failure.[26] By 2022, over 80 uterine transplant procedures had been performed, resulting in more than 40 live births.[26]

PENIS VCA

Severe penile injury may result from combat injury, traumatic loss, cancer, and amputation following ritual circumcision. Total penile reconstruction aims to restore functional abilities such as voiding and sexual function, while also prioritizing aesthetic appearance and patient satisfaction. To date, 5 cases have been reported.[31] The first penile transplant was performed in China in 2006; however, the graft had to be removed 14 days after operation due to psychological rejection by the patient and his wife, highlighting the importance of preoperative psychological counselling.[31] The surgery involves anastomosis of the corpora cavernosa, urethra, dorsal nerves, arteries, and veins. The blood supply to the penis consists of the dorsal, cavernosal, and external pudendal arteries[32]; anastomosing both the superficial and the deep dorsal veins helps reduce graft congestion. The common complications include hematoma, skin partial loss, infection, urinary retention, and psychological rejection.[32,33] The three successful cases demonstrated sensation recovery between 7 to 12 months, while urinary function restoration ranged from a few days to several weeks. Erectile function returned as early as 3 weeks to up to a year.[31]

CHALLENGE OF MULTIPLE COMPONENT VCA RECONSTRUCTION

There are significant challenges that need to be solved in VCA. In facial and upper extremity transplantation cases, the overall rate of surgical complications was reported at 23%. Acute rejection was observed in 89% of recipients, while chronic rejection was seen in 11%. Additionally, 58% of patients experienced opportunistic infections and 19% suffered partial or complete loss of the allograft.[34] As the defect size increases, the greater blood loss, prolonged surgical time, hypovolemia, and increased hypothermia during reperfusion create additional challenges.[35] For example, a case in France involving a face and bilateral hand transplant resulted in extensive graft necrosis, infection, and death due to hypoxic cardiac arrest.[35] Similarly, a triple-limb transplant case ended in multiple organ failure, while a quadruple-extremity allotransplantation case resulted in death due to challenges in maintaining resuscitation and electrolyte balance during surgery.[36]

In addition to concomitant VCA transplant, lower limb transplantation remains a subject of debate, largely due to the availability of advanced prosthetic options. Despite these reservations, successful cases have been described.[37]

CURRENT IMMUNOSUPPRESSANTS – BLOCKADE AND COMPLICATIONS

Given that most VCA includes skin, a highly immunogenic tissue, an effective immunosuppression regimen is crucial (Figure 36.4). Several challenges include

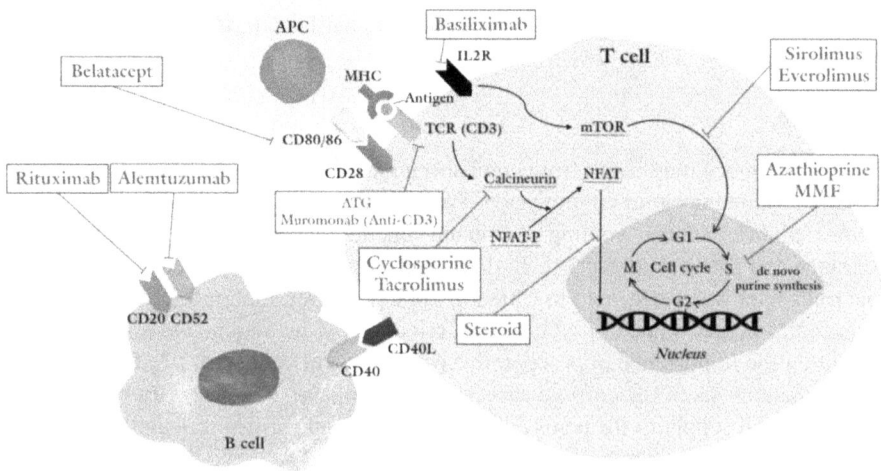

Figure 36.4 General scheme of physiological mechanisms related to induction and maintenance immunosuppression regimens commonly used during postoperative course of VCA. (ATG, Anti-thymocyte globulin; MMF, Mycophenolate mofetil; MHC, Major histocompatibility complex; APC, Antigen-presenting cell; TCR, T cell receptor.)

sensitization, acute rejection, and chronic rejection. Sensitization can be induced by substantial blood transfusions prior to surgery. Acute rejection occurs in over 80% of VCA cases,[38] highlighting the importance of the immunosuppressive induction phase to reduce innate immune activation. This phase commonly involves a regimen including corticosteroids, interleukin-2 receptor antagonists (such as basiliximab), antithymocyte globulin (ATG), and anti-CD52 antibodies (such as alemtuzumab)[38] (Table 36.1). For recipients of face, upper limb, uterus, and laryngeal transplants, the induction regimen typically includes a combination of ATG and steroids.[39] In contrast, abdominal wall VCA usually involves alemtuzumab or daclizumab,[21] while penile VCA commonly includes daclizumab, steroids, and alemtuzumab.[39] The maintenance phase generally includes tacrolimus, mycophenolate mofetil (MMF), and prednisolone. Specifically, for face, upper limb, penile, and laryngeal VCA, the maintenance regimen typically consists of tacrolimus, MMF, and prednisolone, while uterus VCA usually involves tacrolimus and azathioprine (Table 36.1). The dosage varied in different cases.

Long-term use of immunosuppressants can lead to cytotoxicity, hypoglycemia, and nephrotoxicity.[40] It has also been linked to oncological complications, including Epstein–Barr virus (EBV)–related post-transplant B-cell lymphomas and Non-Hodgkin lymphomas. Additionally, it may predispose patients to opportunistic infections, such as herpes simplex virus, cytomegalovirus (CMV), EBV, *Verruconis gallopava*, and *Pneumocystis jirovecii*, as well as an increased risk of organ failure.[40,41] A case of avascular necrosis of the hip, resulting from bone infarction after the use of systemic immunosuppression, has also been reported.[42] Due to its cytotoxicity, new modalities are sought as alternative immunomodulatory agents.[43]

FUTURE STRATEGIES IN IMMUNOMODULATION

New Pharmaceutical Strategy

Novel pharmaceutical regimens are being explored to reduce toxicity in transplantation. For instance, rapamycin (sirolimus), an mTOR inhibitor, promotes regulatory T cell (Treg) differentiation and reduces nephrotoxicity.[44] Eculizumab, a monoclonal antibody targeting complement component 5, has also been evaluated in solid organ transplantation.[45] Additionally, the combination of CTLA4-Ig and tofacitinib has demonstrated immunomodulatory efficacy in solid organ transplantation.[46] These novel pharmaceutical regimens offer new insights and opportunities for advancing VCA transplantation.

BONE MARROW CELL TRANSFUSION

To decrease the use of pharmaceutical immunosuppressant, bone marrow cell transfusions have been proposed. Vascularized bone marrow components can facilitate the tolerance of vascularized allografts. To minimize pharmaceutical maintenance regimen, bone marrow transplants have been used concomitantly with low-dose tacrolimus monotherapy.[47]

Table 36.1 The demographic data, including gender, etiology, and immunosuppression regimens, of different types of VCAs operation

		Face	(%)	Upper limbs	(%)	Uterus	(%)	Pebile	(%)	Trachea/ Larynx	(%)
Sex	M	41	80.4	74	76.3	0	0.0	5	100.0	14	73.7
	F	10	19.6	23	23.7	84	100.0	0	0.0	5	26.3
	NIA	0	0.0	0	0.0	0	0.0	0	0.0	0	0.0
Etiology	Trauma/Burn	41	80.4	76	78.4	0	0.0	4	80.0	0	0.0
	Congenital Anomalies	0	0.0	0	0.0	72	85.7	0	0.0	0	0.0
	Malignancy/Tumor	7	13.7	0	0.0	3	3.6	1	20.0	9	47.4
	Infection	0	0.0	18	18.6	0	0.0	0	0.0	0	0.0
	Others (Iatrogenic)		5.9	0	0.0	0	0.0	0	0.0	10	52.6
	NIA	0	0.0	14	14.4	9	10.7	0	0.0	0	0.0
	ATG	5	9.8	17	15.7	11	13.1		0.0	0	0.0
	ATG + Steroid	33	64.7	21	41.2	43	51.2		20.0	3	15.8
	ATG + Steroid + Bailiximab	0	0.0	6	11.8	0	0.0		0.0	0	0.0
	ATG + Steroid + Alemtuzumab + Basiliximab	0	0.0	6	11.8	0	0.0		0.0	0	0.0
Induction	ATG + Rituximab	4	7.8	0	0.0	0	0.0	0	0.0	0	0.0
	Steroid	0	0.0	1	2.0	0	0.0	0	0.0	9	47.4
	Steroid + Basiliximab		2.0	15	29.4	8	9.5	0	0.0	0	0.0
	Steroid + Alemtuzumab		2.0	19	37.3	0	0.0		60.0	0	0.0
	Others and NIA		13.7	23	45.1	22	26.2		20.0	7	36.8
	Tacrolimus + MMF	1	2.1	0	0.0	14	16.7	0	0.0	1	5.3
	Tacrolimus + Azathioprine	0	0.0	0	0.0	34	40.5	0	0.0	0	0.0
Maintenance	Tacrolimus + MMF + Steroid	45	93.8	56	61.5	10	11.9	3	60.0	11	57.9
	Tacrolimus + MMF + Steroid + MPA	0	0.0	8	8.8	0	0.0	0	0.0	0	0.0
	Others and NIA	2	4.2	27	29.7	26	31.0	2	40.0	7	36.8

Note: Except for uterus transplantation, the majority of VCA recipients were male and suffered from traumatic or burn injury. The most common immunosuppression regimens of induction and maintenance therapy were "ATG plus steroid" and "Tacrolimus, MMF, plus steroid," respectively.

Abbreviations: M, Male; F, Female; N/A, Not Applicable; ATG, Anti-thymocyte globulin; MMF, Mycophenolate mofetil; MPA, Mycophenolic acid.

IMMUNE CELL THERAPY AND ADJUNCTIVE REGIMEN

Cell therapy has also been developed as an alternative immunomodulatory treatment. It encompasses both immune cell therapy and stem cell therapy, which aim to enhance immunosuppressive regulators while reducing immunoreactive cytokines. Immune cell therapy involves modulators of innate immunity, including tolerogenic dendritic cells, regulatory macrophages, and invariant natural killer T cells, as well as modulators of adaptive immunity, such as regulatory T cells and regulatory B cells.[48] Stem cell therapy involves the transplantation of hematopoietic stem and progenitor cells, as well as mesenchymal stem cells (MSCs), which can promote allograft tolerance.[12, 48] Further studies have investigated light therapy,[49] and extracellular vesicles (EVs) derived from MSCs[50] as adjunctive treatments. Several clinical trials have been initiated.[43]

CONCLUSION

VCA has emerged as a viable clinical option for the reconstruction of complex and extensive defects. Despite its potential, the procedure is accompanied by various morbidities and challenges, particularly related to the use of immunosuppressants. To enhance the success and sustainability of VCA, future advancements should focus on the development of novel immunotherapeutic strategies and cell-based therapies, which may reduce complications and improve long-term outcomes for recipients.

REFERENCES

1. Diaz-Siso JR, Bueno EM, Sisk GC, Marty FM, Pomahac B, Tullius SG. Vascularized composite tissue allotransplantation: state of the art. *Clin Transplant.* 2013;27(3):330–337.
2. Dubernard JM, Owen E, Herzberg G, Lanzetta M, Martin X, Kapila H, *et al.* Human hand allograft: report on first 6 months. *Lancet.* 1999;353(9161):1315–1320.
3. Devauchelle B, Badet L, Lengelé B, Morelon E, Testelin S, Michallet M, *et al.* First human face allograft: early report. *Lancet.* 2006;368(9531):203–209.
4. Wells MW, Rampazzo A, Papay F, Gharb BB. Two decades of hand transplantation: a systematic review of outcomes. *Ann Plast Surg.* 2022;88(3):335–344.
5. Mendenhall SD, Brown S, Ben-Amotz O, Neumeister MW, Levin LS. Building a hand and upper extremity transplantation program: lessons learned from the first 20 years of vascularized composite allotransplantation. *Hand NY.* 2020;15(2):224–233.
6. Shores JT, Malek V, Lee WPA, Brandacher G. Outcomes after hand and upper extremity transplantation. *J Mater Sci Mater Med.* 2017;28(5):72.
7. Elliott RM, Tintle SM, Levin LS. Upper extremity transplantation: current concepts and challenges in an emerging field. *Curr Rev Musculoskelet Med.* 2014;7(1):83–88.
8. Shores JT, Malek V, Lee WPA, Brandacher G. Outcomes after hand and upper extremity transplantation. *J Mater Sci Mater Med.* 2017;28(5):72.
9. Dorante MI, Wang AT, Kollar B, Perry BJ, Ertosun MG, Lindford AJ, *et al.* Facial expression after face transplant: an international face transplant cohort comparison. *Plast Reconstr Surg.* 2023;152(2):315e–325e.
10. Kantar RS, Alfonso AR, Diep GK, Berman ZP, Rifkin WJ, Diaz-Siso JR, *et al.* Facial transplantation: principles and evolving concepts. *Plast Reconstr Surg.* 2021;147(6):1022e–1038e.
11. Mohan R, Borsuk DE, Dorafshar AH, Wang HD, Bojovic B, Christy MR, *et al.* Aesthetic and functional facial transplantation: a classification system and treatment algorithm. *Plast Reconstr Surg.* 2014;133(2):386–397.

12. Huang CH, Kuo YR, Wu YC, Lee HC, Lee SS. Modified Le Fort II approach with adequate vascularization preservation in midface allotransplantation: mock surgery. *Asian J Surg.* 2022;45(6):1259–1262.
13. Shanmugarajah K, Hettiaratchy S, Butler PE. Facial transplantation. *Curr Opin Otolaryngol Head Neck Surg.* 2012;20(4):291–297.
14. Pomahac B, Pribaz J, Eriksson E, Annino D, Caterson S, Sampson C, *et al.* Restoration of facial form and function after severe disfigurement from burn injury by a composite facial allograft. *Am J Transplant.* 2011;11(2):386–393.
15. Homsy P, Huelsboemer L, Barret JP, Blondeel P, Borsuk DE, Bula D, *et al.* An update on the survival of the first 50 face transplants worldwide. *JAMA Surg.* 2024;159(12):1339–1345.
16. Longo B, Pomahac B, Giacalone M, Cardillo M, Cervelli V. 18 years of face transplantation: adverse outcomes and challenges. *J Plast Reconstr Aesthet Surg.* 2023;87:187–199.
17. Strome M, Stein J, Esclamado R, Hicks D, Lorenz RR, Braun W, *et al.* Laryngeal transplantation and 40-month follow-up. *N Engl J Med.* 2001;344(22):1676–1679.
18. Candelo E, Belafsky PC, Corrales M, Farwell DG, Gonzales LF, Grajek M, *et al.* The global experience of laryngeal transplantation: series of eleven patients in three continents. *Laryngoscope.* 2024;134(10):4313–4320.
19. Farwell DG, Birchall MA, Macchiarini P, Luu QC, de Mattos AM, Gallay BJ, *et al.* Laryngotracheal transplantation: technical modifications and functional outcomes. *Laryngoscope.* 2013;123(10):2502–2508.
20. Grajek M, Maciejewski A, Giebel S, Krakowczyk Ł, Ulczok R, Szymczyk C, *et al.* First complex allotransplantation of neck organs: larynx, trachea, pharynx, esophagus, thyroid, parathyroid glands, and anterior cervical wall: a case report. *Ann Surg.* 2017;266(2):e19–e24.
21. Levi DM, Tzakis AG, Kato T, Madariaga J, Mittal NK, Nery J, *et al.* Transplantation of the abdominal wall. *Lancet.* 2003;361(9376):2173–2176.
22. Light D, Kundu N, Djohan R, Quintini C, Gandhi N, Gastman BR, *et al.* Total abdominal wall transplantation: an anatomical study and classification system. *Plast Reconstr Surg.* 2017;139(6):1466–1473.
23. Atia A, Hollins A, Shammas R, Phillips BT, Ravindra KV, Sudan DL, *et al.* Surgical techniques for revascularization in abdominal wall transplantation. *J Reconstr Microsurg.* 2020;36(7):522–527.
24. Giele H, Vaidya A, Reddy S, Vrakas G, Friend P. Current state of abdominal wall transplantation. *Curr Opin Organ Transplant.* 2016;21(2):159–164.
25. De Winkel NV, Muylle E, Canovai E, Amin I, Vianna RM, Farinelli P, *et al.* 67: Long-term outcome after non-vascularized rectus fascia transplantation in solid organ transplantation: a global multi-center IRTA survey. *Transplantation.* 2023;107(7S):39.
26. Brännström M, Racowsky C, Carbonnel M, Wu J, Gargiulo A, Adashi EY, *et al.* Uterus transplantation: from research, through human trials and into the future. *Hum Reprod Update.* 2023;29(5):521–544.
27. Brännström M. Uterus transplantation. *Curr Opin Organ Transplant.* 2015;20(6):621–628.
28. Fageeh W, Raffa H, Jabbad H, Marzouki A. Transplantation of the human uterus. *Int J Gynaecol Obstet.* 2002;76(3):245–251.
29. Ozkan O, Akar ME, Ozkan O, Erdogan O, Hadimioglu N, Yilmaz M, *et al.* Preliminary results of the first human uterus transplantation from a multiorgan donor. *Fertil Steril.* 2013;99(2):470–476.e5.
30. Ozkan O, Dogan NU, Ozkan O, Mendilcioglu I, Dogan S, Aydinuraz B, *et al.* Uterus transplantation: from animal models through the first heart beating pregnancy to the first human live birth. *Womens Health (Lond).* 2016;12(4):442–449.
31. Lake IV, Girard AO, Lopez CD, Cooney DS, Burnett AL, Brandacher G, *et al.* Penile transplantation: lessons learned and technical considerations. *J Urol.* 2022;207(5):960–968.
32. Szafran AA, Redett R, Burnett AL. Penile transplantation: the US experience and institutional program set-up. *Transl Androl Urol.* 2018;7(4):639–645.
33. Hu W, Lu J, Zhang L, Wu W, Nie H, Zhu Y, *et al.* A preliminary report of penile transplantation. *Eur Urol.* 2006;50(4):851–853.
34. Milek D, Reed LT, Echternacht SR, Shanmugarajah K, Cetrulo CL, Jr., Lellouch AG, *et al.* A systematic review of the reported complications related to facial and upper extremity vascularized composite allotransplantation. *J Surg Res.* 2023;281:164–175.
35. Carty MJ, Hivelin M, Dumontier C, Talbot SG, Benjoar MD, Pribaz JJ, *et al.* Lessons learned from simultaneous face and bilateral hand allotransplantation. *Plast Reconstr Surg.* 2013;132(2):423–432.

36. Swanson E, Cheng H-T, Lough D, Lee W, Shores J, Brandacher G. Lower extremity allotransplantation: are we ready for prime time? *Vascular Composit Allotransplant*. 2015;2:37–46.

37. Cavadas PC, Thione A, Carballeira A, Blanes M. Bilateral transfemoral lower extremity transplantation: result at 1 year. *Am J Transplant*. 2013;13(5):1343–1349.

38. Fischer S, Lian CG, Kueckelhaus M, Strom TB, Edelman ER, Clark RA, *et al*. Acute rejection in vascularized composite allotransplantation. *Curr Opin Organ Transplant*. 2014;19(6):531–544. doi: 10.1097/MOT.0000000000000140. PMID: 25333831.

39. Van Dieren L, Tawa P, Coppens M, Naenen L, Dogan O, Quisenaerts T, *et al*. Acute rejection rates in vascularized composite allografts: a systematic review of case reports. *J Surg Res*. 2024;298:137–148.

40. Iske J, Nian Y, Maenosono R, Maurer M, Sauer IM, Tullius SG. Composite tissue allotransplantation: opportunities and challenges. *Cell Mol Immunol*. 2019;16(4):343–349.

41. Tsai YT, Lu PL, Lee KM, Kuo YR. Lung and brain abscesses in an upper extremity allotransplantation recipient. *Clin Infect Dis*. 2022;75(3):545–548.

42. Kuo YR, Chen CC, Wang JW, Chang JK, Huang YC, Pan CC, *et al*. Bone infarction of the hip after hand allotransplantation: a case report. *Microsurgery*. 2019;39(4):349–353.

43. Anggelia MR, Cheng HY, Lai PC, Hsieh YH, Lin CH, Lin CH. Cell therapy in vascularized composite allotransplantation. *Biomed J*. 2022;45(3):454–464.

44. Sutter D, Dzhonova DV, Prost JC, Bovet C, Banz Y, Rahnfeld L, *et al*. Delivery of rapamycin using in situ forming implants promotes immunoregulation and vascularized composite allograft survival. *Sci Rep*. 2019;9(1):9269.

45. Schinstock CA, Bentall AJ, Smith BH, Cornell LD, Everly M, Gandhi MJ, *et al*. Long-term outcomes of eculizumab-treated positive crossmatch recipients: Allograft survival, histologic findings, and natural history of the donor-specific antibodies. *Am J Transplant*. 2019;19(6):1671–1683.

46. Iglesias M, Khalifian S, Oh BC, Zhang Y, Miller D, Beck S, *et al*. A short course of tofacitinib sustains the immunoregulatory effect of CTLA4-Ig in the presence of inflammatory cytokines and promotes long-term survival of murine cardiac allografts. *Am J Transplant*. 2021;21(8):2675–2687.

47. Schneeberger S, Gorantla VS, Brandacher G, Zeevi A, Demetris AJ, Lunz JG, *et al*. Upper-extremity transplantation using a cell-based protocol to minimize immunosuppression. *Ann Surg*. 2013;257(2):345–351.

48. Huang CH, Chen WY, Chen RF, Ramachandran S, Liu KF, Kuo YR. Cell therapies and its derivatives as immunomodulators in vascularized composite allotransplantation. *Asian J Surg*. 2024;47(10):4251–4259.

49. Liu KF, Ramachandran S, Chang CW, Chen RF, Huang CH, Huang HT, *et al*. The synergistic effect of full-spectrum light therapy and transient immunosuppressants prolonged allotransplant survival. *Plast Reconstr Surg*. 2024;154(4):775–783.

50. Kang M, Huang CC, Gajendrareddy P, Lu Y, Shirazi S, Ravindran S, *et al*. Extracellular vesicles from TNFα preconditioned MSCs: effects on immunomodulation and bone regeneration. *Front Immunol*. 2022;13:878194.

AUTHOR COMMENTARY

Savitha Ramachandran

The paper "Cell Therapies and Its Derivatives as Immunomodulators in Vascularized Composite Allotransplantation (VCA)," provides a detailed review of the emerging role of cell-based therapies in enhancing the outcomes of VCA. VCA, which involves the transplantation of multiple tissues, including skin, muscles, bone, nerves, and blood vessels, is the next significant frontier in reconstructive as well as transplant medicine. It is important to note that, to date, 85% of VCA recipients have experienced rejection within the first year after transplantation, a rate greatly exceeding all other transplanted organs, and that all VCA recipients have experienced toxicity associated with traditional calcineurin inhibitor (CNIs) and steroid-based regimes for immunosuppression. As VCA is life enhancing as opposed to life saving, alternatives to CNIs and steroids are necessary. This paper addresses this challenge by exploring innovative strategies involving cell-based therapies and their potential to modulate the immune response, which can potentially reduce reliance on current calcineurin and steroid-based immunosuppression regimes.

KEY INSIGHTS AND CONTRIBUTIONS

The paper provides a detailed summary of all animal and clinical studies using cell therapy to induce post-transplant immune tolerance. It discusses the various forms of cell therapy that modulate both adaptive and innate immune systems, such as mesenchymal stem cells (MSCs), regulatory T cells (Tregs), and dendritic cells (DCs). It provides detailed analysis of the mechanisms by which these cells interact with the immune system to prevent graft rejection and their roles in both the adaptive and the innate immune systems. For example, MSCs are shown to modulate both innate and adaptive immune responses by secreting immunosuppressive factors, promoting tissue repair, and inducing tolerance. This paper also highlights that Tregs, which are pivotal in maintaining immune homeostasis and preventing autoimmunity, have shown promising results in solid organ transplant.

The role of cell therapy derivatives, such as exosomes and cytokine-based treatments, as potential immunomodulatory agents are also reviewed in this article as a less invasive alternative to traditional cellular therapies. The paper draws attention to the growing body of evidence suggesting that exosomes derived from MSCs, for example, can carry therapeutic molecules that modulate the immune response, reduce inflammation, and promote tissue regeneration. This focus on cell-derived products is innovative and aligns with the trend toward more targeted, less invasive therapeutic modalities in transplant medicine.

The paper concludes by acknowledging the challenges faced in scaling these therapies for human use, including issues related to cell sourcing, standardization of protocols, and the long-term safety and efficacy of these approaches. It also summarizes future directions and challenges, among which are the need for better understanding of the mechanisms of immune tolerance in VCA, the optimization of cell-based therapies for clinical use, and the integration of these therapies into a personalized, multidisciplinary approach to VCA. Finally, the paper also highlights the importance of addressing the ethical and regulatory hurdles associated with the use of cellular and genetic therapies in transplant medicine.

CONCLUSION

This paper offers an important contribution to the field of vascularized composite allotransplantation by highlighting the potential of cell-based therapies and cell derivatives as immunomodulators for inducing immune tolerance and reducing reliance of current CNI-based treatments that have significant on and off target side effects. It also discusses current outcomes in the literature and future directions for research in this growing field.

EDITOR COMMENTARY

Current VCA depends on "conventional" immunosuppression that is associated with significant long-term side effects, yet 85% of recipients of VCA have had rejection episodes in the first year despite being on therapy. Improvements that can facilitate the safer use of VCA would be a significant step in the wider use of this life-changing therapy. Face transplants offer by far and away the best aesthetic result in major facial deformity, such as gunshot wounds and chemical burn assault sequelae. Furthermore, some patients are too debilitated for "full" immunosuppression, e.g., the first cases of transplantation of hearts of genetically modified pigs.

As of 2023, there have been 10 deaths and 7 VCA losses in the 48 (known) face transplantations that have been performed worldwide (Longo et al., 2023). Furthermore, chronic rejection, which is not treatable and was once thought to be rare, has been increasingly reported in VCA.

The greatest challenges in VCA lie not in the surgery itself, but in the prevention of rejection as well as the psychosocial difficulties. The value of the paper lies in the discussion of the potential for cell therapies to induce tolerance in VCA patients, which is at the cutting edge of a complex topic.

REFERENCE

Longo B, Pomahac B, Giacalone M, Cardillo M, Cervelli V. 18 years of face transplantation: adverse outcomes and challenges. *J Plast Reconstr Aesthet Surg.* 2023 Dec;87:187–199. doi: 10.1016/j.bjps.2023.09.043.

CHAPTER 37

Functional Quadriceps Reconstruction: 3D Gait Analysis, EMG and Environmental Simulator Outcomes

Lo S, Childs C, Mahendra A, Young P, Carse B. *J Plast Reconstr Aesthet Surg.* 2022 Nov;75(11):3924–3937
doi: 10.1016/j.bjps.2022.08.009. Epub 2022 Aug 6. PMID: 36117134

EXPERT COMMENTARY

Eldon Mah

Current Challenges

The limb salvage approach to lower limb sarcoma management has been the gold standard for at least the last two decades. The addition of radiotherapy (neo-adjuvant or adjuvant) and the advances in reconstructive procedures for wound coverage has greatly increased the rate of successful limb salvage and increased patient satisfaction Telehealth Satisfaction Scale (TeSS).

However, a salvaged limb is not always a functional limb. Correlation between the extent of tumour resection, resultant functional deficit, and impact of functional reconstruction are not well understood nor have they been extensively studied. With ongoing refinement and development of surgical technique in muscle- and or nerve-transfers, the next frontier in reconstructive sarcoma surgery lies in improving patient's (disease-free) quality of life by broadening the goal of reconstruction to include restoration of function and/or minimization of functional deficit(s).

Functional considerations in lower limb reconstruction post-sarcoma evolves around three main clinical questions. What is the expected functional deficit after tumour resection? What is the predicted improvement with functional reconstruction? What is the difference between reconstructive techniques? It is obvious, then, that the first crucial step in developing a deeper appreciation of function and to address these clinical questions is to have an objective, reproducible, reliable measure for lower limb function. I commend the author of this paper for the application of 3D gait analysis in his endeavour to objectively measure lower limb function post-sarcoma reconstruction and the comparative study on patients who underwent functional muscle reconstruction versus those without.

DOI: 10.1201/9781003413738-37

Objective Functional Outcome Measures

Subjective measures, such as MRC grading, have limited use in the assessment of patients after functional muscle transfer. In addition to assessor bias and the inconsistent interpretation of strength, a higher grading does not directly correlate to higher function. The ideal measure of function would be one that is objective and best reflects the daily activities of patients.

The use of 3D gait analysis in the post–lower limb sarcoma resection/reconstruction patient cohort marks an important step towards better understanding of the patients' functional recovery. It allows consistent, reproducible, and comparable measures of post-resection functional deficit(s) and the outcome of functional reconstructions with different surgical techniques. The addition of environmental simulators to the gait analysis gives further relevance to the study and allows insight into the true daily function of patients.

Several other functional assessment measures have been described, including those that we have instituted: stair climb test, 4 × 10 meters walk test, and 30 seconds sit-to-stand tests. These assessments are less sophisticated than gait analysis, but they are sensitive, validated, and relatively easy to perform, requiring little in the way of additional resources or additional training for the physiotherapists. Each of these assesses the strength and balance of the patients, and the results are a reasonable reflection of the true daily functional level.

Indications for Muscle Transfer

The clinical indication(s) for functional reconstruction is still mostly guided by anecdotal reports or case series, or they are determined by the individual surgeon's personal experience, preference, and expertise. This is largely due to the limited understanding of the correlation between the postoperative functional impact with the degree of muscle resection and a lack of accurate comparative measures on the efficacy of functional reconstruction. The infrequent need for functional transfer, the variability in choice of muscle flaps (e.g., free or local), and differences in surgical technique also cloud the decision-making process.

Using 3D gait analysis, the authors of this paper demonstrate that patients with functional reconstruction score significantly better compared with a similar cohort of patients who did not have functional reconstruction. In both groups, the number of muscles resected ranged from a single muscle to all 4 muscles. The average number of quadricep components resected were 2.58 in the functional group and 2.85 in the non-functional group. The clinical indications or method of patient selection for functional reconstruction was not discussed in detail in the paper, but the findings from this study suggest that muscle transfer is efficacious in all degrees of muscle resection. The author noted in the discussion that the findings of this paper have led to the clinical decision to offer functional muscle transfer in *all* cases with quadricep resection.

However, the study population seems slightly skewed towards greater amounts of muscle resection – 11/24 patients in the reconstructive group had 3 or more muscles resected whilst only 3/24 patients had single muscle resection. Thus, the benefit of muscle transfer as seen perhaps reflects the effect in patients with greater muscle resection. This differs slightly from the indications for functional muscle transfer adopted at our institution, with our focus more on patients with greater degrees of muscle resection. Objective functional assessment performed on patients with single muscle resection without reconstruction did not show significant functional deficit; hence, muscle transfer surgery is usually not offered (Gu et al., 2023). All patients with 3 or more muscle resected in the quadricep compartment would be offered free muscle transfer.

In my view, the group that most requires further investigation and comparative study are patients with resection of 2 out of 4 quadricep muscles. In our experience, postoperative functional assessment in this group showed significant variation – some are significantly debilitated, whilst some are not and have acceptable daily function.

Choice of Functional Muscle Transfer

Currently there is no consensus on the ideal muscle transfer in this patient group. The heterogeneity of sarcoma defects, timing of radiotherapy, and variety of surgical techniques in muscle transfer all make comparative studies difficult. The majority of patients included in this paper received regional muscle flaps, i.e., long head of biceps femoris and sartorius transfers, with occasional free muscle transfer. At our institution, the majority of patients undergoing functional reconstruction would have free muscle transfer (usually latissimus dorsi myocutaneous flap), with occasional use of gracilis muscle transfer to VM defects. Differences in defect characteristics and the rate of neoadjuvant radiotherapy use is likely to have contributed in part to this difference.

Despite the significant differences in choice of functional muscle transfer, at our institution we observe similar clinical outcomes to those presented in this paper, i.e., patients who received functional reconstruction can return to activities of daily living. Unfortunately, comparative studies between different functional muscle flaps is definitely lacking and will be difficult to achieve. It is worth noting that the choice of muscle flap and the power of the muscle transfer per se may not be as critical to the functional gain as we may think, as functional muscles can be "trained up" with exercise over time. Rather, it is the vector of pull and balance of forces crossing the joint that are more relevant. In simple terms, free muscle transfer (usually of a larger muscle complex/mass) may be more appropriate in cases of more significant muscle loss, with local regional transfer (usually of isolated muscles) more appropriate for defects with lesser muscle loss.

CONCLUSION

The goal of reconstruction is to restore form and function. This paper elegantly illustrates the value of functional muscle transfer after quadriceps compartment sarcoma tumour resection. The introduction of 3D gait analysis objectively measures the functional return and allows future comparative studies. I congratulate the authors on their ongoing effort to push the boundaries of reconstruction and for objectively reviewing their results for better patient care.

REFERENCE

Gu X, Ricketts S, Mah E. Functional outcomes after single quadriceps muscle resection in patients with soft tissue sarcoma of the anterior compartment of the thigh. *ANZ J Surg.* 2023 Jan;93(1–2):288–293. doi: 10.1111/ans.18205.

EDITOR COMMENTARY

Functional quadriceps reconstruction has been quite the hot topic recently.

In 2012, Professor Lo cowrote a paper with surgeons from Singapore and Taipei that stated that the contribution of functional muscle transfer is likely to be "over-emphasised in many studies." That in cases with total loss, reconstruction performs poorly, whilst in lesser loss, minimal impairment of function means that functional reconstruction may not be warranted. In their view, reconstruction for quadriceps resection means that small resections with residual function are overtreated, whilst larger resections are undertreated with single techniques, suggesting combined muscle transfers, e.g., LD and sartorius as described by Marco Innocenti (2009).

In this paper, 10 years later, with the benefit of objective tools such as gait analysis, there has been a change in practice and Professor Lo recommends that all patients with quadriceps resection (total or partial) should have a functional transfer. The holy grail is to decide treatment based on evidence.

This paper described the first use of objective data to support functional restoration. Data was collected prospectively from PROMs. Additional prospective studies designed specifically to compare different reconstructive strategies will further guide best practices.

BIBLIOGRAPHY

Innocenti M, Abed YY, Beltrami G, Delcroix L, Balatri A, Capanna R. Quadriceps muscle reconstruction with free functioning latissimus dorsi muscle flap after oncological resection. *Microsurgery.* 2009;29(3):189–198. doi: 10.1002/micr.20607.

Lo SJ, Yeo M, Puhaindran M, Hsu CC, Wei FC. A reappraisal of functional reconstruction of extension of the knee following quadriceps resection or loss. *J Bone Joint Surg Br.* 2012;94-B(8):1016–1023. doi: 10.1302/0301-620X.94B8.29033

CHAPTER 38

Targeted Muscle Reinnervation: A Novel Approach to Postamputation Neuroma Pain

Souza JM, Cheesborough JE, Ko JH, Cho MS, Kuiken TA, Dumanian GA.
Clin Orthop Relat Res. 2014 Oct;472(10):2984–2990

EXPERT COMMENTARY

Jeannette Ting

Targeted muscle reinnervation (TMR) and regenerative peripheral nerve interfaces (RPNI) are two emerging techniques that can be used to manage neuroma pain. They are often grouped and discussed together and although there are some fundamental similarities, they are, in fact, quite different techniques. The basic principle for both TMR and RPNI is the same – to give the severed nerve a purpose. Otherwise, much like bored toddlers, the nerves grow haphazardly looking for something to do. Until TMR and RPNI, the surgical management of severed nerves has mainly been to bury or wrap it – whether it be nerves, flaps, muscle, bone, or synthetic material.

This paper is considered the landmark paper for the use of TMR for neuroma pain. The first published use of TMR in the literature came from Kuiken et al. (2009) for powering of myoelectric prostheses. Kuiken is one of the co-authors of this landmark paper and has published extensively in the TMR literature since.

This paper is a retrospective study of 26 patients over 10 years between 2002 and 2012 where it was noted that patients fitted with TMR-powered myoelectric prosthesis also reported reduced neuroma pain. A total of 15 of the 26 patients had reportable neuroma pain with 87% having complete or significant improvement in their neuroma pain. The paper also described how TMR was performed, allowing surgeons reading the paper to replicate it for themselves. The technique may appear ludicrous at first – coapting a very large severed nerve to a significantly smaller motor nerve. However, subsequent papers inspired by this study have shown similarly positive results. This includes a prospective study by Dumanian et al. (2019) following 28 amputees, showing statistically improvement in phantom limb pain and residual limb pain after TMR compared to standard treatment (burying transected nerve ending in innervated muscle). A systematic review published in 2024 (ElAbd et al., 2024) compared 449 TMR to 716 control patients and found that patients with TMR had decreased pain medication requirements and improved pain measures.

DOI: 10.1201/9781003413738-38

RPNI was first described almost a decade later than TMR in 2012, and so there are fewer papers describing it. The idea is similar – to give the nerve something to do. The severed nerves are wrapped in small muscle graft, which is buried in more muscle. The muscle degenerates and subsequently regenerates and with neurotization by the severed nerve. It is significantly easier to perform than TMR, taking 7–10 minutes in general. The pilot study in 2016 (Woo et al., 2016) had 46 RPNI performed in 16 amputees with 71% reduction in neuroma pain and 53% reduction in phantom pain at an average of 7.5 months follow-up. The team of Woo, Kung, Cederna, and Urbanchek have continued to lead the way in research of RPNI in the literature.

To date, there has been no paper testing RPNI against TMR although there was a paper published in 2022 that looked at both techniques together in a rat model (Saltzman et al., 2022). The results thus far have been promising as the future for patients with neuroma pain seems to be more optimistic than a decade ago.

REFERENCES

Dumanian GA, Potter BK, Mioton LM, Ko JH, Cheesborough JE, Souza JM, Ertl WJ, Tintle SM, Nanos GP, Valerio IL, Kuiken TA, Apkarian AV, Porter K, Jordan SW. Targeted muscle reinnervation treats neuroma and phantom pain in major limb amputees: a randomized clinical trial. *Ann Surg.* 2019 Aug;270(2):238–246. doi: 10.1097/SLA.0000000000003088.

ElAbd R, Dow T, Jabori S, Alhalabi B, Lin SJ, Dowlatshahi S. Pain and functional outcomes following targeted muscle reinnervation: a systematic review. *Plast Reconstr Surg.* 2024 Feb 1;153(2):494–508. doi: 10.1097/PRS.0000000000010598.

Kuiken TA, Li G, Lock BA, Lipschutz RD, Miller LA, Stubblefield KA, Englehart KB. Targeted muscle reinnervation for real-time myoelectric control of multifunction artificial arms. *JAMA.* 2009 Feb 11;301(6):619–628. doi: 10.1001/jama.2009.116.

Saltzman C, Staidl N, Roth E, Weihrauch D, Hoben GM. Targeted muscle reinnervation and regenerative peripheral nerve interface support similar quantities of sensory neurons but vary in motor neuron regeneration in a rat model. *Plast Reconstr Surg Global Open.* 2022 Oct;10(10S):23–24. doi: 10.1097/01. GOX.0000898428.87031.60.

Woo SL, Kung TA, Brown DL, Leonard JA, Kelly BM, Cederna PS. Regenerative peripheral nerve interfaces for the treatment of postamputation neuroma pain: a pilot study. *Plast Reconstr Surg Glob Open.* 2016 Dec 27;4(12):e1038. doi: 10.1097/GOX.0000000000001038.

EDITOR COMMENTARY

Pain after amputation is a reasonably common sequela of amputation; regenerative sprouting from severed nerves that fail to reach an end organ target continue to grow blindly. The overwhelming majority of neuromas are asymptomatic, with estimates of 75%–96% (upper limb) and 68%–89% (lower limb). Over 150 techniques have been described to treat neuromas, often meaning that none are completely satisfactory. The most common techniques involve either reconstruction of nerve continuity, burying the nerve (into muscle/ bone), and ligation or capping of the nerve end.

In TMR, nerves and muscles that no longer serve motor function in the residual limb after amputation, are "repurposed" to provide EMG signals for more intuitive prosthetic control. Nerves were given "somewhere to go and something to do." Histological studies found that the structure resembled preamputation nerves more than neuromas (Kim et al. 2012). This paper is a retrospective study that found TMR intended for control of prostheses also reduced neuroma pain/residual limb pain. Since then, there have been over 100 papers on TMR for pain including the multicentre, single-blinded RCT by Dumanian et al. (2019).

RPNI is a novel creative solution designed originally as an interface to amplify action potentials for the control of prostheses by burying nerve endings into a free muscle graft from expendable muscle and then burying in soft tissue. The muscle would degenerate and then revascularize and become reneurotized. It is simple and does not require microsurgery skills. After finding that RPNI also reduced neuromas, it was also co-opted for use in treating pain.

There have been no RCTs of RPNI yet. Kubiak et al. (2019) retrospectively reviewed the outcomes of 90 patients who underwent limb amputation with and without prophylactic RPNI implantation. The latter group included traditional approaches, such as burying/ ligating/capping the nerves. The two groups were well matched for sex and level of amputation and were followed for at least 12 months postoperatively. A total of 0% in the RPNI group developed symptomatic neuromas during the study period compared to 13.3% in the control group.

There have been no comparative studies of TMR versus RPNI yet, but they should be imminent. De Lange et al. (2022) reviewed the use of TMR and RPNI to prevent neuropathic pain, whilst Mauch et al. (2023) reviewed the use of TMR and RPNI for both pain treatment and prophylaxis.

REFERENCES

Kim PS, et al. The effects of targeted muscle reinnervation on neuromas in a rabbit rectus abdominis f lap model. *J Hand Surg Am.* 2012;37:1609–1616.
Kubiak CA, Kemp SWP, Cederna PS, Kung TA. Prophylactic regenerative peripheral nerve interfaces to prevent postamputation pain. *Plast Reconstr Surg.* 2019 Sep;144(3):421e–430e. doi: 10.1097/ PRS.0000000000005922.
de Lange JWD, Hundepool CA, Power DM, Rajaratnam V, Duraku LS, Zuidam JM. Prevention is better than cure: Surgical methods for neuropathic pain prevention following amputation: a systematic review. *J Plast Reconstr Aesthet Surg.* 2022 Mar;75(3):948–959. doi: 10.1016/j.bjps.2021.11.076.
Mauch JT, Kao DS, Friedly JL, Liu Y. Targeted muscle reinnervation and regenerative peripheral nerve interfaces for pain prophylaxis and treatment: a systematic review. *PM R.* 2023 Nov;15(11):1457–1465. doi: 10.1002/pmrj.12972.

CHAPTER 39

The Economy in Autologous Tissue Transfer: Part 1. The Kiss Flap Technique

Zhang YX, Hayakawa TJ, Levin LS, Hallock GG, Lazzeri D. *Plast Reconstr Surg.* 2016 Mar;137(3):1018–1030 doi: 10.1097/01.prs.0000479971.99309.21

EDITOR COMMENTARY

Yixin and I were faculty together at the 2018 ICPF course in Bogotá. He gave an elegant demonstration of harvesting a relatively large medial SCIP/groin flap, then he went on to use a higher SCIP propeller flap to close the first defect. It was very well executed and one of the highlights of the live surgery sessions. During the subsequent cadaveric workshop, I had constant requests to demonstrate this by delegates who I found out later mistook me for Yixin Zhang.

Professor Zhang elegantly demonstrates how multiple small skin paddles allow direct closure of the donor site whilst still providing a large amount of tissue for transfer. The smaller flaps form pieces of a larger jigsaw; two rectangles/triangles, etc., can be assembled to form a larger square – the large square flap could have been harvested directly, but the donor site would not have been amenable to direct closure.

Free flap transfer for reconstruction is a reliable technique. With more complex reconstructions, the problems of limited donor sites and donor site morbidity become greater. The emphasis on optimizing the donor site represents a higher level at the top of the conventional reconstructive ladder. This philosophy is referred to as the "kiss flap technique" by the authors and in the literature as "kiss flaps" or used as a prefix, e.g., "kiss DIEP" (Luo Z et al., 2019). Those of us familiar with perforator flaps will have probably done something similar to reconstruct selected defects, e.g., to close skin and mucosal defects with separate islands. Others have called it a "split paddle design" (Marsh and Chana, 2010) or "efficient use" (Chang NJ et al., 2011; Scaglioni MR et al., 2019; Bag and Das, 2024). It could be argued that the KISS principle is additionally/ more focused on the donor site, but more significantly it provides a catchy name for the concept. Zhang is immersed in this philosophy and uses it almost daily to reduce the necessity of using skin grafts to close flap donor sites, and to optimize both donor sites and the flap – taken to the nth degree.

The authors describe a classification of different kiss flaps, which can be free or pedicled. The most useful patterns are chimeric flaps with the same pedicle, and thus a single anastomosis. Some situations may need 2 separate anastomoses (in parallel) or in series. Kiss flaps are most often harvested from areas with well-defined branching, e.g., LCFA, subscapular, etc. It can also be applied to a single branch, e.g., posterior interosseus artery reverse flow/pedicled for hand defects (Zhang YX et al., 2013).

It could be said that having two perforators perfuse their own smaller areas may offer improved vascularity compared to using one perforator for a larger square area. However, the flipside is that dividing a flap between two perforators does have some risks, e.g., direct damage to perfusion, or it may introduce other potential problems, such as twisting of pedicles. Particular caution is needed with possible complications when aiming for the next level or trying anything new in general.

There is an extra suture line which will result in an additional scar at the reconstructed site; this scar can be placed along a natural anatomical border/crease where possible or limited to situations where an extra scar would be less of an issue, e.g., scalp reconstruction (Xiong L et al., 2018). However, for a neophallus, for example, having the extra scar on the ventral scar may be regarded by some as (aesthetically) unacceptable, whilst in situations such as circumferential pharyngectomy, it may significantly increase the risk of leakage/fistulae.

Planning (and experience) is crucial. The design comes from analysis of the wider donor site by pinch testing and definition of the perforators, e.g., with color Doppler ultrasound (CDU) or CTA. Good preoperative imaging is important and successful application of Kiss depends on the configuration of the perforator permitting it; however, a level of awareness with constant reevaluation and adaptability is still necessary.

Another related concept from the author is that of "sequential flaps" where the (second) local perforator flap instead of being combined with the primary flap into a "kiss flap" is instead used to close the donor site of the primary flap (ICPF example described above). This is particularly useful for closure of flap donor sites, e.g., the defect after harvest of (small) radial forearm flaps can be closed with (bilobed) flaps based on perforators from the ulnar artery (Jeng and Tan, 2012), and the closure of LD (Wang Y et al., 2018) and leg propeller flaps donor sites (Ran X et al., 2022). We have used Keystone flaps to close large ALT donor sites (presented at WSRM 2009, Okinawa). You could say that these represent sequential flaps versus the parallel (kiss) flaps.

That was Part 1. I believe that Part 2 is in progress and should be worth the wait.

REFERENCES

Bag SK, Das C. Tailoring of ALT flap for optimizing donor site morbidity. *Indian J Plast Surg.* 2024 May 30;57(3):223–226. doi: 10.1055/s-0044-1787056.

Chang NJ, Waughlock N, Kao D, Lin CH, Lin CH, Hsu CC. Efficient design of split anterolateral thigh flap in extremity reconstruction. *Plast Reconstr Surg.* 2011 Dec;128(6):1242–1249. doi: 10.1097/PRS.0b013e318230c868.

Jeng SF, Tan NC. Optimizing aesthetic and functional outcomes at donor sites. *Chang Gung Med J.* 2012 May–Jun;35(3):219–230. doi: 10.4103/2319-4170.106150.

Luo Z, Qing L, Zhou Z, Wu P, Yu F, Tang J. Reconstruction of large soft tissue defects of the extremities in children using the kiss deep inferior epigastric artery perforator flap to achieve primary closure of donor site. *Ann Plast Surg.* 2019;82(1):64–70. doi: 10.1097/sap.0000000000001659.

Marsh DJ, Chana JS. Reconstruction of very large defects: a novel application of the double skin paddle anterolateral thigh flap design provides for primary donor-site closure. *J Plast Reconstr Aesthet Surg.* 2010;63:120–125.

Ran X, Liu Y, Yang R, Zang M. Application of perforator propeller flap sequential transfer technique in repair of soft tissue defect of distal lower extremity. *Zhongguo Xiu Fu Chong Jian Wai Ke Za Zhi.* 2022 Apr 15;36(4):451–455. doi: 10.7507/1002-1892.202111047.

Scaglioni MF, Barth AA, Giovanoli P. Reconstruction of an upper posterior thigh extensive defect with a free split-anterolateral thigh (s-ALT) flap by perforator-to-perforator anastomosis: a case report. *Microsurgery.* 2019 Jan;39(1):91–94. doi: 10.1002/micr.30295.

Wang Y, Ren Z, Xue J, Guo L, Gao D, Hao Q, Gao F, Yang J. Effectiveness of posterior intercostal artery perforator flap in repair of donor defect after latissimus dorsi myocutaneous flap transfer. *Zhongguo Xiu Fu Chong Jian Wai Ke Za Zhi.* 2018 Sep 15;32(9):1187–1191. doi: 10.7507/1002-1892.201803046.

Xiong L, Guo N, Gazyakan E, Kneser U, Hirche C. The anterolateral thigh flap with kiss technique for microsurgical reconstruction of oncological scalp defects. *J Plast Reconstr Aesthe Surg.* 2018;71(2):273–276. doi: 10.1016/j.bjps.2017.10.018.

Zhang YX, Qian Y, Pu Z, Ong YS, Messmer C, Li Q, Agostini T, Erdmann D, Levin LS, Lazzeri D. Reverse bipaddle posterior interosseous artery perforator flap. *Plast Reconstr Surg.* 2013 Apr;131(4):552e–562e. doi: 10.1097/PRS.0b013e31828275d9.

CHAPTER 40

Body Contouring by Lipolysis: A 5-Year Experience with over 3,000 Cases

Illouz YG. *Plast Reconstr Surg.* 1983 Nov;72(5):591–597
doi: 10.1097/00006534-198311000-00001 PMID: 6622564

EDITOR COMMENTARY

The study includes a large number of 3,447 procedures on 1,326 patients with liposuction with infiltration. Illouz used a hypotonic "wetting" solution composed of 100 mL NS, 20 mL water, and 1,000 units of hyaluronidase. Areas were tunnelled and suctioned until reasonable aesthetic contours were achieved. The author limited removal of fat to 6 pounds to avoid shock; if more than 4 pounds of fat were removed, then fluid resuscitation may be necessary. Drains were sometimes used and removed after 48 hours. There were no haematomas reported. The most commonly treated areas were "saddlebags," knees, gluteal folds, buttocks, hips. and abdomen.

There are several weaknesses to note – no specific outcomes are measured, there were apparently no significant complications, and no specific follow-up was mentioned. Furthermore, it is a single surgeon experience with potential observer bias and a lack of a control group. However, as a descriptive paper of a surgeon's vast experience of a (relatively) novel procedure, it was a true landmark paper in the development of modern safe liposuction. This particular issue of *Plastic and Reconstructive Surgery* had several other articles on liposuction, which was popularized in Europe well before in the United States.

Yves-Gerard Illouz (1929–2015) was a French plastic surgeon (he qualified first as a general surgeon in 1968 and received his specialist certification only after a long battle in 1989). His main innovations were using blunt cannula (of 3 different sizes, which were smaller and cheaper than expensive instruments used by the Fischers) and fluid infiltration that he called "dissecting hydrotomy." This paved the way eventually for the tumescent technique by Jeffrey Klein (1993), a dermatologist who developed his technique to allow liposuction without general anaesthesia by gradually changing his formula in vivo.

Before this, various techniques for fat reduction had been intermittently reported in the latter half of 20th century, mostly using sharp instruments such as curettes (Schrudde 1980; Kesselring 1978). but the often-prolonged postoperative recovery deterred

DOI: 10.1201/9781003413738-40

wider uptake. A major development came from the father and son team, Arpad and Giorgio Fischer, in Rome, who added suction to a variety of blunt cannula of their own design (some early prototypes had motor-driven rotating blades inside), initially using this "liposculpture" technique to treat trochanteric lipodystrophy that previously had most commonly been treated with "Pitanguy's technique" of open en bloc resection. They also described an early form of cross tunnelling (1976, conference abstracts). Their techniques were effective and seemed to be associated with fewer complications, such as haematoma, but, in turn, they were associated with the rare but serious complication of persistent lymphorrhoea. Fournier invited Giorgio Fischer to Paris (in 1976) when Dr. Lawrence Field, a dermatologist, was visiting, and the latter became one of the first Americans to learn the technique of blunt liposuction.

Illouz discovered his wet technique liposuction in 1977 ostensibly to fulfill a request from a friend (who also happened to be a famous actress) for removal of a large lipoma of the shoulder/back without leaving a scar. He had described the technique in French journals before this particular article. Fournier, who worked with Illouz, had developed a "dry technique" (1983) that he preferred for "precision," but he later changed to infiltration with local anaesthesia. Hetter added adrenaline to the infiltration in 1984, which reduced the drop in haematocrit.

Dr. Norman Martin, an otololaryngologist, visited Ilouz in 1980 and took the technique back to Los Angeles. This prompted more doctors to visit Fournier and Illouz; there was an instructional course in Paris in 1982, followed by an invitation for Illouz to speak at the American Society of Plastic and Reconstructive Surgeons (ASPRS) meeting (forerunner of the American Society of Plastic Surgeons [ASPS]) later in the same year in Hawaii, which attracted even more attention. Liposuction in America exploded. The ASPRS tried to control/ monopolize the field by asking Illouz and Fournier to sign a contract to teach plastic surgeons exclusively; Illouz signed but Fournier did not.

If we look further back in history, there is the infamous case involving Charles Dujarier, a French "osteoarticular" surgeon, of some renown and titles. In 1928, he operated on Suzanne Geoffre, who has been variously described as a ballerina or dancer at the Folies Bergère, and who, at the time, was a model for the couturier Paul Poiret. She was due to be married soon and had just opened up her own fashion house. She found her calves to be too fat for the emerging fashion of dresses ending at the knee, supposedly threatening to shoot herself unless Dujarier treated her. For some reason, Dujarier agreed to perform the surgery in a local hospital for free, apparently underplaying the risks and complexity of the surgery. It was said that he used a curette to remove fat, then excised too much skin and various complications led eventually to one leg needing to be amputated; however, no operative notes have been published. The patient sued and won a contentious widely reported lawsuit; this has been reported as the first lawsuit in plastic surgery, though there are at least two prior reports for cosmetic surgery in France in 1913. Dujarier appealed successfully, ostensibly because he did the surgery for free, for "scientific purposes," but he died a few months after. There was significant backlash and cosmetic surgery had a poor reputation in France for decades.

REFERENCES

Fournier PF, Otteni FM. Lipodissection in body sculpturing: the dry procedure. *Plast Reconstr Surg.* 1983 Nov;72(5):598–609. doi: 10.1097/00006534-198311000-00002.

Hetter GP. The effect of low-dose epinephrine on the hematocrit drop following lipolysis. *Aesthetic Plast Surg.* 1984;8(1):19–21. doi: 10.1007/BF01572780.

Kesselring UK, Meyer R. A suction curette for removal of excessive local deposits of subcutaneous fat. *Plast Reconstr Surg.* 1978 Aug;62(2):305–6. doi: 10.1097/00006534-197808000-00040. PMID: 674424.

Klein JA. Tumescent technique for local anesthesia improves safety in large-volume liposuction. *Plast Reconstr Surg.* 1993 Nov;92(6):1085–1098.

Schrudde J. Lipexeresis as a means of eliminating local adiposity. *Aesthetic Plast Surg.* 1980 Dec;4(1):215–26. doi: 10.1007/BF01575221. PMID: 24174084.

CHAPTER 41

"Components Separation" Method for Closure of Abdominal Wall Defects: An Anatomic and Clinical Study

Ramirez OM, Ruas E, Dellon AL. *Plast Reconstr Surg.* 1990 Sep;86(3):519–526
doi: 10.1097/00006534-199009000-00023 PMID: 2143588

EDITOR COMMENTARY

The aim of abdominal wall reconstruction (AWR) is to close the abdominal defect in a manner that offers functional dynamic muscle support without excessive tension closure. True defects with tissue loss may occur after trauma, infection, or surgery. Incisional ventral herniae (IVH) are true defects in the fascia or musculature through which intra-abdominal contents can protrude, with the risk of incarceration and strangulation. In contrast, with diastasis of the recti (or divarication) the recti become lateralized due to weakening/stretching of the linea alba without an actual fascial defect per se.

Until the late 19th century, the usual way to repair IVH involved mobilizing the abdominal wall muscle/fascia in various ways, including "aponeuroplasties" and muscle transposition (Ger R, 1983) that do not offer a dynamic repair. For larger defects, a bridging mesh was usually used, but mesh could become infected and would then have to be removed. Skin grafting over granulation is often used to "control" a dire situation but is wholly inadequate as a long-term option.

Ramirez suggested that it was the multiple muscle layers of the lateral abdominal wall with different orientations that made en bloc movement difficult. The novel concept in component separation (CS) was that creation of an intermusculofascial plane between the layers in conjunction with a relaxing incision of the fascia allowed medial mobilization of the rectus abdominis complex sufficient for midline closure. The existence of multiple layers imbues some degree of redundancy to the structure of the lateral abdominal wall so clinically relevant weakness is usually not seen when a single layer, such as the external oblique (EO), is disrupted.

In their landmark study, the authors dissected the abdominal walls of 10 fresh cadavers and reported on the ability to mobilize musculofascial tissue with various maneuvers. They noted that the EO muscle/fascia was the major restriction to medialization of the rectus due to its fascial rigidity and its attachments to the rib cage and iliac crest. By incising the EO aponeurosis 1 cm lateral to the arcus semilunaris and freeing the rectus muscle from its posterior sheath, each rectus could be advanced medially up to 5, 10, and 3 cm at the superior, middle, and inferior thirds of the abdomen, respectively. The layer between the external and internal obliques (IO) is relatively avascular and easy to dissect. The nerves lie mostly in the layer between the IO and transversalis abdominis (TA); motor nerves from the intercostals pierce the TA fascia at the back whilst sensory nerves to the lower abdomen, groin, and scrotum (ilioinguinal and iliohypogastric) also pierce the TA to gain access to this layer. The rectus moves with the IO/TA and the muscles remain innervated as the nerves to the rectus lie deep to the IO.

They applied these techniques to 11 patients with ventral hernia (of various etiologies) and successfully reconstructed defects of up to 15 × 25 cm without the need for autologous flaps. The layers were closed with non-dissolvable interrupted sutures, then the skin flaps were closed in layers with drains.

Although CS has been largely attributed to Ramirez, some argue that the work is derivative of Donald Young (Halvorson EG, 2009). In 1961, Young described the use of relaxing incisions in the EO; the detachment/ disconnection of the EO from the rectus was performed in a slightly different manner – Young was more focused on epigastric herniae and emphasized the attachments to the costal margin. Undoubtedly CS as described by Ramirez et al. is an evolutionary step of prior techniques, including Young, that also evolved from others, especially Gibson CL (1916). However this study reports on significant advancements in technique that basically revolutionized AWR. The strengths include the design: Anatomical findings in cadavers were validated through a prospective clinical study with 11 cases. The major limitations were the small sample size and variable and short follow-up (ranging from 4 months to 3.5 years). Since this study, component separation has evolved with significant modifications to become less traumatic with fewer complications.

The use of innervated muscle for AWR in CS allows more robust reconstruction; CS is preferable to flaps that tend to lack muscle or have muscle that is denervated, or mesh which has issues, particularly when used in bridge mode. Meshes have risks of infection, extrusion, and fistulae formation. Recurrence is the most important outcome measure, and, although Ramirez et al. reported zero recurrences, their data was insufficient to draw long-term conclusions. Subsequent studies found recurrence rates of between 8.7% and 32%, depending on patient comorbidities, use of mesh, length of follow-up, and the exact surgical technique itself.

With increased adoption of CS came better appreciation of the best indications and contraindications as multiple limitations were found. The "radical" approach by Ramirez et al. involved significant mobilization of tissues, resulting in a large wound and spaces involving most of the central abdominal wall, predisposing it to complications such as hematomas, seromas (about 2%), and infections, which in some studies were as high as 20%, reflecting the fact that many AWR surgeries are performed under contaminated conditions. Drainage can be prolonged, and some suggest the use of glue, sutures, and or compression. In addition, the wide transection of perforators through the recti reduces the perfusion to the central abdominal skin that becomes more reliant on intercostal perforators, leading to potential midline skin necrosis (5%) usually below umbilicus and wound dehiscence. Bulging could occur at the site of EO incisions whilst rupture could damage neurovasular bundles, potentially denervating the rectus.

The technique has been continually modified largely to reduce morbidity. Shestak KC et al. (2000) used a less radical technique to accelerate recovery. They achieved slightly less unilateral mobility with:

- 4 cm above umbo
- 8 cm below umbo at waist
- 3 cm in lower abdomen.

Similarly, they found that an additional 2 cm movement could be gained by elevating the rectus off posterior sheath entirely compared to 3/5/3 cm by Ramirez et al. This posterior dissection is relatively easy in "virgin" abdomens (the anterior sheath has the tendinous intersections), but this layer can be quite fibrotic after prior surgery, and dissection may damage muscle, which is counterproductive.

Some make an additional distinction in CS, calling it anterior component separation (ACS) when dividing the EO aponeurosis and dissecting between the EO and IO muscles. Posterior component separation (PCS), on the other hand, involves division of the posterior lamella of the IO as well as the TA muscle and dissecting between the muscle and transversalis fascia (or peritoneum). The plane between IO and TA is more difficult to dissect.

Saulis and Dumanian (2002) described "perforator-sparing" soft tissue dissection, which reduced wound necrosis and infection from 20% to 2%. Maas SM et al. (1999) used lateral skin incisions to preserve perfusion to the medial skin; whilst this modification has not been that popular, it is potentially useful in cases with stoma, a situation which makes it difficult to use CS otherwise. Milburn (2007) Others have used endoscopic assistance to make lateral counter-incisions and balloon dissectors. In general, minimally invasive CS that avoids extensive skin undermining can reduce complications but at the expense of the extent of advancement. Heller L et al. (2012) limited skin elevation to about 5 cm lateral to the arcus. The fascial incision was made 1–2 cm from arcus, from inguinal ligament to the costal margin, with superior extension through the EO over the chest wall. The intermuscular plane was dissected as far back as possible to the midaxillary line, taking care to avoid trauma to IO and rectus with extra caution at the Spigelian fascia.

In 2009 Ibarra-Hurtado et al. used botulinum toxin A (BTXA, off-label) to inject the lateral muscles to facilitate hernia closure. In a prospective series in 12 patients, there was a 5.25 cm mean reduction in the defect width after 4 weeks followed by successful open repair with EO release/ CS in six. Some call this a "chemical component separation," some have used BTXA to "optimize" the patient for anticipated difficult closures even with CS, whilst others use it as an alternative to CS. An analysis of a prospective hernia database of patients undergoing AWR by Marturano et al. (2023) compared CS with ultrasound-guided injections of BTXA alone and found that the muscle relaxation/elongation with the toxin was sufficient to allow a subset of patient to have AWR without CS with non-inferior outcomes. BTXA seems least useful for subxiphoid (M1) herniae (Polcz ME et al., 2025). Similarly, some have used preoperative progressive pneumoperitoneum (PPP) by repeated insufflation of gas into the peritoneal cavity for preoperative "optimization," but there are major risks of significant complications.

The first author recognizes the main limitations of CS being the size of the defect and the blood supply of the skin. In subsequent articles, he recommends limiting the skin separation from muscle/fascia as per modern abdominoplasty, leaving the lateral parts intact. He also recommends a graduated step-wise approach to CS – larger defects may need more relaxing incisions in EO, which can be reinforced with mesh. With all these variants, the best CS repair technique is unclear; comparison between the different techniques is largely impossible. Studies have been retrospective mostly with one RCT.

In the acute situation, techniques such as NPWT in combination with tension sutures such as the VADER technique (van der Velde M, 2005), which can also be achieved with commercial devices such as Dermaclose (Synovis Micro), can help particularly where there is an element of tissue/bowel oedema. Subcutaneous NPWT has been used in combination with CS to aid the skin closure and reduce soft tissue complications (Sato T et al., 2018) whilst incisional NPWT for high-risk AWR incisions is reasonably well established though the benefits are not wholly clear (Leuchter M et al., 2021).

REFERENCES

Celdrán Á, Fraile MJ, Georgiev-Hristov T, González-Ayora S. A stepwise approach based on a rational use of components separation and double mesh prosthesis for incisional hernia repair. *Hernia.* 2016 Apr;20(2):201–207. doi: 10.1007/s10029-015-1438-6.

Ger R, Duboys E. The prevention and repair of large abdominal-wall defects by muscle transposition: a preliminary communication. *Plast Reconstr Surg.* 1983 Aug;72(2):170–178. doi: 10.1097/00006534-198308000-00008.

Gibson CL. Post-operative intestinal obstruction. *Ann Surg.* 1916 Apr;63(4):442–51. doi: 10.1097/00000658-191604000-00006. PMID: 17863520; PMCID: PMC1406860.

Halvorson EG. On the origins of components separation. *Plast Reconstr Surg.* 2009;124:1545–1549.

Heller L, McNichols CH, Ramirez OM. Component separations. *Semin Plast Surg.* 2012 Feb;26(1):25–28. doi: 10.1055/s-0032-1302462.

Ibarra-Hurtado TR, Nuño-Guzmán CM, EcheagarayHerrera JE, *et al.* Use of botulinum toxin type a before abdominal wall hernia reconstruction. *World J Surg.* 2009;33:2553–2556.

Leuchter M, Hitzbleck M, Schafmayer C, Philipp M. Use of incisional preventive negative pressure wound therapy in open incisional hernia repair: who benefits? *Wound Repair Regen.* 2021 Sep;29(5):759–765. doi: 10.1111/wrr.12948.

Lowe JB, Garza JR, Bowman JL, *et al.* Endoscopically assisted "components separation" for closure of abdominal wall defects. *Plast Reconstr Surg.* 2000;105:720–729.

Maas SM, van Engeland M, Leeksma NG, Bleichrodt RP. A modification of the "components separation" technique for closure of abdominal wall defects in the presence of an enterostomy. *J Am Coll Surg.* 1999 Jul;189(1):138–140. doi: 10.1016/s1072-7515(99)00067-8.

Marturano MN, Ayuso SA, Ku D, Raible R, Lopez R, Scarola GT, Gersin K, Colavita PD, Augenstein VA, Heniford BT. Preoperative botulinum toxin A (BTA) injection versus component separation techniques (CST) in complex abdominal wall reconstruction (AWR): a propensity-scored matched study. *Surgery.* 2023 Mar;173(3):756–764. doi: 10.1016/j.surg.2022.07.034.

Milburn ML, Shah PK, Friedman EB, *et al.* Laparoscopically assisted components separation technique for ventral incisional hernia repair. *Hernia.* 2007;11:157–161.

Polcz ME, Holland AM, Lorenz WR, *et al.* Preoperative Botulinum Toxin A (BTA) injection in abdominal wall reconstruction for subxiphoid (M1) hernias. *Hernia.* 2025;29:96. doi: 10.1007/s10029-025-03290-2.

Sato T, Fujita M, Kushimoto S. Ventral herniorrhaphy with the combined use of component separation technique and negative pressure wound therapy in patient with complex abdominal wall hernia complicated with parastomal hernia: a case report. *Nihon Gekakei Rengo Gakkaishi (Journal of Japanese College of Surgeons).* 2018;43:295–299. doi: 10.4030/jjcs.43.295.

Saulis AS, Dumanian GA. Periumbilical rectus abdominis perforator preservation significantly reduces superficial wound complications in "separation of parts" hernia repairs. *Plast Reconstr Surg.* 2002 Jun;109(7):2275–2280. doi: 10.1097/00006534-200206000-00016.

Shestak KC, Edington HJ, Johnson RR. The separation of anatomic components technique for the reconstruction of massive midline abdominal wall defects: anatomy, surgical technique, applications, and limitations revisited. *Plast Reconstr Surg.* 2000 Feb;105(2):731–738. doi: 10.1097/00006534-200002000-00041.

Van der Velde M, Hudson DA. VADER (vacuum-assisted dermal recruitment): a new method of wound closure. *Ann Plast Surg.* 2005 Dec;55(6):660–604. doi: 10.1097/01.sap.0000187181.59748.19.

Young D. Repair of epigastric incisional hernia. *Br J Surg.* 1961;48:514–516.

CHAPTER 42

Adjuvant Ipilimumab versus Placebo after Complete Resection of High-Risk Stage III Melanoma (EORTC 18071): A Randomised, Double-Blind, Phase 3 Trial

Eggermont AM, Chiarion-Sileni V, Grob JJ, Dummer R, Wolchok JD, Schmidt H, Hamid O, Robert C, Ascierto PA, Richards JM, Lebbé C, Ferraresi V, Smylie M, Weber JS, Maio M, Konto C, Hoos A, de Pril V, Gurunath RK, de Schaetzen G, Suciu S, Testori A. *Lancet Oncol.* 2015 May;16(5):522–530

EDITOR COMMENTARY

Stage III melanoma is associated with a high risk of distant metastasis and death; the 5-year and 10-year melanoma-specific survival is 77% and 69%, respectively, for these patients, according to the *AJCC* 8th edition (2017), dipping further to 32% and 24% in the stage IIID subgroup. The aim of this trial (EORTC 18071) was to assess whether adjuvant ipilimumab (anti-CTLA-4) could improve survival in patients with resected, high-risk stage III melanoma.

Ipilimumab is an immune checkpoint inhibitor (ICI). (Immune) checkpoints in this context are proteins made by some immune cells and cancer cells that regulate/inhibit the immune response, thus limiting the ability of T cells to kill cancer cells and include cytotoxic T lymphocyte antigen 4 (CTLA-4) and programmed death-1 receptor (PD-1) and PD-L1, its ligand. ICIs block these proteins from binding with their targets; thus, as a type of immunotherapy, they boost the anti-cancer immune response.

With the demonstrated efficacy of ICIs and molecularly targeted therapy (e.g., BRAF and MEK inhibitors) in the management of unresectable and metastatic melanoma, these were then applied as adjuvant therapy for patients with high-risk stage III disease in this study. This was an international, randomised, prospective trial with a reasonably large sample size (n = 951) that was initiated in 2008. The median follow-up was 6.9 years by the final analysis of the data in 2019 (Eggermont AMM et al., 2019). There was significantly prolonged median recurrence-free survival (RFS) in patients treated with adjuvant ipilimumab as compared to placebo (26.1 vs 17.1 months).

Further analysis published a year later demonstrated improved 5-year RFS (40.8% vs 30.3%) and 5-year overall survival (65.4% vs 54.4%) in patients treated with adjuvant

DOI: 10.1201/9781003413738-42

ipilimumab (Eggermont, 2016). However, 41.6% of patients in the ipilimumab group experienced immune-related adverse effects of grade 3 or 4 (vs 2.7% in the placebo group), with 5 deaths (1.1%) reported in the ipilimumab group. This was a significant downside with more than half of patients (53.3%) having to stop treatment. This study does not address whether maintenance treatment with ipilimumab is needed.

Despite these disadvantages, the EORTC 18071 trial was a breakthrough being the first phase III trial to establish a significant survival benefit with adjuvant ICI therapy. It was the beginning of significant changes in the management of high-risk resected melanoma, and subsequent trials with different drugs demonstrated better responses. Most notably:

- Nivolumab (anti-PD-1, Checkmate 238 trial Weber J et al., 2017). Patients with stage IIB–IV melanoma treated with adjuvant nivolumab had better 4-year RFS compared to ipilimumab (51.7% vs 41.2%). Furthermore, patient tolerance was better with fewer having to stop treatment (9.7% vs 42.6%).
  - The combined use of nivolumab and ipilimumab further increased 5-year overall survival rates (Larkin, 2019). Ba H et al. (2003) confirmed that the combination conferred the best disease-free survival and overall survival, but had significant risk of grade 3–5 adverse events.
- Pembrolizumab (also anti-PD-1, KEYNOTE 054 trial, Eggermont, 2018). Patients with stage III disease treated with adjuvant pembrolizumab had better 1-year RFS (75.4% vs 61.0%) compared to placebo.
  - The systematic review by Ba H et al. (2023) confirmed the improved efficacy and tolerability of anti-PD-1 immunotherapy over ipilimumab.
- BRAF and MEK inhibitors. The COMBI-AD trial (Dummer, 2020) demonstrated better 3-year RFS (58% vs 39%) and 3-year overall survival (86% vs 77%) with adjuvant dabrafenib–trametinib compared to placebo in patients with stage III melanoma who had specific mutations (BRAF V600E or V600K mutations).

Adjuvant anti-PD-1 and BRAF-targeted therapies are accepted as standard of care in patients with high-risk resected melanoma. Although the superiority of one over the other, or in combination within the adjuvant setting, has not been established, available evidence suggests that regardless of BRAF-mutation status, anti-PD-1 immunotherapy tends to yield more durable responses. Phase III clinical trials (Robert C et al., 2019) demonstrated acquired resistance to targeted therapies that limited progression-free survival associated with BRAF/MEK inhibitors compared to nivolumab in advanced melanoma, even in the BRAF-mutation subgroup.

Neoadjuvant Immunotherapy

It was suggested that upfront neoadjuvant immunotherapy with these drugs could stimulate stronger immune responses against the tumour than adjuvant therapy with the same and may downstage the tumour and facilitate resection. Versluis JM et al. (2023, OpACIN trial) found that patients with stage III melanoma given neoadjuvant combined ipilimumab–nivolumab had better 5-year RFS (70% vs 60%) and 5-overall survival

(90% vs 70%) compared to adjuvant therapy. Further work is aimed at the determination of optimal combinations and dosing regimens.

Another advantage was found after analysis of pooled data of 6 trials by Menzies AM et al. (2021), it was found that the pathologic response to neoadjuvant systemic therapy was a strong indicator of survival and could potentially direct further treatment. Reijers ILM et al. (2022, PRADO trial) showed that the pathological response of the index lymph node alone (ILN, the largest lymph node metastasis at baseline) could be used to provide response-directed management for the individual. This protocol enabled de-escalation of treatment for 55/60 patients achieving major pathologic response (MPR) to neoadjuvant therapy (seen in 66% of the patients with high-risk stage III melanoma in this trial). Patients could be spared adjuvant therapy and/or TLND with improved quality of life, without compromise of RFS or distant metastasis-free survival (DMFS). Reijers ILM et al. (2025) went on to compare the OpACIN-neo and PRADO trials, which looked at the neoadjuvant ipilimumab-nivolumab in stage III disease – in the former all patients had therapeutic node dissection without adjuvant therapy whilst in the latter further management was determined by MPR. They concluded that the pathologic response to neoadjuvant ICI was associated with survival outcomes and TLND could be potentially omitted in most with MPR. Additional adjuvant systemic treatment seems to be redundant in those with MPR, but may improve outcomes in those with pathologic non-response (pNR). It is a potentially significant development to be able to proscribe more nuanced and personalised approaches that can minimise treatment morbidity without compromising oncological efficacy.

It has been gratifying to see the progress made in the 10 years that I have been editing *Stone's Plastic Surgery Facts and Figures* from the 3rd Edition (2011), 4th Edition (2018), and the in-press 5th Edition. I first reported a situation where the established options of cytokines IFN alpha and IL-2 offered little impact but immunotherapy showed promise and then reported on the survival benefits seen with this landmark paper with ICI up to the present where ICIs are almost a standard of care with more developments inevitable.

REFERENCES

Ba H, *et al.* Comparison of efficacy and tolerability of adjuvant ther apy for resected high-risk stage III-IV cutane ous melanoma: a systemic review and Bayesian network meta-analysis. *Ther Adv Med Oncol.* 2023;15:17588359221148918.

Dummer R, *et al.* Five-year analysis of adjuvant Dabrafenib plus Trametinib in stage III melanoma. *N Engl J Med.* 2020;383:1139–1148.

Eggermont AMM, *et al.* Adjuvant ipilimumab versus placebo after complete resection of high risk stage III melanoma (EORTC 18071): a ran domised, double- blind, phase 3 trial. *Lancet Oncol.* 2015;16:522–530.

Eggermont AMM, *et al.* Prolonged survival in stage III melanoma with Ipilimumab adjuvant therapy. *N Engl J Med.* 2016;375:1845–1855.

Eggermont AMM, *et al.* Adjuvant pembrolizumab versus placebo in resected stage III Melanoma. *N Engl J Med.* 2018 May 10;378(19):1789–1801. doi: 10.1056/NEJMoa1802357.

Eggermont AMM, *et al.* Ipilimumab versus placebo after complete resection of stage III melanoma: long-term follow-up results the EORTC 18071 double-blind phase 3 randomized trial. *J Clin Oncol.* 2019;37:2512.

Larkin J, *et al*. Five-Year Survival with Combined Nivolumab and Ipilimumab in Advanced Melanoma. *N Engl J Med*. 2019 Oct;17;381(16):1535–1546. doi: 10.1056/NEJMoa1910836. Epub 2019 Sep 28. PMID: 31562797.

Menzies AM, *et al*. Pathological response and sur vival with neoadjuvant therapy in melanoma: a pooled analysis from the international Neoadjuvant melanoma consortium (INMC). *Nat Med*. 2021;27:301–309.

Reijers ILM, *et al*. Personalized response-directed surgery and adjuvant therapy after neoadjuvant ipilimumab and nivolumab in high-risk stage III melanoma: the PRADO trial. *Nat Med*. 2022;28:1178–1188.

Reijers ILM, *et al*. Impact of personalized response-directed surgery and adjuvant therapy on survival after neoadjuvant immunotherapy in stage III melanoma: comparison of 3-year data from PRADO and OpA-CIN-neo. *Eur J Cancer*. 2025 Jan;214:115141. doi: 10.1016/j.ejca.2024.115141.

Robert C, *et al*. Five-year outcomes with Dabrafenib plus Trametinib in metastatic melanoma. *N Engl J Med*. 2019;381:626–636.

Versluis JM, *et al*. Survival update of neoadjuvant ipilimumab plus nivolumab in macroscopic stage III melanoma in the OpACIN and OpACIN-neo trials. *Ann Oncol*. 2023;34:420–430.

Weber J, *et al*. Adjuvant nivolumab versus ipilimumab in resected stage III or IV Melanoma. *N Engl J Med*. 2017 Nov 9;377(19):1824–1835. doi: 10.1056/NEJMoa1709030.

CHAPTER 43

Primary Repair of Flexor Tendons

Kleinert HE, Kutz JE, Atasoy E, Stormo A. *Orthop Clin North Am.* 1973 Oct;4(4):865–876
PMID: 4598164

EDITOR COMMENTARY

Galen thought tendons had nerve fibres making them sensitive and thus should "never be pricked." Some have interpreted this as saying that he advised against tendon repair, which was probably untrue as there are reports that he repaired the tendons of gladiators.

It is not difficult to suture tendons and prepare the ground for sound union; the real problem is to obtain a freely sliding tendon capable of restoring good function.

Guy Pulvertaft, 1948

Flexor tendon injuries in zone II, which extends from the proximal A1 pulley to the flexor digitorum superficialis (FDS) insertion distally are recognized as the most challenging injuries to repair, and primary repair was routinely avoided due to unacceptably high rates of complications, including infections, adhesions, and contractures. Bunnell first used the term "No man's land" (NML) in parentheses in the legend to a diagram in the second edition of his book *Surgery of the Hand* (Lippincott, 1948). He was likely alluding to the dire situation in the trenches of the Great War – he was part of the neurosurgical team in Beaune, France, in 1917–1919 – but the precise reason for the analogy is unclear. He described the NML as the region "between distal crease in palm and middle crease of the finger." This is often taken to mean the area where flexor digitorum profundus (FDP) and FDS tendons change position relative to one another, where repair often led to adhesions which significantly reduce finger mobility; thus, Bunnell's admonition was never to repair both tendons. He first advocated tendon grafting over repair, then he excised the FDS tendon to allow better gliding of the profundus tendon, which was repaired with fine sutures. He described "suture at a distance" with a stainless-steel wire pull out in the proximal tendon to take tension off the primary repair. In a similar way, Verdan used transfixion needles that were removed after 3 weeks.

Boyes called zone II the "critical zone," where primary repair would always result in poor motion. He felt that infection was often the most common cause of failure (1947) and was a great advocate of grafting over repair. Despite this prevailing opinion, there were sporadic reports of reasonable results with repair from the 1950s onwards (Siler,

                                  DOI: 10.1201/9781003413738-43

1950; Posch, 1956). Verdan, who had defined zone 2, presented his results with primary repair at the 1959 annual meeting of the American Society for Surgery of the Hand (ASSH).

A 1967 citation is often promoted as a landmark paper; however, it is a brief abstract from the Proceedings of the 22nd Annual Meeting of the ASSH, San Francisco, in that year. Whilst it was an important presentation that stimulated much contentious discussion, it was never published. The abstract itself includes few details but these were elaborated upon in the 1973 publication in *Orthopedic Clinics of North America* that has been chosen as the landmark paper. Apologies are needed in advance – it will be difficult to find – I had to read it in microfiche form. In this article, the authors describe 358 primary repairs of flexor tendons with 225 of these lying in NML. The main features of their repair protocol were:

- Careful cleaning and tourniquet control; meticulous haemostasis to avoid haematomas that will exacerbate pain and swelling in the short term and fibrosis/stiffness in the long term.
- Midlateral or zigzag extensions for exposure.
- Minimal tissue trauma with "no-touch technique" for tendon handling. Transfixion is used to bring tendon ends together for repair rather than relying on the sutures to draw them together.
- 5'0 primary suture (2 strand Bunnell core, later changed to various modifications of Kessler) with 6'0/7'0 running paratenon suture. Both FDS and FSP tendons were repaired.
- Dorsal dynamic splint for 3–3.5 weeks with wrist, hand, and finger in partial flexion. After surgery, the patient is asked to extend the fingers against the resistance of the rubber bands as far as the dorsal splint. The splint permits active extension to zero degrees – during finger extension the flexor muscle relaxes by synergistic reaction. This was confirmed with early EMG studies (Lister GD et al., 1977) though later studies showed some inconsistent flexor relaxation. On attempted flexion, the rubber band immediately flexes the finger and removes tension.
- Graded exercise regime after cast removed

Dynamic splinting reduces stiffness and contractures by passive flexion of digits through rubber bands and pulleys (that point to the wrist rather than the palm, as opposed to the later McGrouther modification with palmar pulleys). Early motion improves healing and reduces adhesions but relies on the repair particularly the suture and the technique used.

In the 1973 paper, the authors presented a 10-year experience as a retrospective case series of patients with flexor tendon injury in zone II who had repair of both FDS and FPS tendons followed by postoperative rehabilitation. Results were deemed good to excellent in 87% of private service patients compared to 76% poor results on teaching service patients. The suggestion that good results could be obtained with a discredited technique, even though Kleinert had stressed the need for an experienced surgeon and patient compliance to avoid poor results, was deemed too controversial even before the presentation. The committee had suggested that Kleinert himself should give the presentation instead of the original speaker, Kutz, who was then not a member of ASSH. There were varying degrees of resistance, particularly from Joseph Boyes, who happened to be the discussant of the presentation. Eventually, at the 1969 meeting, Kleinert suggested that the doubters should go to Louisville to see for themselves, and a special ASSH committee headed by William Littler went to review the results. Famously, he remarked: "If I injure a flexor tendon in a finger, I am getting on a plane and flying to Louisville." Committee members presented their findings at a 1970 meeting, where the discussion was not so heated – it seemed evident that a paradigm shift in hand surgery had occurred. "No-man's land" became "skilled-man's land."

Prior to this article, the accepted wisdom was that it was unsafe to commence motion before 3 weeks. This was based on the work of Mason and Allen on dogs (1941), which found that motion very early after repair, when the repair site is soft and weak with reduced tensile strength, could be harmful, but, after 3 weeks, motion was beneficial to repair during remodelling stage. By the 1960s, surgeons, including Bunnell, began to realize that postoperative management of these injuries was also integral to the overall functional outcomes. However, surgeons before this time lacked the appropriate materials (and techniques) needed for early motion. Examples of necessary improvements included the Kessler secure grasping suture that allowed early motion (Urbaniak modification 1972/1973 of original Kessler, 1969).

The Kleinert et al. report of controlled passive motion was followed by Duran and Houser in 1975, who promoted controlled passive motion 2 to 5 days after surgery with intermittent passive flexion and active extension of digits, with better results than that of Kleinert. The modified Duran approach described by Strickland and Glogovac (1980) is still in common use. James Small et al. (1989) in Belfast adopted controlled early active mobilization for all flexor tendon injuries in the hand and wrist. The Belfast regime, as it became known, was found to be a safe and effective protocol for rehabilitation. Subsequent randomized controlled studies comparing early active range of motion and passive range of motion have since demonstrated a significant increase in range of motion with the active protocol without an increased rupture rate. Of course, EAM protocols required evolutions in the technique, including increasing the strength of the core sutures (number of strands) and peripheral sutures (improve gliding, though some advocate for fewer peripheral sutures as the number of core sutures increase). There are a number of different EAM protocols and none of them can be called a "gold standard" for all.

This paper was important because it was one of the first to break the "thou shalt not repair both tendons" barrier. Primary repair of both tendons and early mobilization is now the standard of care. The use of WALANT for flexor repair may also have its own set of benefits, but this matter lacks definitive studies at the moment.

As for Harold Kleinert (1921–2013) himself, who was also known as HEK, his other major contribution was to mentor and train hundreds of hand surgeons from around the world. His legacy is found in his statement:

as teachers ... we are successful only if our pupils become far better than their teachers.

REFERENCES

Boyes JH. Immediate vs delayed repair of the digital flexor tendons. *Ann West Med Surg.* 1947 Jun;1(4):145–52. PMID: 20250033.

Bunnell S. *Surgery of the Hand*, 1st edn. Philadelphia: JB: Lippincott; 1944.

Kessler I, Nissim F. Primary repair without immobilization of flexor tendon division within the flexor sheath. *Acta Orthop Scand.* 1969;40:587–601.

Kleinert HE, Kutz JE, Ashbell TS, Martinez E. Primary repair of lacerated flexor tendons in "No Man's Land". *J Bone Joint Surg Am.* 1967;49A:577.

Lister GD, Kleinert HE, Kutz JE, Atasoy E. Primary flexor tendon repair followed by immediate controlled mobilization. *J Hand Surg Am.* 1977 Nov;2(6):441–51. doi: 10.1016/s0363-5023(77)80025-7. PMID: 336675.

Mason JL, Allen HS. The rate of healing tendons: an experimental study of tensile strength. *Ann Surg.* 1941;113(3):424–459.

Newmeyer WL 3rd, Manske PR. No man's land revisited: the primary flexor tendon repair controversy. *J Hand Surg Am.* 2004 Jan;29(1):1–5. doi: 10.1016/s0363-5023(03)00381-2.

Posch JL. Primary tenorrhaphies and tendon grafting proce dures in hand Injuries. *AMA Arch Surg.* 1956;73:609–624.

Siler VE. Primary tenorrhaphy of the flexor tendons in the hand. *J Bone Joint Surg.* 1950;32A:218–224.

Small JO, Brennan MD, Colville J. Early active mobilisation following flexor tendon repair in zone 2. *J Hand Surg.* 1989;14(4):388–391.

Verdan CE. Primary repair of flexor tendons. *J Bone Joint Surg.* 1960;42A:647–657.

CHAPTER 44

Ultrastructural Observations of Lymphatic Vessels in Lymphedema in Human Extremities

Koshima I, Kawada S, Moriguchi T, Kajiwara Y. *Plast Reconstr Surg.*
1996 Feb;97(2):397–405; discussion 406–407
doi: 10.1097/00006534-199602000-00018 PMID: 8559823

EXPERT COMMENTARY

Jaume Masia

This article, "Ultrastructural Observations of Lymphatic Vessels in Lymphedema in Human Extremities" by Koshima et al. is a cornerstone in the field of lymphatic surgery, offering groundbreaking insights into the pathophysiology of lymphedema. The study's significance lies in its detailed ultrastructural analysis of lymphatic vessels in lymphedematous tissues, providing essential information for understanding disease mechanisms and advancing surgical approaches.

Key Reasons for Its Importance

1. **Microscopic Insights into Lymphatic Dysfunction**
   The authors utilize advanced ultrastructural techniques, such as electron micros-copy, to reveal critical abnormalities in lymphatic vessel walls, valve structures, and surrounding tissues in lymphedematous extremities. These observations underpin our understanding of how chronic lymph stasis contributes to vessel degeneration and dysfunction.

2. **Foundational Evidence for Supermicrosurgery**
   The study supports the rationale for developing supermicrosurgical techniques, in particular lymphovenous anastomosis (LVA). By demonstrating the structural viability of lymphatic vessels in early stages of lymphedema, it provides evidence that surgical intervention can restore function and mitigate disease progression.

3. **Pathophysiological Framework**
   This research clarifies how fibrosis, inflammation, and secondary changes in lymphatic vessels exacerbate lymphedema. These findings have influenced the design of combined therapies, including surgical and conservative interventions, targeting both mechanical and inflammatory components of the disease.

DOI: 10.1201/9781003413738-44

4. **Pioneering Work by Renowned Authors**
   Professor Isao Koshima is a leading figure in reconstructive microsurgery, and this study reflects the precision and vision that have shaped modern lymphatic surgery. It bridges basic science and clinical practice, offering a foundation for the evolution of lymphatic surgery techniques.

In conclusion, this article is seminal for its role in advancing our understanding of lymphedema's ultrastructural pathology and influencing the development of innovative surgical strategies that continue to transform patient care.

EDITOR COMMENTARY

This is a retrospective study of 14 patients who had extremity LVAs (6 upper limbs, 8 lower limbs) for lymphoedema resistant to conservative treatment. Follow-up averaged 25.5 months for the upper limb and 23.4 months for the lower limb. The outcome measures recorded were a little basic and incomplete, particularly for the lower limb, but the results seem to support a trend to size reduction.

During these surgeries, lymphatic tissue was taken for light and electron microscopy. These results were more enlightening, particularly with the hypothetical sequence of changes with lymphoedema. Degeneration of smooth muscle and occlusion of lymphatics seem to start from the proximal parts of the extremities, meaning that the distal parts could potentially be used for bypass.

After I Koshima moved to Tokyo, his new team published a follow-up of sorts (Hara et al., 2013), using indocyanine green to look at the lymphatics in lymphedematous limbs and the effect of LVA on 43 limbs in 25 patients. The ICG findings were related to the changes in collecting lymph vessels that had been classified as Normal (no hardening or dilatation), Ectasis (dilatation but no hardening), Contraction (hardening but no narrowing), Sclerosis types (narrowing) (NECST Classification, Mihara 2012). They found that in:

- Linear ICG pattern, there were approximately equal proportions of N, E, and C. No S type seen.
- Stardust, there were almost equal proportions of S, C, and E/N combined.
- Diffuse, almost half were composed of S type and less than 10% N type.

The suggestion was that the ICG findings could be used to predict the types of lymphatic abnormalities likely to be encountered intraoperatively during LVA. That where possible, LVAs should be attempted in regions with linear>splash>diffuse ICG patterns to increase the chances of finding good lymphatics. They injected the ICG the day before surgery (15–22 hours), which some have critiqued would give a good, generalized overview but would be less useful for discrimination of individual lymphatics as candidates for anastomosis than, say, injecting the ICG just before surgery on the operating table. There is some evidence that LVAs performed in limbs that have more functioning lymphatics work better.

This study laid the foundation for the development of (the modern) LVA for lymphoedema, but it lacked statistical analysis to support the somewhat general conclusions.

REFERENCES

Chang DW, Suami H, Skoracki R. A prospective analysis of 100 consecutive lymphovenous bypass cases for treatment of extremity lymphedema. *Plast Reconstr Surg.* 2013 Nov;132(5):1305–1314. doi: 10.1097/PRS.0b013e3182a4d626.

Hara H, Mihara M, Seki Y, Todokoro T, Iida T, Koshima I. Comparison of indocyanine green lymphographic findings with the conditions of collecting lymphatic vessels of limbs in patients with lymphedema. *Plast Reconstr Surg.* 2013 Dec;132(6):1612–1618. doi: 10.1097/PRS.0b013e3182a97edc.

Mihara M, Hara H, Hayashi Y, Narushima M, Yamamoto T, Todokoro T, Iida T, Sawamoto N, Araki J, Kikuchi K, Murai N, Okitsu T, Kisu I, Koshima I. Pathological steps of cancer-related lymphedema: histological changes in the collecting lymphatic vessels after lymphadenectomy. *PLOS ONE.* 2012;7(7):e41126. doi: 10.1371/journal.pone.0041126. Erratum in: *PLOS ONE.* 2013;8(5). doi: 10.1371/annotation/6fff4d28-3f99-44eb-82d6-ccd885a1ba11.

CHAPTER 45

Cleft Palate Repair by Double Opposing Z-Plasty

Furlow LT Jr. *Plast Reconstr Surg.* 1986;78(6):724–738

EDITOR COMMENTARY

The aim of cleft palate surgery is to repair the cleft whilst reconstructing the dynamic sphincter mechanism seen in the normal palate – particularly the action of the levator veli palatini. This muscle originates at the cranial base and descends to insert into the transverse aponeurosis of the soft palate to form a muscular sling. In cleft palates, the abnormal muscle is attenuated, oriented sagittally/longitudinally and inserts into the posterior border of the (cleft) hard palate (Kriens O, 1969, 1975). Otto Kriens stressed the need to correct this with intra-velar veloplasty (IVV), releasing the muscle from its abnormal attachments with midline repair. However, the extent of mobilization achieved was often limited and from his experience with a large series of revision surgeries Brian Sommerlad (2003) advocated an "anatomical repair" through extensive "radical" circumferential dissection of the levator muscle, separation from the mucosa, the palatal depressors and the abnormal attachments to be repaired in a transverse orientation using high power magnification (i.e., microscope, though modern high power loupes can also be used). Some suggest that it would be better described as "extensive" rather than "radical"; the midline scar may limit palatal movement. The hard palate cleft was dealt with at the time of lip repair with a single layer vomerine flap. Court Cutting independently described a form of radical IVV in 1995.

Leonard Furlow Jr (1930–2024) found that the standard practice of von Lagenbeck repair with IVV was associated with a high rate of VPI (over half). Consequently, he proposed a radically different approach to cleft palate repair using a Z-plasty of the oral mucosa of the soft palate with an opposing Z-plasty of the nasal mucosa. The hard palate is repaired by mucoperiosteal flaps elevated and sutured in the midline. This technique will lengthen the soft palate like Z-plasties elsewhere, with the flipside being that would not be so useful for wide clefts. The anteriorly based flaps are composed of mucosa only, whilst the inclusion of muscle in the posteriorly based flaps means that upon completion of the transposition, the velar muscles become transversely orientated with some overlap whilst also elongating the soft palate. Although there is overlap, the palatal depressor muscles (palatoglossus and palatopharyngeus) actually lie in between the levators. Furthermore, the relative position of the muscles to the Z-plasty design cannot be predicted with this technique; thus, results of the muscle transposition will vary.

DOI: 10.1201/9781003413738-45

Postoperative videofluoroscopy (Lipira AB et al., 2011) has shown some twisting motion of the muscles reflecting its "non-anatomic" repair (one of the main criticisms). MRI imaging may help ameliorate this by allowing some preoperative planning.

With only three cases, Furlow first reported on his new approach in 1978 at the annual meeting of the Southeastern Society of Plastic Surgeons. This technique was quickly adopted by many who saw its potential, including Peter Randall, who was one of the first to publish a large series (106 cases, 1986). This article by Furlow in 1986 is a retrospective case series that reviewed 22 patients with this double Z-plasty soft palate repair. The limitations of the study include the small sample size and the statistical analysis being largely descriptive only. There was speech assessment with velopharyngeal assessment in 20 patients and formal speech evaluation in 16 of these (in contrast to the careful assessment of speech in Sommerlad's paper 2003). The median follow-up period was 3.75 years. The author reported that complications were uncommon with one case of fistula, one case of postoperative stridor, and one with fever. It is a single surgeon's experience.

This technique became commonly known as "Furlow palatoplasty" or just "Furlows." Furlows is more commonly used in North America whilst Sommerlad's IVVP is more commonly used in the United Kingdom. Proponents of Furlow's technique say that the overlap tightens the sphincter and improves function, whilst critics say this type of repair is non-anatomic and may actually limit muscle excursion.

The seemingly simple yet clever technique can elongate the soft palate whilst avoiding longitudinal scar that could be prone to contracture and velar shortening (i.e., IVV). The main advantage seems to be better speech outcomes compared to prior techniques, which has been confirmed by subsequent larger case series that demonstrated favorable outcomes for speech, as well as midfacial growth, and rates of secondary surgery (Kirschner RE, 1999; Jackson O, 2013; LaRossa D et al., 2004). A systematic review (Timbang MR et al., 2014) reported lower odds of VPI and secondary surgery relative to straight line palatoplasty (SL-IVV), though some criticized the review for not including studies with "radical" IVV and other evolutions of the original technique. The Cleft Outcomes Registry/Research Network (CORNET) Speech and Surgery study is a prospective, multi-center study that will compare the Furlow palatoplasty versus other techniques involving IVV with the primary outcome measures being hypernasality/ speech at 3 years and with secondary outcomes being fistula rate, measures of speech produce, and QOL. Recruitment finished in February 2023, with the end of the study activities expected in early 2025.

In addition, several case series support the use of the Furlow technique as a secondary procedure to treat VPI after prior palatoplasty (Dailey, 2006; Kurnik, 2020). The ongoing VPI-OPS study is a prospective multi-center observational study comparing revision Furlow palatoplasty to pharyngoplasty (sphincter or pharyngeal flap) in the treatment of VPI. This study began recruitment in 2021 and is expected to continue into 2025.

The main limitation of the Furlow palatoplasty is the increased propensity to fistulae. One RCT reported high fistula rates with the Furlow technique compared to von Langenback–IVV palatoplasty (Williams WN et al., 2011). Fistulas can have significant impact on patients as they can affect speech, hygiene, and oral function, whilst treatment may result in additional scars that can impair growth and make future surgery more difficult. Some advocate avoiding the technique in wider clefts to reduce fistula rate (Losken HW, 2011), whilst others have tried to compensate for the higher risk of fistulae by combining it with buccal myomucosal flaps (Mann RJ, 2017) or buccal fat (Denadai R, 2023). Many modifications exist, including use of relaxing incisions suggested by Randall (Children's Hospital of Pennsylvania, sometimes called the CHOP, Li et al., 2014) which is probably the most common variation. VY closure is another strategy used by some but may tend to shorten the AP distance.

It is said that when a Furlow palatoplasty fails, it often fails in a "spectacular" fashion that can be difficult to salvage, which is the biggest downside to the technique.

REFERENCES

Cutting CB, Rosenbaum J, Rovati L. The technique of muscle repair in the cleft soft palate. *Oper Tech Plast Reconstr Surg.* 1995;2:215–222.

Dailey SA, Karnell MP, Karnell LH, Canady JW. Comparison of resonance outcomes after pha ryngeal flap and Furlow double-opposing Z-plasty for surgical management of velopharyngeal incom petence. *Cleft Palate Craniofac J.* 2006;43(1): 38–43.

Denadai R, Chou PY, Lo LJ. Reinforcing the modified double-opposing Z-plasty approach using the pedi-cled buccal fat flap as an interpositional layer for cleft palate repair. *Cleft Palate Craniofac J.* 2023 Apr;60(4):503–508. doi: 10.1177/10556656211064769.

Jackson O, Stransky CA, Jawad AF, *et al.* The Children's Hospital of Philadelphia modification of the Furlow double-opposing Z-palatoplasty: 30-year experience and long-term speech outcomes. *Plast Reconstr Surg.* 2013;132(3):613–622.

Kriens OB. An anatomical approach to veloplasty. *Plast Reconstr Surg.* 1969 Jan;43(1):29–41. doi: 10.1097/00006534-196901000-00006.

Kriens OB. Anatomy of the velopharyngeal area in cleft palate. *Clin Plast Surg.* 1975 Apr;2(2):261–288.

Kirschner RE, Wang P, Jawad AF, *et al.* Cleft-palate repair by modified Furlow double-opposing Z-plasty: the Children's Hospital of Philadelphia experience. *Plast Reconstr Surg.* 1999;104(7):1998–2010.

Kurnik NM, Weidler EM, Lien KM, *et al.* The effec tiveness of palate re-repair for treating velopharyngeal insufficiency: a systematic review and meta-analysis. *Cleft Palate Craniofac J.* 2020;57(7):860–871.

LaRossa D, Jackson OH, Kirschner RE, *et al.* The Children's Hospital of Philadelphia modification of the Furlow double-opposing z-palatoplasty: long- term speech and growth results. *Clin Plast Surg.* 2004;31(2):243–249.

Li C, Shi J, Zheng Q, Shi B. The children's hospital of philadelphia modification of the furlow double-opposing Z-palatoplasty. *Plast Reconstr Surg.* 2014;133(3):429e–431e. doi: 10.1097/prs.0000000000000157.

Lipira AB, Grames LM, Molter D, *et al.* Videofluoroscopic and nasendoscopic correlates of speech in velopha-ryngeal dysfunction. *Cleft Palate Craniofac J.* 2011;48:550–560.

Losken HW, van Aalst JA, Teotia SS, *et al.* Achieving low cleft palate fistula rates: surgical results and tech-niques. *Cleft Palate Craniofac J.* 2011;48:312–320.

Mann RJ, Martin MD, Eichhorn MG, Neaman KC, Sierzant CG, Polley JW, Girotto JA. The double opposing Z-plasty plus or minus buccal flap approach for repair of cleft palate: a review of 505 consecutive cases. *Plast Reconstr Surg.* 2017 Mar;139(3):735e–744e. doi: 10.1097/PRS.0000000000003127.

Randall P, LaRossa D, Solomon M, Cohen M. Experience with the Furlow double-reversing Z-plasty for cleft palate repair. *Plast Reconstr Surg.* 1986;77:569–576.

Sommerlad BC. A technique for cleft palate repair. *Plast Reconstr Surg.* 2003;112:1542–1548.

Timbang MR, Gharb BB, Rampazzo A, Papay F, Zins J, Doumit G. A systematic review comparing Furlow double-opposing Z-plasty and straight-line intravelar veloplasty methods of cleft palate repair. *Plast Reconstr Surg.* 2014 Nov;134(5):1014–1022. doi: 10.1097/PRS.0000000000000637.

Williams WN, Seagle MB, Pegoraro-Krook MI, *et al.* Prospective clinical trial comparing outcome measures between Furlow and von Langenbeck palatoplasties for UCLP. *Ann Plast Surg.* 2011;66(2):154–163.

CHAPTER 46

Clinical Application of the Tension-Stress Effect for Limb Lengthening

Ilizarov GA. *Clin Orthop Relat Res.* 1990 Jan;(250):8–26
PMID: 2403497

EDITOR COMMENTARY

Ilizarov is the name that we all associate with distraction osteogenesis (DI), but he was not the first to attempt bone lengthening by distraction nor was he the first to use external fixation. There had been reports of the use of distraction for limb lengthening even before the underlying principles were properly understood. Codivilla from Bologna reported on femoral lengthening in 1905 using "sudden and intense force" whilst his protégé, Putti (1921) chose gradual distraction as he understood the dangers and drawbacks of excessive force. Similarly, a German surgeon, Wagner, used an external fixator (1970–1980s) for distraction, but it was associated with many complications and patients often needed grafting and plating after removal of the fixator, probably due to the rapid distraction rate. De Bastiani et al. (1987) limited periosteal stripping and distracted at 1 mm/day after 10–15 days of "callostasis." What set Ilizarov apart was the amount of basic and clinical research he did to support his theories and develop his protocol, which was more central to successful DI than the hardware.

This series of three seminal articles were the only articles that Ilizarov published in the English language peer-reviewed literature (they were edited by Stuart Green). Any one of these could be chosen for discussion here as a "landmark" article.

- Ilizarov GA. The tension-stress effect on the genesis and growth of tissues: Part I, the influence of stability of fixation and soft tissue preservation. *Clin Orthop Rel Res* 1989a;238:249–281.

- Ilizarov GA. The tension-stress effect on the genesis and growth of tissues: Part II, the influence of the rate and frequency of distraction. *Clin Orthop Rel Res* 1989b;239:263–285.

- Ilizarov GA. Clinical application of the tension-stress effect for limb lengthening. *Clin Orthop Rel Res* 1990;250:8–26.

The paper describes the experimental background with animal studies (canine tibia) that demonstrated:

- Increasing stability of the fixator frame reduced malunion and allowed more direct osteogenesis without intervening cartilage.
- Increasing damage to the marrow with the osteotomy decreased new bone formation. It was important to avoid disrupting the periosteal blood supply.
- Fractionating the distraction more yielded better outcomes for bone and soft tissue. In the absence of automatic distraction, it was suggested to distract at least 4 times a day.

The author then described their clinical experience in lengthening limbs that were abnormal due to prior disease, e.g., childhood osteomyelitis, or in achondroplastic dwarves:

- Wires should be introduced to the bone slowly to reduce thermal damage.
- Skill and experience were needed in setting up the frame – wires were inserted before the rings; otherwise, there would displacement and tissue necrosis.
- Stability requires proper tensioning of the wires.

The paper is largely descriptive with summaries of the experimental work and clinical experience. It is very informative, but there are no comparative studies and no quantitative analyses.

The biography of the man is worth recounting. Gavriil Abramovich Ilizarov (1921–1992) was born in Belarus a year before his "official" birth year. Upon graduation in 1944 he had to treat many war wounded. "I have worked for five years, all of them at once." He sought new ways to treat these individuals, including designing new instruments. In 1952, he received a patent for his circular external fixator. The story that he used bicycle parts to create his external fixator is apparently apocryphal; Ilizarov was supposedly inspired by the apparatus of horse carriages.

Although the fixator was originally used to fixate fractures, its design allowed it to manipulate bones segments, including the index case (possibly another myth). Apparently, Ilizarov went on vacation sometime in 1956 and the apparatus on a patient having treatment for an ankylosed knee was apparently turned the wrong way, causing distraction instead of compression. Upon his return, he noticed the bone production, i.e., osteogenesis between bone ends. Given that his location behind the Iron Curtain in a town far from the "big" centres, it is unclear if he knew about other attempts to elongate bone, e.g., Codivilla and Putti. As mentioned previously, he was not the first to describe osteogenesis by distraction, but he carried out a large amount of animal and clinical research into optimal parameters. He combined extensive experimental work with his clinical work, and he developed the concept of "transosseus compression distraction osteosynthesis," which became known as the "Ilizarov technique." He elucidated the importance of the tension stress in stimulating "biosynthetic activity in tissues" with proper control of blood supply, loading, and lengthening. He also developed a versatile external fixation system.

He developed and popularized his technique for the gradual lengthening of bone in the 1960s and 1970s, with his first publication in Russian in 1965. The amount of his work was so large that not only did he receive his PhD in 1968, but also the thesis was accepted for a DSc, conferred the following year. Although Ilizarov became chief surgeon at Kurgan, Siberia, in what was then the USSR (now in Russia just north of Khazakhstan) in 1955, his views were still opposed by the orthodoxy, particularly by those at the "big" centres in Moscow and Leningrad, and he was often derided at conferences. Things changed in 1967 when he successful treated Valeriy Brumel, a Soviet high jump gold medallist (1964) who had endured years of unsuccessful multiple surgeries for leg fractures resulting from a motorcycle accident – at one point amputation was considered. After treatment by Ilizarov, Brumel even returned briefly to competing, though at a lower level, and he retired in 1970. In 1968, Ilizarov treated the polio deformities of Shostakovich. He began to be treated as a Soviet hero, and he was called the "Magician of Kurgan."

News of his successful treatment of Brumel reached the Western press around 1972 and inspired visits by Western surgeons, including J Hellinger from Dresden who was the first to describe the method of "Ilisarov" in a Western journal in 1973. Spinelli, a young surgeon from Rome, had been under instructions from his boss, Professor Monticelli, to research distraction osteogenesis following interest by the media, and he visited Ilizarov in 1980. Apparently, the team in Rome did not credit Ilizarov when presenting their research, which upset Ilizarov and made him suspicious of the "West" for a long time.

Italians play an important role in the story of Ilizarov. What made Ilizarov truly famous internationally was his successful correction of the tibial malunion of Carlo Mauri. Mauri was an Italian "adventurer" who had travelled with Thor Heyerdahl despite fracturing his leg years earlier whilst working as a ski instructor in 1961. He suffered from chronic tibial infection, leg length discrepancy, and foot deformity. It was whilst he was on the Tigris expedition in 1977 that a fellow adventurer on the trip, a Russian doctor, Senkevic, introduced him to Ilizarov. (Mauri had his operation in 1980 when Spinelli was in Kurgan.) Mauri also happened to be a photojournalist and was a good friend of Dr. Angelo Villa, an orthopaedic surgeon from Lecco. When he returned to Italy, Mauri appeared before the media and also gave lectures to the hospital of Dr. Villa, where Dr. Catteneo from Lecco and Bianchi Maiocchi from Milan, who happened to be president of AO Italy at the time, were in attendance. Carlo Mauri died of a heart attack in 1982 whilst training for his next adventure.

Ilizarov's work was not that well known outside of the USSR but that was about to change. The Italian surgeons invited Ilizarov to be guest speaker at an AO meeting in Bellagio in 1981, his first outside of the Iron Curtain, where he received a 10-minute standing ovation. Bianchi Maiocchi visited Kurgan and was pivotal in getting the rights to manufacture and distribute the apparatus in Italy and many other counties. The international version was made of medical grade stainless steel and did not rust, unlike the Russian one. This was a pivotal step in bringing ilizarov to the world, and the first course in the West was held in 1983 near Lecco. Dr. Paley was a young resident from Canada when he visited Lecco in 1985, and he then went on to visit Kurgan in 1986 and again in 1987, where he became immersed in the work of Ilizarov. Paley, who published his classic paper in 1988, and Blair of Richards Medical were central to the wider uptake of the technique in North America and the United Kingdom. Stuart Green from California also visited Kurgan in 1987 and formed a good relationship with Ilizarov, and he was invited by the Russian to edit his English-language papers, including this one.

Remarkably, Ilizarov still faced significant politicking at home. Before his death in 1992, he never secured election to the USSR Academy of Medical Sciences. He has an asteroid that orbits the sun named after him in 1982, which is named 3750 Ilizarov.

Distraction osteogenesis has also been important in craniofacial surgery. Attempts to lengthen the mandible with distraction had been described in 1927 by Rosenthal with a tooth-borne appliance and then in 1937 by Kazanjian, using an appliance over the face to provide gradual distraction. Surgeons saw the potential of Ilizarov distraction in the treatment of micrognathia with sleep apnea and upper airway obstruction. Snyder (1973) was the first to report on the use of the Ilizarov technique in mandible in a canine model. It took until 1992 before McCarthy et al. (1992) reported on extraoral distraction in 4 children with congenital anomalies. This lengthened the pediatric mandible without a need for bone grafting or intermaxillary fixation. Development of internal distractors and resorbable devices has meant that distraction has replaced rib graft reconstruction in the treatment of Pruzansky type II mandibles. Distraction is also used in midfacial and cranial vault expansion procedures often needed in patients with craniosynotoses. The ability to simultaneously lengthen soft tissues without muscle or nerve dysfunction makes distraction osteogenesis a very powerful tool with less tendency to relapse.

REFERENCES

De Bastiani G, Aldegheri R, Renzi-Brivio L, Trivella G. Limb lengthening by callus distraction (callotasis). *J Pediatr Orthop.* 1987 Mar–Apr;7(2):129–134. doi: 10.1097/01241398-198703000-00002.

McCarthy JG, Schreiber J, Karp N, Thorne CH, Grayson BH. Lengthening the human mandible by gradual distraction. *Plast Reconstr Surg.* 1992 Jan;89(1):1–8.

Paley D. Current techniques of limb lengthening. *J Pediatr Orthop.* 1988 Jan–Feb;8(1):73–92. doi: 10.1097/01241398-198801000-00018.

Snyder CC, Levine GA, Swanson HM, Browne EZ Jr. Mandibular lengthening by gradual distraction: a preliminary report. *Plast Reconstr Surg.* 1973;51:506–508.

CHAPTER 47

A 10-Year Experience in Nasal Reconstruction with the Three-Stage Forehead Flap

Menick FJ. *Plast Reconstr Surg.* 2002 May;109(6):1839–1855; discussion 1856–1861 doi: 10.1097/00006534-200205000-00010 PMID: 11994582

EDITOR COMMENTARY

In historical descriptions of nasal reconstruction, two names are always mentioned, Sushruta and Tagliocozzi. Sushruta is usually said to have lived at around *c.*600 BCE, but varying reports have put him anywhere within a 1,000-year span; Sushruta described a staged pedicled cheek flap for nose reconstruction in his text, the *Sushruta Samhita.* Then about two thousand years later we have Gaspare Tagliocozzi (1545–1599) describing a staged flap from the biceps area, requiring the arm to be bandaged to the head for several weeks.

Much has been written about the historical aspects of how the technique of the forehead flap in nasal reconstruction came to the English-speaking world. It might be easier to start "somewhere in the middle" with the infamous 1794 October edition of *The Gentleman's Magazine.* On page 891 there is a description from "B.L." of an operation on an Indian cart driver who worked for the British Army near "Poonah" (now Pune, in the state of Maharashtra in western India) by a local potter (of the Koomas caste) which was witnessed by two English doctors, James Trindlay (possibly Findlay) and Thomas Cruso. I have a copy of the book (it is more commonplace than you would expect for a book from the 18th century), and it does say "Trindlay" but apparently this was a typographical/ transcription error from the original report in India. The patient, called Cowasjee, had been living without a nose for about a year after it (as well as a hand) had been chopped off by the local forces of Tipu Sultan as punishment for working for the British forces. Then one day, one of the local officials, Sir Charles Mallet, saw a merchant with a scar on his nose, and, upon inquiry, he was told that the nose had been reconstructed by a local potter using his forehead. This potter/surgeon was then summoned to reconstruct the nose for Cowasjee (and 4 soldiers), and the story eventually found its way into the pages of *The Gentleman's Magazine.* This sort of surgery *nasikasadhana* had been practiced by a few families for centuries as hereditary knowledge since the time of Sushruta; the techniques were generally not taught outside the family. The British doctors were in the right place at the right time.

On page 1093 of the 1794 *The Gentleman's Magazine* (December issue), there was a response from "T.J.," who was rather indignant about the statement that the surgery was unknown in Europe. T.J. mentioned that "Taliacotius/Talicautius" and others had described similar methods of reconstruction. He was presumably referring to the aforementioned Gaspare Tagliacozzi, who described the technique in his book *De Curtorum Chirurgia per insitionem* (On the Surgery of Mutilation by Grafting), published in 1597. This involved a delayed distally based arm flap (for 40 days), with 6 stages over 4 months. Tagliacozzi was a professor of surgery in Bologna, and, in his book, he described the surgery that the Branca family from Catania, Sicily, had kept secret since the 1400s (they kept no records). According to records by the Neapolitan royal historian Fazio (1400–1457), Gustavo Branca used the 'Indian method' with the cheek *c.*1400, but the son, Antonius, chose to use the arm, giving rise possibly to the "Italian method." Tagliocozzi credited predecessors including Branca whilst ironically also criticized their secrecy. He may have learnt the technique from Fioravanti, another Bolognese surgeon who managed to observe 5 surgeries *c.*1549 under somewhat false pretences (and without declaring himself to be a doctor) by the (Pietro and Paolo) Vianeo family of Calabria, who were then the main practitioners of the Italian method (until the last son died in 1571), possibly having learnt it from the Branca family themselves. Carpue believes that Tagliacozzi performed the surgery having taught himself by amassing previous descriptions. For a variety of reasons, the description of Tagliocozzi's method disappeared from view for several centuries after his death in 1599, despite the early interest, as the book was quickly plagiarized by Meietti and went into at least 4 editions. Tagliocozzi's image serves as the symbol of the American Board of Plastic Surgeons, whilst the American Association of Plastic Surgeons (AAPS) uses the "classic" surgical image.

It was said that nasal reconstruction techniques had been closely guarded "secrets," which made piecing the history difficult. Bavarian army surgeon Heinrich von Pfalzpaint (1415–1465) had described a 2-stage method using the arm. He possibly learnt it from the younger Branca or one of his pupils. Apparently, Pfalzpaint said: "If one comes to you with a cut off nose, let no one watch and make him swear to tell nobody how you cured him." Despite this entreaty, he supposedly passed on the technique to 2 colleagues and reported on his method of nose reconstruction in 1460, though the manuscript was lost until one of the few copies was found and printed again in 1868. His method was even unknown to fellow German surgeon von Grafe, who described a "German method" in 1818 after learning about Carpue's work (for which he wrote a foreword, see below).

Joseph Constantine Carpue (1764–1846) was said to have been inspired by the article in *The Gentleman's Magazine* and had corresponded with several people involved in the matter, including Sir Charles Mallet and Cowasjee's superior, Lieutenant Colonel Ward, who had witnessed the surgery. He gathered all the information that he could and analyzed both the Italian and the Indian methods. He chose the latter and prepared himself with 11 cadaveric dissections, and like buses, after waiting 15 years to perform the surgery, he had two patients in quick succession and performed the surgery (the first in Britain) in 1814 and 1815. He described it in meticulous detail his 1816 book, and the surgery became widely disseminated in Europe as the "Indian Method." You will have noticed that at some point the Indian practitioners transitioned from using the cheek to using the forehead, though it is unclear when this happened. Some say that it was a student of Sushruta who is unnamed (and unknown). Manuzzi, an adventurer from Venice, described the Indian forehead method in his 1702 book after seeing it c.1686. This came to light after discovery and translation of manuscripts in 1907. Tribhovandas Motichand Shah, chief medical officer of Junagadh State in India, wrote an article about use of the (median) forehead flap for nose reconstruction in the Indian Medical Gazette in 1888 followed by a monograph the next year.

The timeline and sequence above may not reflect what actually happened; hence, the liberal use of "probably" and "possibly." There has been much debate on the topic, including the identity of "B.L" in the literature. There are also some dubious stories floating around on websites; in particular, one involving Sir Eyre Coote (1726–1783), who supposedly was captured by Indian forces in 1781, had his nose cut off, and then reconstructed so well that he showed it off to everyone when he returned home. The problem is that there is no mention of this anywhere else, including in his biographies (of which there are two).

Of course, Harold Gillies used the pedicled arm flap (as well as the forehead flap, i.e., the "up and down flap" in 1935). According to an account by Millard in *A Rhinoplasty Tetralogy* (1996), during World War I a patient called George had the initial surgery and then had the flap divided just before he was moved to make room for a massive influx of casualties. The story (which may be apocryphal) was that the patient then strode into Gillies's clinic 15 years later, remarking that he had made his packet as "an elephant man in a sideshow" and wanted to retire with a "fine nose."

For various reasons, like Carpue, most modern surgeons have preferred the forehead flap over the arm flap (and the cheek flap). The classic Indian flap used midline tissue on paired arteries and was based at or above the level of the eyebrows, which means less forehead to use and a higher arc of rotation that is more liable to cause kinking. There have been numerous modifications, including bringing the incisions closer to the medial canthus to lower the point of rotation. McCarthy et al. (1985) performed the first anatomic study to delineate the redundancy in blood supply to the forehead flap, building on Kazanjian's median forehead flap (1946) and Millard's paramedian forehead flap (1964, 1974). Millard demonstrated that bilateral pedicles were not needed; in addition, the angular artery (from the facial artery) could provide sufficient vascularity to support the forehead flap independent of the supraorbital and supratrochlear arteries. This allowed the lower incisions to be lowered to gain additional length. Burget and Menick proposed a narrower base/pedicle for the paramedian flap. Supratrochlear vessels have anastomoses with facial arteries (Kelly CP et al., 2008).

This landmark study from Menick is a retrospective review of 90 patients undergoing the three-stage forehead flap technique for reconstruction. The paper provides an extremely detailed description of the author's technique and philosophy.

- In the first stage, the forehead flap is elevated without thinning except for the columellar portion. If a vascularized intranasal lining is present, primary cartilage grafts are placed. Otherwise, missing lining is constructed using a variety of means, e.g., folded forehead flap, intranasal flaps, or skin grafts. Primary cartilage grafts are not placed without vascularized cover.
  - The donor site is closed primarily or allowed to heal with secondary intention.
- In the second stage 3 weeks later, the now-delayed forehead flap is elevated with 3 to 4 mm of subcutaneous fat except for the columella, which remains attached, and the underlying construct including subcutaneous fat and frontalis muscle of forehead is thinned and sculpted. Delayed primary cartilage grafting can now be performed during this stage if needed. The cover skin is then replaced.
- In the third stage 3 weeks later, the pedicle is divided. The most distal parts of the flap can be elevated again with 3 to 4 mm of subcutaneous fat, and the underlying construct is thinned and sculpted as needed to create the expected subunit contours, defining the dorsal lines, alar crease, and sidewall junction, in particular.

It is a very pragmatic approach with a clear description of the reconstructive priorities.

- The skin and lining take priority – closure of wounds reduces infections and contraction/scarring.
- Support is important, but cartilage grafts should be postponed to a second stage if they cannot be completely covered by vascularized soft tissue in the first stage. If first-stage grafts/flap have failed leaving unhealed wounds at the second stage, they should be grafted and healed before cartilage is used.
- The nasal contour is achieved by meticulous debulking and shaping. but this will only be evident if the overlying (forehead) skin. which is a bit stiff and thick. is thinned out significantly. The soft tissue envelope can be re-elevated as a thin supple layer, having been effectively delayed. In theory, this can be repeated if the shape is not satisfactory by adding another step for more debulking or more cartilage before the final stage of pedicle division.
  - Millard emphasized this sculpturing to avoid "blob(bing) up" – "only a slob is satisfied with a blob."
  - In 1985, Burget and Menick published their landmark description of the subunits of the nose, often described as the most cited rhinoplasty article.

In this paper, Menick used various strategies for lining, most commonly:

- Intranasal lining flaps in 15 patients
- Prelaminated forehead flaps with full-thickness skin grafts for lining in 11 others, including:
  - Folded forehead flaps in 3
  - Turnover flaps in 5
  - Prefabricated flaps in 4
  - Free flaps in 2

According to Menick, the aesthetic results are improved "approaching normal," with the need for later revisions minimized. There was no necrosis of the forehead flap; one case had infection that was related to lining loss. In patients with full-thickness defects, one major revision or more than two minor revisions were required in less than 5%.

As detailed as it is, this is primarily a technique paper with little emphasis on objective results or follow-up. Despite the suggestion and the author's justifications that it is superior to a two-stage procedure, there is no direct comparison with a two-stage forehead flap group. The rate of minor revisions is not mentioned.

Menick provides further practical details in subsequent papers:

- A stated preference for using folded flaps over skin grafts, which were regarded more as a "salvage" option. They would often harvest a larger forehead flap to use the extra in the "dog ear" region as lining, trimming away excess in the intermediate stages.
- Timing to ensure that local problems have been controlled and tissues are stable.
- Exact templates based on contralateral/normal subunit(s) using paper tape and foil.
- Instead of keeping the columella portion connected (as bipedicle), the flap is completely elevated during the second stage for complete exposure.

Menick's 2012 article, in particular, provides useful insights on how to manage a "failed" reconstruction is enlightening. Minor contouring for "finesse definition" should be performed through direct incisions according to the subunit principles (and then quilted down onto the recipient bed), whilst major debulking probably should be performed via a full degloving along the peripheral incisions – up to 80% can be re-elevated after pedicle division. If a problem area cannot be reached, then it can be approached several months later along a different border.

Nose reconstruction, like ear reconstruction, has benefited from the meticulous work of the pioneers. Much practice is needed to get results resembling those of Menick and Burget, but, by following the guiding principles, surgeons may be able to give their patients decent results. In the future, if the problems of immunosuppression can be solved, nasal transplants may be an option, but, currently, forehead flaps will remain at the top of the ladder for nasal reconstruction.

BIBLIOGRAPHY

Gillies, H. D. Experiences with the tubed pedicle flaps. *Surg Gynecol Obstet.* 1935;60:291.

Kazanjian, V. H. The repair of nasal defects with the median forehead flap; primary closure of forehead wound. *Surg Gynecol Obstet.* 1946 Jul;83:37-49. PMID: 20988036.

Kelly CP, Yavuzer R, Keskin M, Bradford M, Govila L, Jackson IT. Functional anastomotic relationship between the supratrochlear and facial arteries: an anatomical study. *Plast Reconstr Surg.* 2008 Feb;121(2):458–465. doi: 10.1097/01.prs.0000297651.52729.ec.

McCarthy JG, Lorenc ZP, Cutting C, Rachesky M. The median forehead flap revisited: the blood supply. *Plast Reconstr Surg.* 1985 Dec;76(6):866–869. doi: 10.1097/00006534-198512000-00012.

Menick FJ. An approach to the late revision of a failed nasal reconstruction. *Plast Reconstr Surg.* 2012 Jan;129(1):92e–103e. doi: 10.1097/PRS.0b013e3182362226.

Millard DR Jr. Forehead flap in immediate repair of head, face and jaw. *Am J Surg.* 1964 Oct;108:508–513. doi: 10.1016/0002-9610(64)90145-x.

Millard DR Jr. Reconstructive rhinoplasty for the lower half of a nose. *Plast Reconstr Surg.* 1974 Feb;53(2):133–139. doi: 10.1097/00006534-197402000-00003.

CHAPTER 48

Supermicrosurgical Lymphaticovenular Anastomosis for the Treatment of Lymphedema in the Upper Extremities

Koshima I, Inagawa K, Urushibara K, Moriguchi T. *J Reconstr Microsurg.* 2000 Aug;16(6):437–442 doi: 10.1055/s-2006-947150 PMID: 10993089

EXPERT COMMENTARY

Valerie Ho Wai Yee

In search of an effective and efficient treatment for secondary lymphedema, which affects more than 150 million people worldwide,[1,2] the authors focused on breast cancer-related lymphoedema (BRCL) in this case series. Lymphaticovenular anastomosis (LVA) was proposed based on the rationale of directing excess lymph fluid in the soft tissue space back to the systemic circulation bypassing the obstruction by connecting lymphatic vessels to the subdermal venular system for the treatment of lymphedema refractory to complete decongestive therapy (CDT).[3] As these vessels were only 0.3 mm to 0.6 mm in diameter in the series, supermicrosurgical techniques were necessary for the anastomoses. Operations were performed under general anaesthesia. To identify the dilated lymphatic vessels, indigocarmine was injected intradermally to dye the lymphatics. Skin incisions were then made to select suitable lymphatics and subdermal venules for anastomosis. The surgical effects and the decrease in circumference were shown to be persistent in the follow-up period of up to 6 years.

There has been continuing development and pursuit of excellence in this procedure, including histological analysis, diagnosis, staging, patient selection, preoperative planning, means of anaesthesia, identification of lymphatic vessels and venules, positioning, supermicrosurgical techniques and adjuncts, ancillary procedures, perioperative decongestive therapy, evaluation of outcomes, and tissue engineering research on regenerative medicine, such as BioBridge™, which is a new biological scaffold for regeneration of lymphatic channels. In recent years, the treatment effect from lymphaticovenous bypass has been observed to have a role in the treatment of Alzheimer's disease, which affects about 35 million people worldwide.

It has been consistently demonstrated in the literature that after LVA, there are reductions in excess limb volume, incidence of cellulitis, and dependence on compression garments, with positive impact on patients' quality of life under the

DOI: 10.1201/9781003413738-48

domains of physical function, mental function, household activities, mobility activities, and life and social activities.[4–7]

The key to success of LVA lies in the three components, i.e., lymphatics, venules, and anastomosis. It is essential to locate the most favourable points for LVA by identifying good functional lymphatic vessels and suitable nearby venules in the preoperative mapping.

Understanding the histopathophysiology of disease and its effects on the lymphatics is fundamental to providing the best personalised treatment for lymphoedema patients. Mihara M. and Hara H. et al. studied the histological changes found in 114 specimens of collecting lymphatic vessels from 37 patients with cancer-related lymphoedema and classified them into normal, ectasis, contractile, and sclerotic types (NECST)[8] as lymphoedema progresses due to the increase in the endolymphatic pressure after lymphadenectomy. Yamamoto T et al. proposed the lymphosclerosis classification, which is either morphological or functional, and it differentiates high-flow lymphatic channels (s0 and s1) from sclerotic, less functional channels (s2 and s3).[9] These classifications have highlighted the importance of intervention at early stages when lymphatic vessels are still functional, such as in the dilatation and contraction stage, to prevent the aggravation of lymphoedema by suppressing the irreversible degenerative changes observed.

Traditionally, the most common methods of lymphatic mapping are lymphoscintigraphy and indocyanine green lymphography (ICG-L). ICG-L is a minimally invasive imaging modality that can not only evaluate the severity of lymphoedema, but also allows real-time visualisation of superficial linear lymphatic vessels before dermal backflow is established.[10–12] However, several limitations include the information provided being only two-dimensional and potential lymphatic vessels for LVA may be masked by dermal backflow patterns, particularly in stardust and diffuse patterns seen in severe lymphedema[13] or if they >1.5–2 cm beneath the skin, which can happen in the thigh or upper arm. ICG-L does not provide information about the venular system and, more importantly, is contraindicated in patients with iodine allergy.

To overcome these limitations, the use of conventional high-frequency ultrasound (CHFUS) and ultra-high-frequency ultrasound (UHFUS) has been reported by Akitatsu et al. as an alternative to ICG-L, particularly in limbs severely affected by lymphoedema.[14–17] The accuracy of UHFUS in detecting lymphatic vessels and in evaluating their degeneration status has been studied with a strong correlation with their histological features.[18] High echoic regions around the lower echoic regions on USG represent degeneration of smooth muscle cells and hyperplasia of collagen fibres in the lymphatic vessels in more severe lymphoedema. The presence of dilated lymphatic vessels with abundant lymph flow is an important factor in determining the likely therapeutic effect of LVA. Yang et al. reported that using a lymphatic vessel with a diameter larger than 0.5 mm in LVA results in better postoperative outcomes. This complies with the principles in fluid dynamics, which states that the diameter has a strong correlation with the amount of flow.[19] Surgeons can select the best lymphatic vessels at each point preoperatively using UHFUS.

UHFUS can also be applied intraoperatively to allow selection of more functional lymphatic vessels. More detailed assessment of the lymphatic vessels, such as the wall thickness, size of lumen, presence of valves, converging point, etc. is actually feasible with laser tomography. With more information, the surgeon can select the more functional lymphatic vessels for LVA for better therapeutic effect.

In the past, LVA was often reserved for patients with early-stage lymphoedema due to the difficulty in identifying functional lymphatic vessels using ICG-L in patients with advanced lymphoedema. However, USG mapping of the entire limb can be technically demanding and time-consuming. Hidehiko Yoshimatsu et al. demonstrated "the milestone-swirl sign" approach by combining the milestone sign from ICG-L with the swirl sign detected via USG to identify functional lymphatic vessels in patients with advanced-stage lymphoedema.[20]

In addition, ultrasonography can also be used to detect venules. LVA is effective only when the pressure gradient at the anastomosis allows lymph to flow into the venule. Visconti G. et al. demonstrated that the recipient venule has an independent impact on the LVA outcomes, regardless of the lymphatic degeneration status. The venule dynamics have been classified by the BSOH classification, i.e., Backflow, Slack, Outlet, and Hydropower[21] with Hydropower being the ideal – the venule has no blood inside because it has been completely cleared by the lymph after LVA. Surgeons should aim to select venules that are close to the lymphatic vessels, have good calibre match, and are reflux-free when using a push-and-release technique in USG colour Doppler mode. Once the exact location of both lymphatic vessels and venules is identified, the incision(s) can be made precisely via a 1.5–2 cm skin incision. The helps to reduce the time required for dissection, rendering LVA a minimally invasive procedure which can be performed under local anaesthesia in the hands of experienced lymphoedema surgeons.

The "Lymphosome concept" should be taken into consideration in performing ICG-L and in the planning for LVA. A lymphosome is defined as a skin territory containing the superficial lymph-collecting vessels connecting to a specific group of sentinel lymph nodes. The whole body can be demarcated into lymphosomes using this concept.[22,23] Compensatory anatomical changes, e.g., lymphangiogenesis and dermal backflow, were observed after lymphadenectomy. It is important to locate precisely the most proximal point of lymphatic degeneration or the confluence point for LVA and saving all the lymphatic trees below. It is the quality and flow of the lymphatic channels that are bypassed in a reflux-free venule that contributes to improvement in lymphoedema, not simply the number of LVAs performed.

There are other alternative imaging technologies that may be useful in staging and in preoperative planning, such as magnetic resonance lymphography (MRL) and photoacoustic imaging (PAI). MRL compensates for some of the weaknesses of lymphoscintigraphy (low resolution) and ICG-L (limited depth). A combination allows for a more comprehensive assessment of the lymphatic morphology and function, providing information on the number, depth, trajectory, and stasis of the lymphatic vessels, thus enabling efficient and effective performance of LVA.[24] However, adverse events at the injection sites for gadolinium-based agents, such as necrosis, haemorrhage, oedema, and inflammation, etc. have been reported. Second, images may be contaminated with venous enhancement due to venous uptake following extravascular injection. Lastly, MRL is more costly compared to ICG-L, hence, increasing the overall treatment cost. PAL can visualise the three-dimensional relationships between lymphatic vessels and veins and evaluate the depth from the skin surface of each. However, it is necessary to superimpose the obtained image onto the patient's extremity precisely in clinical practice. Methods such as multiple markings and using augmented reality were proposed by Suzuki et al. to improve the accuracy and facilitate preoperative planning.[25]

The field and scope of lymphoedema surgery has been expanding over the last two decades and will certainly continue to expand as the application nowadays is not limited to only treating lymphedema, but also has a potential role in treating medical conditions such as Alzheimer's disease. More and more research is ongoing to evaluate the long-term efficacy and cost-effectiveness. Readers are encouraged to keep an eye and mind open to the updates and to be actively involved in research to find answers.

REFERENCES

1. Rockson SG, Rivera KK. Estimating the population burden of lymphedema. *Ann N Y Acad Sci.* 2008;1131:147–154.
2. Chang DW, Masia J, Garza R 3rd, Skoracki R, Neligan PC. Lymphedema: surgical and medical therapy. *Plast Reconstr Surg.* 2016 Sep;138(3):209s–218s.
3. O'Brien BM, Sykes P, Threlfall GN, Browning FS. Microlymphaticovenous anastomoses for obstructive lymphedema. *Plast Reconstr Surg.* 1977 Aug;60(2):197–211
4. Gasteratos K, Morsi-Yeroyannis A, Vlachopoulos NC, Spyropoulou GA, Del Corral G, Chaiyasate K. Microsurgical techniques in the treatment of breast cancer-related lymphedema: a systematic review of efficacy and patient outcomes. *Breast Cancer.* 2021;28(5):1002–1015.
5. Coriddi M, Dayan J, Sobti N, Nash D, Goldberg J, Klassen A, Pusic A, Mehrara B. Systematic review of patient-reported outcomes following surgical treatment of lymphedema. *Cancers (Basel).* 2020;12(3):565.
6. Chang DW, Suami H, Skoracki R. A prospective analysis of 100 consecutive lymphovenous bypass cases for treatment of extremity lymphedema. *Plast Reconstr Surg.* 2013;132:1305–1314.
7. Cornelissen AJM, Kool M, Lopez Penha TR, Keuter XHA, Piatkowski AA, Heuts E, van der Hulst RRWJ, Qiu SS. Lymphaticovenous anastomosis as treatment for breast cancer-related lymphedema: a prospective study on quality of life. *Breast Cancer Res Treat.* 2017 Jun;163(2):281–286.
8. Mihara M, Hara H, Hayashi Y, Narushima M, Yamamoto T, Todokoro T, Iida T, Sawamoto N, Araki J, Kikuchi K, Murai N, Okitsu T, Kisu I, Koshima I. Pathological steps of cancer-related lymphedema: histological changes in the collecting lymphatic vessels after lymphadenectomy. *PLOS ONE.* 2012;7(7):e41126.
9. Yamamoto T, Yamamoto N, Yoshimatsu H, Narushima M, Koshima I. Factors associated with lymphosclerosis: an analysis on 962 lymphatic vessels. *Plast Reconstr Surg.* 2017;140(4):734–741.
10. Yamamoto T, Narushima M, Doi K, *et al.* Characteristic indocyanine green lymphography findings in lower extremity lymphedema: the generation of a novel lymphedema severity staging system using dermal backflow patterns. *Plast Reconstr Surg.* 2011;127:1979–1986.
11. Yamamoto T, Matsuda N, Doi K, *et al.* The earliest finding of indocyanine green lymphography in asymptomatic limbs of lower extremity lymph-edema patients secondary to cancer treatment: the modified dermal backflow stage and concept of subclinical lymphedema. *Plast Reconstr Surg.* 2011;128:314e–21e.

12. Yamamoto T, Yamamoto N, Doi K, *et al.* Indocyanine green-enhanced lymphography for upper extremity lymphedema: a novel severity staging system using dermal backflow patterns. *Plast Reconstr Surg.* 2011;128:941.

13. Ogata F, Narushima M, Mihara M, *et al.* Intraoperative lymphography using indocyanine green dye for near- infrared fluorescence labeling in lymphedema. *Ann Plast Surg.* 2007;59:180–184.

14. Hayashi A, Yamamoto T, Yoshimatsu H, *et al.* Ultrasound visualization of the lymphatic vessels in the lower leg. *Microsurgery.* 2016;36:397–401.

15. Hayashi A, Hayashi N, Yoshimatsu H, *et al.* Effective and efficient lymphaticovenular anastomosis using preoperative ultrasound detection technique of lymphatic vessels in lower extremity lymphedema. *J Surg Oncol.* 2018;117:290–298.

16. Hayashi A, Giacalone G, Yamamoto T, *et al.* Comparative study of ultra high-frequency ultrasonographic imaging with 70 MHz scanner for visualization of the superficial lymphatic vessels in extremities. *Plast Reconstr Surg Global Open.* 2019;7(1):e2086. doi: 10.1097/ GOX.0000000000002086.

17. Visconti G, Yamamoto T, Hayashi A, *et al.* Ultrasound- assisted lymphaticovenular anastomosis for the treatment of peripheral lymphedema. *Plast Reconstr Surg.* 2017;139:1380e–1e.

18. Bianchi A, Visconti G, Hayashi A, Santoro A, Longo V, Salgarello M. Ultra-high frequency ultrasound imaging of lymphatic channels correlates with their histological features: a step forward in lymphatic surgery. *J Plast Reconstr Aesthet Surg.* 2020;73(9):1622–1629.

19. Yang JC, Wu SC, Hayashi A, *et al.* Selection of optimal functional lymphatic vessel cutoff size in supermicrosurgical lymphaticovenous anastomosis in lower extremity lymphedema. *Plast Reconstr Surg.* 2022 Jan 1;149(1):237–246.

20. Yoshimatsu H, Cho M-J, Inoue K, Karakawa R, Fuse Y, Hayashi A, Yano T. Combining indocyanine green lymphography and ultrasonography findings to identify lymphatic vessels in advanced-stage lymphedema: the milestone and swirl sign approach. *J Plast Reconstr Aesthet Surg.* 2025;102:134–141.

21. Visconti G, Salgarello M, Hayashi A. The recipient venule in supermicrosurgical lymphaticovenular anastomosis: flow dynamic classification and correlation with surgical outcomes. *J Reconstr Microsurg.* 2018;34(8):581–589.

22. Suami H. Lymphosome concept: anatomical study of the lymphatic system. *J Surg Oncol.* 2017;115:13–17.

23. Suami H, Scaglioni MF. Anatomy of the lymphatic system and the Lymphosome concept with reference to lymphedema. *Semin Plast Surg.* 2018;32:5–11.

24. Pons G, Clavero JA, Alomar X, Rodríguez-Bauza E, Tom LK, Masia J. Preoperative planning of lymphaticovenous anastomosis: the use of magnetic resonance lymphangiography as a complement to indocyanine green lymphography. *J Plast Reconstr Aesthet Surg.* 2019;72(6):884–891.

25. Suzuki Y, Kajita H, Watanabe S, Otaki M, Okabe K, Sakuma H, *et al.* Surgical applications of lymphatic vessel visualization using photoacoustic imaging and augmented reality. *J Clin Med.* 2021;11:194.

EDITOR COMMENTARY

This is a relatively small retrospective study (12 patients in each arm). However, it is a controlled study well designed to compare surgery with a new technique (supermicrosurgical LVA) with non-surgery patients. Supermicrosurgery (<0.8 mm) and LVAs are interwined – Isao Koshima reasoned that lower pressure venous vessels needed to be used to avoid the shortcomings of older procedures (such as O'Brien et al.), but the vessels involved would then be much smaller, necessitating changes in philosophy and technique. This paper introduces the new approach to the modern LVA, and the general principles have been widely adopted.

In this study, the surgeons used indigocarmine to stain the lymphatics, which has significant drawbacks but was one of few options until the advent of ICG-L (Ogata et al., 2007). As mentioned in the expert commentary, ICG-L has its own set of limitations, and other modalities, such as ultrasound (particularly ultra-high-frequency ultrasound), are increasingly being used, often in a complementary/ supplementary fashion, particularly in advanced staged disease (Cha HG et al., 2021).

The wider uptake of supermicrosurgery has been accompanied by other advancements, such as microscopes, instruments, and sutures. These techniques have been successfully applied to problems other than lymphoedema/LVA. Apart from size reduction, one of the most important and measurable benefits of LVA/lymphatic surgery is the considerable reduction in the rate of soft tissue infections. Plant extracts that have anti-LTB4 activity have also reduced the rate of infections without surgery (Chiu T et al., 2020).

Various prophylactic strategies, e.g., LYMPHA (Boccardo F et al., 2014), BLAST (Masia J et al., 2016), and others without a snappy acronym (Johnson AR et al., 2021), that perform LVA at the time of lymph node dissection are being trialled. Selecting the subset that would benefit the most is the challenge.

REFERENCES

Boccardo F, Casabona F, De Cian F, Friedman D, Murelli F, Puglisi M, Campisi CC, Molinari L, Spinaci S, Dessalvi S, Campisi C. Lymphatic microsurgical preventing healing approach (LYMPHA) for primary surgical prevention of breast cancer-related lymphedema: over 4 years follow-up. *Microsurgery.* 2014 Sep;34(6):421–424. doi: 10.1002/micr.22254. Erratum in: *Microsurgery.* 2015 Jan;35(1):83.

Cha HG, Oh TM, Cho MJ, Pak CSJ, Suh HP, Jeon JY, Hong JP. Changing the paradigm: lymphovenous anastomosis in advanced stage lower extremity lymphedema. *Plast Reconstr Surg.* 2021 Jan 1;147(1):199–207. doi: 10.1097/PRS.0000000000007507.

Chiu TW, Kong SL, Cheng KF, Leung PC. Treatment of post-mastectomy lymphedema with herbal medicine: an innovative pilot study. *Plast Reconstr Surg Glob Open.* 2020 Jun 24;8(6):e2915. doi: 10.1097/ GOX.0000000000002915.

Johnson AR, Fleishman A, Granoff MD, Shillue K, Houlihan MJ, Sharma R, Kansal KJ, Teller P, James TA, Lee BT, Singhal D. Evaluating the Impact of Immediate Lymphatic Reconstruction for the Surgical Prevention of Lymphedema. *Plast Reconstr Surg.* 2021 Mar 1;147(3):373e–381e. doi: 10.1097/ PRS.0000000000007636. PMID: 33620920.

Ogata F, Azuma R, Kikuchi M, Koshima I, Morimoto Y. Novel lymphography using indocyanine green dye for near-infrared fluorescence labeling. *Ann Plast Surg.* 2007 Jun;58(6):652–655. doi: 10.1097/01.sap .0000250896.42800.a2.

Masià J, Pons G, Rodríguez-Bauzà E. Barcelona lymphedema algorithm for surgical treatment in breast cancer-related lymphedema. *J Reconstr Microsurg.* 2016 Jun;32(5):329–335. doi: 10.1055/s-0036-1578814.

Ogata F, Narushima M, Mihara M, Azuma R, Morimoto Y, Koshima I. Intraoperative lymphography using indocyanine green dye for near-infrared fluorescence labeling in lymphedema. *Ann Plast Surg.* 2007 Aug;59(2):180–184. doi: 10.1097/01.sap.0000253341.70866.54.

CHAPTER 49

A New Concept in the Early Excision and Immediate Grafting of Burns

Z Janzekovic. *J Trauma*. 1970;10:1103–1108

EDITOR COMMENTARY

In addition to the development of fluid resuscitation formulae, one of the most significant advances in burn management has been the early tangential excision of the burn wound followed by immediate skin grafting. This development occurred purposefully, methodically, and quietly in Maribor, which was part of Yugoslavia then and is now in Slovenia.

At that point, "conventional" therapy was quite literally to wait for the eschar to slough off and for the wounds to granulate before grafting whilst partial-thickness burns even when deeper would be left to heal spontaneously. Whilst waiting (about 6 weeks or more), wounds would inevitably become infected, and patients become emaciated, exhausted and anaemic. Early reports of early surgery from the United Kingdom and the United States had not been particularly successful with similar mortality and only slightly shorter healing times (Jackson DM, 1969; MacMillan BC, 1958, 1962). This was ascribed to several reasons: most grafts failed to take due to one, the radical (depth) of excision leaving little or no dermal remnants and two, only full-thickness burns were debrided – neighbouring areas that were not obviously full thickness would usually be left to heal spontaneously and, inevitably, infection would spread from these areas to involve the grafts.

Dr. Janzekovic began in 1959 with smaller full-thickness burns, allowing excision in an all or nothing manner to remove all dead tissue from the patient. Using magnification and Blair knives, they shaved down to bleeding dermis during the first 2 weeks after injury (usually around day 5) and then covered the wounds with grafts. Wounds were checked the next day – clots or collections would be evacuated and raw areas covered with stored skin. They would be rewarded with near to 100% take of skin grafts.

After this exploratory period, they adopted a systematic program of "early excision" and grafting from February 1961. After a few years, word of the good results got out and visitors came from far and wide, including Carroll from the United States and Wallace from Scotland (who was then, in 1964, the general secretary of the ISBI). Their methods and results (with 1,300 patients) were first presented to an international audience in 1968 at a symposium hosted by the Yugoslav Association for Plastic and Maxillofacial

DOI: 10.1201/9781003413738-49

Surgery in Maribor, where they were met with some scepticism. Professor Derganc, the organizer of the plastic program and with whom Zora had collaborated for the first two papers in English, had invited prominent burn surgeons, including Burke, Jackson, Evans, and Wallace. From then on – 1968 to 1984 – she hosted more than 200 burn surgeons from around the world.

Autografts (covered with chloromycetin compresses) were used for burns under 20%, whilst for larger burns "homografts" (from living donors) were also used for temporary coverage – these would be rejected by day 8 to 12, whilst donor sites heal for reharvesting. Meshing was not a common practice at the time and so larger burns could not be as efficiently covered with autografts. Thus, whilst most patients with smaller burns healed well and could be discharged after 10 days, larger burns remained problematic. They found that in extensive injuries, deep dermal burns would be converted into full thickness over the following days if the patient did not have early surgery. Early surgery would actually not sacrifice healthy tissue (an early concern); rather, it would "save" potentially salvageable damaged tissue and prevent/reduce contractures.

In this paper, the author described the technique and its evolution. A retrospective review presented in 1975 (Janzekovic Z, 1975) added details. A total of 2,615 of 4,370 burns admitted were treated with surgery between 1961 and 1974. The length of hospital stay was shortened from 18.7 to 12.4 days with an actual mortality rate of 19 deaths compared to a predicted 30.5 (according to the Bull Probability Grid). This was not the first attempt to use early excision, but this was the first to show improved healing – the important concepts were complete burn excision and immediate grafting. Furthermore, they observed that bleeding was more profuse after 3 days; tourniquets were used where possible, shaving to white moist dermis or bright yellow fat. Thrombosed or haemoglobin-stained areas, grey/ brown tissue were also removed. There were significant problems that were discussed, including the issue of overgrafting, which led to keratin collections and pustules.

Extensive burns constituted 5% of their patients. They described that in their small number of "critical burns" (over 50%) they would "change blood," i.e., exchange transfusion prior to surgery. Adult patients with burns over 60% would die despite surgery, whilst paediatric mortality was zero in the 8 years reported upon.

Douglas Jackson (of Jackson's burn zones, 1953) from Birmingham, UK, was inspired by Janzekovic's work to have "second thoughts" on the zone of stasis, which he previously considered to be avascular but was then found to bleed on tangential shaving. With partial-thickness burns, even of a deeper extent, the prevailing opinion was that there was little reason to graft what would heal in 3–6 weeks. After visiting Janzekovic, Jackson moved from advocating what Derganc called a "medical conservative approach to deeply damaged dermis" to early excision. He limited early excision and grafting to "analgesic burns" (that were usually deep partial or full thickness). Another observation he made was that after debridement, viable wound beds would become dry and brown and would slough if they were exposed by gaps between grafts, that is, grafting "saved" the wound bed from further damage. Jackson gave the Evans lecture in 1969, describing what he had learned from Maribor, and, when that was subsequently published, it actually predated this paper from Janzekovic.

It is fascinating to see how recently we arrived at what we currently regard as modern burns care. Wider acceptance was slow despite the early work of Zora Janzekovic and contemporaries, including non-randomized retrospective studies from Burke (1974 and 1976). The turning point came with studies of comparative outcomes and controls, namely, David Herndon's 1989 paper. This prospective randomised trial provided stronger evidence of the benefits of early excision and grafting, specifically that there was a mortality benefit with early intervention. The results in 85 adults were compared to 259 children supposedly used as positive treatment controls as they were all treated with early excision whilst the adults were randomized to traditional conservative treatment (daily dressings until eschar separated, followed by homografting) versus fascial excision within 72 hours with either homograft (cadaveric) or autografting. Early surgery reduced mortality from 45% to 9% ($p < 0.05$) in those without inhalation injury in patients between 17 and 30 years of age. Older patients and those with inhalational injuries showed comparable results despite the different treatments.

Zora Janzekovic was manoeuvred into retiring in 1984. She was never given the recognition in her native country by doctors and public alike compared to overseas. She had a long retirement, being particularly interested in art. She spent her last days in a nursing home, where one of the staff was a woman whose life she had saved some 60 years earlier.

REFERENCES

Jackson DM. Second thoughts on the burn wound. *J Trauma Inj Infect Critical Care.* 1969;9(10):839–862.
Janzekovic Z. The burn wound from the surgical point of view. *J Trauma.* 1975 Jan;15(1):42–62.
Herndon DN, Barrow RE, Rutan RL, Rutan TC, Desai MH, Abston S. A comparison of conservative versus early excision: therapies in severely burned patients. *Ann Surg.* 1989;209:547–553.

CHAPTER 50

A Novel Reconstructive Technique after Endoscopic Expanded Endonasal Approaches: Vascular Pedicle Nasoseptal Flap

Hadad G, Bassagasteguy L, Carrau RL, Mataza JC, Kassam A,
Snyderman CH, Mintz A. *Laryngoscope.* 2006 Oct;116(10):1882–1886
doi: 10.1097/01.mlg.0000234933.37779.e4 PMID: 17003708

EDITOR COMMENTARY

Skull base defects leading to CSF leaks can be due to idiopathic, traumatic, or iatrogenic causes. Defects under 1 cm in size are usually closed with non-vascularized techniques with varying degrees of success.

In the 1960s after the development of microscopic and endoscopic techniques, there was a resurgence of the transsphenoidal approach to the pituitary first introduced in the early 20th century (Schloffre 1907, Cushing 1909 though he later preferred a transfrontal approach). With improvements to the transsphenoidal approach, it slowly gained acceptance over the conventional transcranial approach. Small dural defects were usually managed with grafts of muscle, fascia, or fat. In the late 1990s. the expanded endonasal approach (EEA) facilitated resection of lesions of the pituitary, anterior skull base, clivus, and odontoid and laterally into infratemporal fossa. This resulted in larger bony and dural defects, with higher flow CSF leaks; use of fat grafts was associated with leakage rates of up to 20%.

This was a retrospective case series that included 43 patients who had "nasoseptal flaps" (NSF) for a variety of pathologies. The surgical technique is described in detail: incisions along the maxillary crest inferiorly and 1 cm below the superior extent of the septum are connected anteriorly to allow elevation of the septal flap in the submucoperichondrial/subperiosteal plane. Posteriorly, the incisions narrow to just below the sphenoid ostium and the superior limit of the choana to include the pedicle that exits the lateral wall of the nose at the sphenopalatine foramen. The authors used multilayer reconstruction with a first layer of collagen matrix (sometimes onlay fascia graft or abdominal fat), then the NSF and fibrin glue with packing or a Foley catheter to keep the flap in place. Silicone splints were used (with antibiotic cover with third-generation cephalosporins until the packing is removed).

DOI: 10.1201/9781003413738-50

The outcome measures are quite basic: CSF leaks occurred in 2 cases (5%), which were remedied with focal fat grafts; otherwise, there was no flap loss (partial/total) and no infections.

In one case there was a posterior nosebleed that needed cautery. The donor site mucosalized within weeks, with no perforations. There were reports of minor synechiae upon follow-up.

The main weaknesses of the study are the relatively small numbers in combination with a mix of patients and techniques, with quite short follow-up at 2 months. There is no control or another cohort for comparisons. However, as a surgical technique paper, it provided a novel reliable technique to reduce the risk of CSF leaks.

The nasoseptal flap (NSF) was first described by Hadad and Bassagasteguy in 2006. There had been earlier reports of narrow rectangular flaps of septal mucosa for the repair of cerebrospinal fluid (CSF) leaks (Hirsch O, 1952), whilst others had described what were essentially rotational flaps. These were generally "random" flaps of inconsistent reliability. The major innovation of the flap of Hadad et al. was that a broad flap designed to include a consistent axial blood vessel(s) (septal branches of the sphenopalatine artery) that provided reliable tissue. With a narrow pedicle, the flap could be designed to pivot/reach either the anterior skull base, the pituitary, and sella region or the clivus. I am unlikely to write a landmark article, but it is somewhat gratifying to have a landmark article cite my anatomical studies that had characterized the arterial supply of the nasal septum (Chiu T, 2006).

EEA reconstruction of defects with avascular grafts can approach 90% success, but with larger defects with higher flow, the chances of success are much lower at 50%–70%. Hadad et al. demonstrated that the NSF effectively reduces the incidence of CSF leak to 5%. In the early days of EEA, CSF leak was reportedly as high as 24%; however, recent studies suggest that with use of the NSF, CSF leaks resulting from EEA are as low as 3% (Horridge, 2013) versus 12.5% for grafts. Similarly, a meta-analysis by Najafabadi et al. (2021) found CSF leakage after skull base meninogoma was reduced to 4% from 22%.

The NSF has become the workhorse option for anterior skull-base reconstruction. Utilization has significantly decreased morbidity for patients with more complex defects who would otherwise require free flap reconstruction or external approaches for other craniofacial-based local flaps. The septal flap is so effective that its use is being revisited for defects, such as traumatic defects, which would have normally been managed with non-vascularized techniques (El-Sayed IH, 2020). We use the NSF in our centre to reconstruct the irradiated NP, e.g., after surgery for recurrent nasopharyngeal carcinoma, reducing the need for a free flap.

Complications were not specifically discussed in this paper. From subsequent studies, bleeding after NSF is quite rare; the Vidian artery may be large and cause bleeding but is typically controlled intraoperatively. Soudry et al. (2015) found that in a series of 121 NFSs there were 4 flap failures, and, with regard to the donor site, there were 16 perforations, 4 with crusting, and saddle nose in 1. The risk of failure increases with prior irradiation, BMI > 30, larger defects and "high-flow" leaks (Ivan ME et al., 2015). Patel et al. (2010) found a 4% leak rate after 150 NSFs with a learning curve of at least 25 flaps. They recommend use of the NSF for defects >1 cm square; when the NSF is not available, then anterior defects can be managed with an endoscopic pericranial flap and posterior/clival defects with inferior turbinate flaps or TPF. The availability of the NSF should be determined preoperatively where possible.

Due to its versatile nature and customisability, the NSF can be utilised for a range of different defects extending from the frontal recess to the low clivus in the sagittal plane. This paper describes the evolution of the NSF, including its uses, modifications, and relevant morbidity.

Numerous papers confirm it to be the workhorse of anterior (endoscopic) skull-base reconstruction. Modifications reported in the literature include the extended NSF and the elongated NSF. Peris-Celda et al. (2013) described a method to increase the amount of nasal mucosa harvested by including part of the nasal floor (extended NSF). Elongation of the NSF pedicle facilitated inset (Pinheiro Neto CD et al., 2019) whilst Shastri et al. (2020) demonstrated that an additional 5–6 cm of reach could be obtained by releasing the flap pedicle from the sphenopalatine foramen and dissecting the maxillary/sphenopalatine artery out of the pterygopalatine fossa. Essentially, the coiled artery in the PPF is "straightened out" (Chiu T, 2009, 2025). Turner (2022) described the use of elongated NSF to cover TORS defects in the oropharynx.

East Asians and females have shorter nasoseptal to anterior skull-base ratios and thus the standard NSF may be less versatile (Gu D, 2022; Jeong CY et al., 2023) – use of elongated and or extended NSF may help. In the future there may be some form of virtual planning with 3D printed models from CT data (Kayastha D et al., 2023), whilst Cradeur et al. (2025) used 3D printing for simulation and training.

REFERENCES

Chiu T. A study of the maxillary and sphenopalatine arteries in the pterygopalatine fossa and at the sphenopalatine foramen. *Rhinology.* 2009;47:264–270. doi: 10.4193/Rhin08.153.

Chiu T. Anatomical basis of the elongated nasoseptal flap. *Acta Otorhinolaryngol Ital.* 2025 Jun;45(3):192-199. doi: 10.14639/0392-100X-N2159. PMID: 40567097; PMCID: PMC12201921.

Chiu T, Shaw Dunn J. An anatomical study of the arteries of the anterior nasal septum. *Otolaryngol Head Neck Surg.* 2006;134:33–36. doi: 10.1016/j.otohns.2005.09.005.

Cradeur A, Knackstedt M, Latour M, Yim M. Modeling nasal septal flap repair of an anterior skull base defect: a pilot simulation study. *Int Forum Allergy Rhinol.* 2025 Feb;15(2):212–214. doi: 10.1002/alr.23500.

El-Sayed IH. Nasal septal flap repair of the skull base. *Handb Clin Neurol.* 2020;170:227–232. doi: 10.1016/B978-0-12-822198-3.00022-7.

Gu D. Radioanatomical study of the skull base and septum in Chinese: implications for using the HBF for endoscopic skull base reconstruction. *Oxid Med Cell Longev.* 2022;2022:9940239.

Hirsch O. Successful closure of cerebrospinal fluid Rhinorrhea by endonasal surgery. *AMA Arch Otolaryngol.* 1952 Jul;56(1):1–12. doi: 10.1001/archotol.1952.00710020018001.

Horridge M, Jesurasa A, Olubajo F, Mirza S, Sinha S. The use of the nasoseptal flap to reduce the rate of post-operative cerebrospinal fluid leaks following endoscopic trans-sphenoidal surgery for pituitary disease. *Br J Neurosurg.* 2013;27:739–741.

Ivan ME, Iorgulescu JB, El-Sayed I, McDermott MW, Parsa AT, Pletcher SD, Jahangiri A, Wagner J, Aghi MK. Risk factors for postoperative cerebrospinal fluid leak and meningitis after expanded endoscopic endonasal surgery. *J Clin Neurosci.* 2015 Jan;22(1):48–54. doi: 10.1016/j.jocn.2014.08.009.

Jeong CY, Cho JH, Park YJ, Kim SW, Park JS, Basurrah MA, Kim DH, Kim SW. Differences in the predicted nasoseptal flap length among races: a propensity score matching analysis. *PLOS ONE.* 2023;18:e0283140.

Kayastha D, Wiznia D, Manes RP, Omay SB, Khoury T, Rimmer R. 3D printing for virtual surgical planning of nasoseptal flap skull-base reconstruction: a proof-of-concept study. *Int Forum Allergy Rhinol.* 2023;13:2073–2075.

Najafabadi AHZ, Khan DZ, Muskens IS. Trends in cerebrospinal fluid leak rates following the extended endoscopic endonasal approach for anterior skull base meningioma: a meta-analysis over the last 20 years. *Acta Neurochir.* 2021;163:711–719.

Patel MR, Stadler ME, Snyderman CH, Carrau RL, Kassam AB, Germanwala AV, Gardner P, Zanation AM. How to choose? Endoscopic skull base reconstructive options and limitations. *Skull Base.* 2010 Nov;20(6):397–404. doi: 10.1055/s-0030-1253573.

Peris-Celda M, Pinheiro-Neto CD, Funaki T, *et al.* The extended nasoseptal flap for skull base reconstruction of the clival region: an anatomical and radiological study. *J Neurol Surg B Skull Base.* 2013;74:369–385. doi: 10.1055/s-0033-1347368.

Pinheiro-Neto CD, Peris-Celda M, Kenning T. Extrapolating the limits of the nasoseptal flap with pedicle dissection to the internal maxillary artery. *Oper Neurosurg.* 2019;16:37–44.

Shastri KS, Leonel LCPC, Patel V, Charles-pereira M, Kenning TJ, Peris-celda M, Pinheiro-neto CD. Lengthening the nasoseptal flap pedicle with extended dissection into the pterygopalatine fossa. *Laryngoscope.* 2020;130:18–24.

Soudry E, Psaltis AJ, Lee KH, Vaezafshar R, Nayak JV, Hwang PH. Complications associated with the pedicled nasoseptal flap for skull base reconstruction. *Laryngoscope.* 2015 Jan;125(1):80–85. doi: 10.1002/lary.24863.

Turner MT, Geltzeiler MN, Ramadan J, *et al.* The nasoseptal flap for reconstruction of lateral oropharyngectomy defects: a clinical series. *Laryngoscope.* 2022;132:53–60. doi: 10.1002/lary.29660.

Index

For Product Safety Concerns and Information please contact our EU
representative GPSR@taylorandfrancis.com
Taylor & Francis Verlag GmbH, Kaufingerstraße 24, 80331 München, Germany